Pluripotent Stem Cell: Current Understanding and Future Directions

Guest Editor
Aline Yen Ling Wang
Center for Vascularized
Composite
Allotransplantation
Chang Gung Memorial
Hospital
Taoyuan
Taiwan

Editorial Office
MDPI AG
Grosspeteranlage 5
4052 Basel, Switzerland

This is a reprint of the Special Issue, published open access by the journal *Biomedicines* (ISSN 2227-9059), freely accessible at: https://www.mdpi.com/journal/biomedicines/special_issues/Stem_Exosomes.

For citation purposes, cite each article independently as indicated on the article page online and as indicated below:

Lastname, A.A.; Lastname, B.B. Article Title. *Journal Name* **Year**, *Volume Number*, Page Range.

ISBN 978-3-7258-3769-4 (Hbk)
ISBN 978-3-7258-3770-0 (PDF)
https://doi.org/10.3390/books978-3-7258-3770-0

© 2025 by the authors. Articles in this book are Open Access and distributed under the Creative Commons Attribution (CC BY) license. The book as a whole is distributed by MDPI under the terms and conditions of the Creative Commons Attribution-NonCommercial-NoDerivs (CC BY-NC-ND) license (https://creativecommons.org/licenses/by-nc-nd/4.0/).

Pluripotent Stem Cell: Current Understanding and Future Directions

Guest Editor
Aline Yen Ling Wang

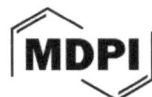

Basel • Beijing • Wuhan • Barcelona • Belgrade • Novi Sad • Cluj • Manchester

Contents

Aline Yen Ling Wang, Ana Elena Aviña, Yen-Yu Liu and Huang-Kai Kao
Pluripotent Stem Cells: Recent Advances and Emerging Trends
Reprinted from: *Biomedicines* 2025, 13, 765, https://doi.org/10.3390/biomedicines13040765 . . . 1

Prince Saini, Sharath Anugula and Yick W. Fong
The Role of ATP-Binding Cassette Proteins in Stem Cell Pluripotency
Reprinted from: *Biomedicines* 2023, 11, 1868, https://doi.org/10.3390/biomedicines11071868 . . 6

Lucas Simões Machado, Camila Martins Borges, Marina Amaro de Lima, Juliano Rodrigues Sangalli, Jacinthe Therrien, Laís Vicari de Figueiredo Pessôa, et al.
Exogenous OCT4 and SOX2 Contribution to In Vitro Reprogramming in Cattle
Reprinted from: *Biomedicines* 2023, 11, 2577, https://doi.org/10.3390/biomedicines11092577 . . 24

Zhenwu Zhang, Xinyu Bao and Chao-Po Lin
Progress and Prospects of Gene Editing in Pluripotent Stem Cells
Reprinted from: *Biomedicines* 2023, 11, 2168, https://doi.org/10.3390/biomedicines11082168 . . 38

Elena S. Yarkova, Elena V. Grigor'eva, Sergey P. Medvedev, Denis A. Tarasevich, Sophia V. Pavlova, Kamila R. Valetdinova, et al.
Detection of ER Stress in iPSC-Derived Neurons Carrying the p.N370S Mutation in the *GBA1* Gene
Reprinted from: *Biomedicines* 2024, 12, 744, https://doi.org/10.3390/biomedicines12040744 . . . 62

Keshi Chung, Malvina Millet, Ludivine Rouillon and Azel Zine
Timing and Graded BMP Signalling Determines Fate of Neural Crest and Ectodermal Placode Derivatives from Pluripotent Stem Cells
Reprinted from: *Biomedicines* 2024, 12, 2262, https://doi.org/10.3390/biomedicines12102262 . . 85

Dong-Hun Lee, Eun Chae Lee, Ji young Lee, Man Ryul Lee, Jae-won Shim and Jae Sang Oh
Neuronal Cell Differentiation of iPSCs for the Clinical Treatment of Neurological Diseases
Reprinted from: *Biomedicines* 2024, 12, 1350, https://doi.org/10.3390/biomedicines12061350 . . 107

Yangwang Jin, Weixin Zhao, Ming Yang, Wenzhuo Fang, Guo Gao, Ying Wang and Qiang Fu
Cell-Based Therapy for Urethral Regeneration: A Narrative Review and Future Perspectives
Reprinted from: *Biomedicines* 2023, 11, 2366, https://doi.org/10.3390/biomedicines11092366 . . 118

Xiaotian Du, Kejiong Liang, Shili Ding and Haifei Shi
Signaling Mechanisms of Stem Cell Therapy for Intervertebral Disc Degeneration
Reprinted from: *Biomedicines* 2023, 11, 2467, https://doi.org/10.3390/biomedicines11092467 . . 138

Razik Bin Abdul Mu-u-min, Abdoulaye Diane, Asma Allouch and Heba Hussain Al-Siddiqi
Immune Evasion in Stem Cell-Based Diabetes Therapy—Current Strategies and Their Application in Clinical Trials
Reprinted from: *Biomedicines* 2025, 13, 383, https://doi.org/10.3390/biomedicines13020383 . . . 156

Ekaterina Vedeneeva, Vitaly Gursky, Maria Samsonova and Irina Neganova
Morphological Signal Processing for Phenotype Recognition of Human Pluripotent Stem Cells Using Machine Learning Methods
Reprinted from: *Biomedicines* 2023, 11, 3005, https://doi.org/10.3390/biomedicines11113005 . . 179

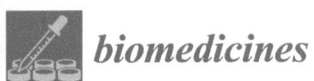

Editorial

Pluripotent Stem Cells: Recent Advances and Emerging Trends

Aline Yen Ling Wang [1,*] Ana Elena Aviña [1,2], Yen-Yu Liu [1] and Huang-Kai Kao [3,4]

1. Center for Vascularized Composite Allotransplantation, Chang Gung Memorial Hospital, Taoyuan 333, Taiwan; 250783@cgmh.org.tw (A.E.A.); louis881128@cgmh.org.tw (Y.-Y.L.)
2. International PhD Program in Medicine, College of Medicine, Taipei Medical University, Taipei 110, Taiwan
3. Department of Plastic and Reconstructive Surgery, Chang Gung Memorial Hospital, Taoyuan 333, Taiwan; kai3488@cgmh.org.tw
4. College of Medicine, Chang Gung University, Taoyuan 333, Taiwan
* Correspondence: aline2355@yahoo.com.tw

The field of induced pluripotent stem cells (iPSCs) continues to evolve, offering unprecedented potential for regenerative medicine, disease modeling, and therapeutic applications. All 10 featured research papers collected in this Special Issue demonstrate the assessment of distinct iPSC features, which include molecular regulations and differentiation protocols, in addition to therapeutic applications, along with genetic editing practices and immune evasion developments. This editorial presents a summary of the essential discoveries within all published works from this issue and establishes their widespread field impact together with upcoming trends. (1) Advances in iPSC-based regenerative medicine by Jin et al. (2023) provides a review of iPSC-based treatments for urethral regeneration, analyzing the drawbacks of conventional graft procedures [1]. The paper by Du et al. (2023) examines stem cell-signaling in treating intervertebral disk degeneration, and demonstrates iPSC-derived therapies as a promising musculoskeletal disorder solution [2]. (2) Molecular and genetic insights in iPSCs by Machado et al. (2023) examines the molecular functions of OCT4 and SOX2 during iPSC reprogramming by exploring their effects on epigenetic modifications while discussing their role in keeping stem cells pluripotent [3]. Zhang et al. (2023) present an extensive review about CRISPR-Cas9 gene editing of iPSCs, which demonstrates both advanced genome precision techniques and promising medical possibilities [4]. Saini et al. (2023) examine ATP-binding cassette proteins together with their regulatory functions for sustaining stem cell pluripotency while demonstrating the importance of intracellular transport systems [5]. (3) Neural differentiation and neurological applications: Neural differentiation research combined with applications in neuroscience by Yarkova et al. (2024) develops a distinct approach to detect endoplasmic reticulum stress in induced pluripotent stem cell-derived neurons for helping model neurodegenerative diseases [6]. Research by Lee et al. (2024) demonstrates how iPSCs can differentiate into neurons, which shows encouraging results in preclinical studies for treating Parkinson's disease [7]. (4) Machine learning and computational applications by Vedeneeva et al. (2023) presents machine learning technology that automatically detects iPSC colonies for high-quality selection enhancement while improving differentiation outcomes [8]. According to Chung et al. in (5) Developmental and signaling pathways (2024), BMP signaling controls the differentiation process of neural crest cells and ectodermal placode cells, which helps advance knowledge of embryological pathways using iPSC technology [9]. (6) Immune evasion strategies in iPSC-based therapies by Mu-u-min et al. (2025) presents immune evasion techniques for stem cell-based diabetes therapy as they review methods including encapsulation, along with genetic modifications to escape immune rejection difficulties [10].

The field of iPSCs has recently made significant improvements in safety together with efficiency and clinical practice readiness [11,12]. Modern reprogramming methods have reduced genomic alterations through the development of safer non-integrative approaches, including messenger RNA (mRNA) transfection and Sendai virus delivery, along with small molecule-based reprogramming to replace traditional viral methods for generating clinical-grade iPSCs [13–16]. The cells receive reprogramming factor genes OCT4, SOX2, KLF4, and c-MYC through transient mRNA transfection procedures, which transiently expresses these factors [13,15,17]. The genome-changing risks during reprogramming are minimized by mRNA transfection because it does not lead to integration. Through this method, scientists obtain controlled gene expression and faster reprogramming kinetics. Sendai virus delivery technique is another powerful tool for reprogramming [18–21]. It is replication-deficient and does not integrate into the host genome, making it safer for generating clinically relevant iPSCs. This method has been widely adopted for generating GMP-compliant (Good Manufacturing Practice) iPSCs for clinical applications. Researchers investigated reprogramming using chemical substances instead of classical transcription factors because these substitutes reduce mutation risks and enhance the process efficiency [22,23]. Simultaneously, the creation of 3D organoid models has taken the power of iPSCs past traditional differentiation methods to produce real-life models of brain and liver together with gastrointestinal system structures that help scientists examine diseases, test new drugs, and develop regenerative medical treatments [24–26]. Scientists can now use CRISPR-Cas9 in combination with iPSC technology to develop personalized regenerative treatments, thanks to recent field revolutionization [27–29]. For example, researcher access to disease mechanisms is enhanced through the gene-editing of iPSCs that come from patients with genetic disorders to produce matching control lines for scientific studies [29,30]. Parkinson's disease-specific neurons derived from iPSCs allow researchers to edit them for disease-progression investigation of key genes [31]. Additionally, CRISPR-based technologies serve as tools to fix genetic errors found in iPSCs extracted from patients before converting these cells into healthy transplantation-ready cells [32,33]. Research has shown that autologous cell therapy could become possible through dystrophin gene correction in Duchenne muscular dystrophy patient-derived iPSCs [34]. Moreover, the latest CRISPR systems, such as base editors and prime editors, enable exact gene modification that produces fewer errors while avoiding double-strand break formation to minimize unintended mutations. Finally, gene-edited iPSCs are now being used to create humanized disease models for drug screening, allowing for the identification of compounds that target disease-specific pathways [35–38]. Additionally, refined differentiation protocols leveraging key signaling pathways, including BMP, Wnt, and TGF-β, have enhanced the efficiency and reproducibility of iPSC-derived cardiomyocytes, neurons, and pancreatic β-cells, accelerating their potential clinical applications [39–41]. However, the main challenge that prevents iPSC-based therapies from implementation is immune rejection. Research teams may employ CRISPR-Cas9 strategies to engineer hypoalloreactive iPSCs by removing HLA class I and II molecules and reducing immune surveillance, while adding PD-L1 regulatory proteins for developing universal cell supplies that would not require immunologic suppressing drugs [42]. Multiple technological developments, together, are accelerating the usage of iPSC technology for translation applications, which is leading medicine toward broad personalization and regeneration at a scale not seen before.

Several issues continue to challenge the advancement of iPSCs, even though research conducted in this Special Issue shows great potential for their use. For example, the obstacles to moving iPSC-derived cell products toward clinical implementation include maintaining reproducibility and scalability. The risk of genetic instability and tumor formation in iPSC-derived cell therapies necessitates stringent safety assessments. Because iPSCs are widely utilized in disease modeling and tissue transplantation methods, the existing ethical rules, together with regulatory procedures, must adapt properly, such as through the implementation of AI with machine learning capabilities in the field of stem cell research. Computational methods described by Vedeneeva et al. (2023) hold great potential to transform current processes for quality checks and cell differentiation protocols [8]. Applied translation of iPSC-based treatments for medical use continues as a key objective that depends on united work between experts in stem cell biology and bioengineering and medical sciences.

The studies assembled in this Special Issue deliver valuable research about pluripotent stem cells together with their potential medical applications. The data proves the versatile nature of iPSCs, as they continue to drive advances in both regenerative medicine and gene therapy together with disease modeling applications. The combination of gene editing along with bioengineering methods and computational technologies will enhance the development process for safe and effective iPSC-based therapeutic options.

As a Guest Editor of this Special Issue, we express heartfelt thanks to all the authors, together with reviewers and researchers who advanced the discipline. iPSC cells have only just begun their path, yet this path leads directly to a new age of regenerative healthcare that will rely heavily on these cells to define its future developments.

Author Contributions: Conceptualization, writing, and reviewing: A.Y.L.W., A.E.A., Y.-Y.L. and H.-K.K. All authors have read and agreed to the published version of the manuscript.

Funding: This research was funded by the National Science and Technology Council, Taiwan (grant number NSTC 112-2314-B-182A-045-MY3), and the Chang Gung Medical Foundation, Chang Gung Memorial Hospital, Taiwan (grant number CMRPG3M0283).

Conflicts of Interest: The authors declare no conflicts of interest.

References

1. Jin, Y.; Zhao, W.; Yang, M.; Fang, W.; Gao, G.; Wang, Y.; Fu, Q. Cell-Based Therapy for Urethral Regeneration: A Narrative Review and Future Perspectives. *Biomedicines* **2023**, *11*, 2366. [CrossRef] [PubMed]
2. Du, X.; Liang, K.; Ding, S.; Shi, H. Signaling Mechanisms of Stem Cell Therapy for Intervertebral Disc Degeneration. *Biomedicines* **2023**, *11*, 2467. [CrossRef] [PubMed]
3. Machado, L.S.; Borges, C.M.; de Lima, M.A.; Sangalli, J.R.; Therrien, J.; Pessoa, L.V.F.; Fantinato Neto, P.; Perecin, F.; Smith, L.C.; Meirelles, F.V.; et al. Exogenous OCT4 and SOX2 Contribution to In Vitro Reprogramming in Cattle. *Biomedicines* **2023**, *11*, 2577. [CrossRef] [PubMed]
4. Zhang, Z.; Bao, X.; Lin, C.P. Progress and Prospects of Gene Editing in Pluripotent Stem Cells. *Biomedicines* **2023**, *11*, 2168. [CrossRef]
5. Saini, P.; Anugula, S.; Fong, Y.W. The Role of ATP-Binding Cassette Proteins in Stem Cell Pluripotency. *Biomedicines* **2023**, *11*, 1868. [CrossRef]
6. Yarkova, E.S.; Grigor'eva, E.V.; Medvedev, S.P.; Tarasevich, D.A.; Pavlova, S.V.; Valetdinova, K.R.; Minina, J.M.; Zakian, S.M.; Malakhova, A.A. Detection of ER Stress in iPSC-Derived Neurons Carrying the p.N370S Mutation in the *GBA1* Gene. *Biomedicines* **2024**, *12*, 744. [CrossRef]
7. Lee, D.H.; Lee, E.C.; Lee, J.Y.; Lee, M.R.; Shim, J.W.; Oh, J.S. Neuronal Cell Differentiation of iPSCs for the Clinical Treatment of Neurological Diseases. *Biomedicines* **2024**, *12*, 1350. [CrossRef]
8. Vedeneeva, E.; Gursky, V.; Samsonova, M.; Neganova, I. Morphological Signal Processing for Phenotype Recognition of Human Pluripotent Stem Cells Using Machine Learning Methods. *Biomedicines* **2023**, *11*, 3005. [CrossRef]
9. Chung, K.; Millet, M.; Rouillon, L.; Zine, A. Timing and Graded BMP Signalling Determines Fate of Neural Crest and Ectodermal Placode Derivatives from Pluripotent Stem Cells. *Biomedicines* **2024**, *12*, 2262. [CrossRef]
10. Mu, U.M.R.B.A.; Diane, A.; Allouch, A.; Al-Siddiqi, H.H. Immune Evasion in Stem Cell-Based Diabetes Therapy-Current Strategies and Their Application in Clinical Trials. *Biomedicines* **2025**, *13*, 383. [CrossRef]
11. Wang, A.Y.L. Human Induced Pluripotent Stem Cell-Derived Exosomes as a New Therapeutic Strategy for Various Diseases. *Int. J. Mol. Sci.* **2021**, *22*, 1769. [CrossRef] [PubMed]

12. Loh, C.Y.; Wang, A.Y.; Kao, H.K.; Cardona, E.; Chuang, S.H.; Wei, F.C. Episomal Induced Pluripotent Stem Cells Promote Functional Recovery of Transected Murine Peripheral Nerve. *PLoS ONE* **2016**, *11*, e0164696. [CrossRef] [PubMed]
13. Warren, L.; Lin, C. mRNA-Based Genetic Reprogramming. *Mol. Ther.* **2019**, *27*, 729–734. [CrossRef] [PubMed]
14. Wang, A.Y.L. Application of Modified mRNA in Somatic Reprogramming to Pluripotency and Directed Conversion of Cell Fate. *Int. J. Mol. Sci.* **2021**, *22*, 8148. [CrossRef]
15. Warren, L.; Manos, P.D.; Ahfeldt, T.; Loh, Y.H.; Li, H.; Lau, F.; Ebina, W.; Mandal, P.K.; Smith, Z.D.; Meissner, A.; et al. Highly efficient reprogramming to pluripotency and directed differentiation of human cells with synthetic modified mRNA. *Cell Stem Cell* **2010**, *7*, 618–630. [CrossRef]
16. Wang, A.Y.L.; Loh, C.Y.Y. Episomal Induced Pluripotent Stem Cells: Functional and Potential Therapeutic Applications. *Cell Transplant.* **2019**, *28*, 112S–131S. [CrossRef]
17. Li, J.; Song, W.; Pan, G.; Zhou, J. Advances in understanding the cell types and approaches used for generating induced pluripotent stem cells. *J. Hematol. Oncol.* **2014**, *7*, 50. [CrossRef]
18. Silva, M.; Daheron, L.; Hurley, H.; Bure, K.; Barker, R.; Carr, A.J.; Williams, D.; Kim, H.W.; French, A.; Coffey, P.J.; et al. Generating iPSCs: Translating cell reprogramming science into scalable and robust biomanufacturing strategies. *Cell Stem Cell* **2015**, *16*, 13–17. [CrossRef]
19. Nishino, K.; Arai, Y.; Takasawa, K.; Toyoda, M.; Yamazaki-Inoue, M.; Sugawara, T.; Akutsu, H.; Nishimura, K.; Ohtaka, M.; Nakanishi, M.; et al. Epigenetic-scale comparison of human iPSCs generated by retrovirus, Sendai virus or episomal vectors. *Regen. Ther.* **2018**, *9*, 71–78. [CrossRef]
20. Nakanishi, M.; Otsu, M. Development of Sendai virus vectors and their potential applications in gene therapy and regenerative medicine. *Curr. Gene Ther.* **2012**, *12*, 410–416. [CrossRef]
21. Trokovic, R.; Weltner, J.; Nishimura, K.; Ohtaka, M.; Nakanishi, M.; Salomaa, V.; Jalanko, A.; Otonkoski, T.; Kyttala, A. Advanced feeder-free generation of induced pluripotent stem cells directly from blood cells. *Stem Cells Transl. Med.* **2014**, *3*, 1402–1409. [CrossRef] [PubMed]
22. Lin, T.; Wu, S. Reprogramming with Small Molecules instead of Exogenous Transcription Factors. *Stem Cells Int.* **2015**, *2015*, 794632. [CrossRef] [PubMed]
23. Wang, J.; Sun, S.; Deng, H. Chemical reprogramming for cell fate manipulation: Methods, applications, and perspectives. *Cell Stem Cell* **2023**, *30*, 1130–1147. [CrossRef] [PubMed]
24. Silva-Pedrosa, R.; Salgado, A.J.; Ferreira, P.E. Revolutionizing Disease Modeling: The Emergence of Organoids in Cellular Systems. *Cells* **2023**, *12*, 930. [CrossRef]
25. Kim, J.; Koo, B.K.; Knoblich, J.A. Human organoids: Model systems for human biology and medicine. *Nat. Rev. Mol. Cell Biol.* **2020**, *21*, 571–584. [CrossRef]
26. Yao, Q.; Cheng, S.; Pan, Q.; Yu, J.; Cao, G.; Li, L.; Cao, H. Organoids: Development and applications in disease models, drug discovery, precision medicine, and regenerative medicine. *MedComm* **2024**, *5*, e735. [CrossRef]
27. Gahwiler, E.K.N.; Motta, S.E.; Martin, M.; Nugraha, B.; Hoerstrup, S.P.; Emmert, M.Y. Human iPSCs and Genome Editing Technologies for Precision Cardiovascular Tissue Engineering. *Front. Cell Dev. Biol.* **2021**, *9*, 639699. [CrossRef]
28. Walsh, C.; Jin, S. Induced Pluripotent Stem Cells and CRISPR-Cas9 Innovations for Treating Alpha-1 Antitrypsin Deficiency and Glycogen Storage Diseases. *Cells* **2024**, *13*, 1052. [CrossRef]
29. McTague, A.; Rossignoli, G.; Ferrini, A.; Barral, S.; Kurian, M.A. Genome Editing in iPSC-Based Neural Systems: From Disease Models to Future Therapeutic Strategies. *Front. Genome Ed.* **2021**, *3*, 630600. [CrossRef]
30. Soldner, F.; Laganiere, J.; Cheng, A.W.; Hockemeyer, D.; Gao, Q.; Alagappan, R.; Khurana, V.; Golbe, L.I.; Myers, R.H.; Lindquist, S.; et al. Generation of isogenic pluripotent stem cells differing exclusively at two early onset Parkinson point mutations. *Cell* **2011**, *146*, 318–331. [CrossRef]
31. Pinjala, P.; Tryphena, K.P.; Prasad, R.; Khatri, D.K.; Sun, W.; Singh, S.B.; Gugulothu, D.; Srivastava, S.; Vora, L. CRISPR/Cas9 assisted stem cell therapy in Parkinson's disease. *Biomater. Res.* **2023**, *27*, 46. [CrossRef] [PubMed]
32. Burnight, E.R.; Gupta, M.; Wiley, L.A.; Anfinson, K.R.; Tran, A.; Triboulet, R.; Hoffmann, J.M.; Klaahsen, D.L.; Andorf, J.L.; Jiao, C.; et al. Using CRISPR-Cas9 to Generate Gene-Corrected Autologous iPSCs for the Treatment of Inherited Retinal Degeneration. *Mol. Ther.* **2017**, *25*, 1999–2013. [CrossRef] [PubMed]
33. Jackow, J.; Guo, Z.; Hansen, C.; Abaci, H.E.; Doucet, Y.S.; Shin, J.U.; Hayashi, R.; DeLorenzo, D.; Kabata, Y.; Shinkuma, S.; et al. CRISPR/Cas9-based targeted genome editing for correction of recessive dystrophic epidermolysis bullosa using iPS cells. *Proc. Natl. Acad. Sci. USA* **2019**, *116*, 26846–26852. [CrossRef] [PubMed]
34. Li, H.L.; Fujimoto, N.; Sasakawa, N.; Shirai, S.; Ohkame, T.; Sakuma, T.; Tanaka, M.; Amano, N.; Watanabe, A.; Sakurai, H.; et al. Precise correction of the dystrophin gene in duchenne muscular dystrophy patient induced pluripotent stem cells by TALEN and CRISPR-Cas9. *Stem Cell Rep.* **2015**, *4*, 143–154. [CrossRef]
35. Bassett, A.R. Editing the genome of hiPSC with CRISPR/Cas9: Disease models. *Mamm. Genome* **2017**, *28*, 348–364. [CrossRef]

36. Shi, Y.; Inoue, H.; Wu, J.C.; Yamanaka, S. Induced pluripotent stem cell technology: A decade of progress. *Nat. Rev. Drug Discov.* **2017**, *16*, 115–130. [CrossRef]
37. Okano, H.; Morimoto, S. iPSC-based disease modeling and drug discovery in cardinal neurodegenerative disorders. *Cell Stem Cell* **2022**, *29*, 189–208. [CrossRef]
38. Cerneckis, J.; Cai, H.; Shi, Y. Induced pluripotent stem cells (iPSCs): Molecular mechanisms of induction and applications. *Signal Transduct. Target. Ther.* **2024**, *9*, 112. [CrossRef]
39. Funa, N.S.; Mjoseng, H.K.; de Lichtenberg, K.H.; Raineri, S.; Esen, D.; Egeskov-Madsen, A.R.; Quaranta, R.; Jorgensen, M.C.; Hansen, M.S.; van Cuyl Kuylenstierna, J.; et al. TGF-beta modulates cell fate in human ES cell-derived foregut endoderm by inhibiting Wnt and BMP signaling. *Stem Cell Rep.* **2024**, *19*, 973–992. [CrossRef]
40. Fujimori, K.; Matsumoto, T.; Kisa, F.; Hattori, N.; Okano, H.; Akamatsu, W. Escape from Pluripotency via Inhibition of TGF-beta/BMP and Activation of Wnt Signaling Accelerates Differentiation and Aging in hPSC Progeny Cells. *Stem Cell Rep.* **2017**, *9*, 1675–1691. [CrossRef]
41. Pushpan, C.K.; Kumar, S.R. iPSC-Derived Cardiomyocytes as a Disease Model to Understand the Biology of Congenital Heart Defects. *Cells* **2024**, *13*, 1430. [CrossRef]
42. Park, H.; Kang, Y.K.; Shim, G. CRISPR/Cas9-Mediated Customizing Strategies for Adoptive T-Cell Therapy. *Pharmaceutics* **2024**, *16*, 346. [CrossRef]

Disclaimer/Publisher's Note: The statements, opinions and data contained in all publications are solely those of the individual author(s) and contributor(s) and not of MDPI and/or the editor(s). MDPI and/or the editor(s) disclaim responsibility for any injury to people or property resulting from any ideas, methods, instructions or products referred to in the content.

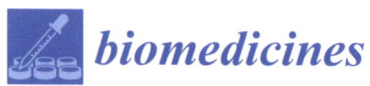 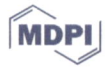

Review

The Role of ATP-Binding Cassette Proteins in Stem Cell Pluripotency

Prince Saini [1,2,3], Sharath Anugula [1,2,3] and Yick W. Fong [1,2,3,*]

- [1] Brigham Regenerative Medicine Center, Brigham and Women's Hospital, Boston, MA 02115, USA; psaini@bwh.harvard.edu (P.S.); sanugula@bwh.harvard.edu (S.A.)
- [2] Department of Medicine, Cardiovascular Medicine Division, Harvard Medical School, Boston, MA 02115, USA
- [3] Harvard Stem Cell Institute, Cambridge, MA 02138, USA
- * Correspondence: yfong@bwh.harvard.edu

Abstract: Pluripotent stem cells (PSCs) are highly proliferative cells that can self-renew indefinitely in vitro. Upon receiving appropriate signals, PSCs undergo differentiation and can generate every cell type in the body. These unique properties of PSCs require specific gene expression patterns that define stem cell identity and dynamic regulation of intracellular metabolism to support cell growth and cell fate transitions. PSCs are prone to DNA damage due to elevated replicative and transcriptional stress. Therefore, mechanisms to prevent deleterious mutations in PSCs that compromise stem cell function or increase the risk of tumor formation from becoming amplified and propagated to progenitor cells are essential for embryonic development and for using PSCs including induced PSCs (iPSCs) as a cell source for regenerative medicine. In this review, we discuss the role of the ATP-binding cassette (ABC) superfamily in maintaining PSC homeostasis, and propose how their activities can influence cellular signaling and stem cell fate decisions. Finally, we highlight recent discoveries that not all ABC family members perform only canonical metabolite and peptide transport functions in PSCs; rather, they can participate in diverse cellular processes from genome surveillance to gene transcription and mRNA translation, which are likely to maintain the pristine state of PSCs.

Keywords: ABC transporters; pluripotency; cell signaling; metabolism; phospholipids; glutathione; reactive oxygen species

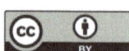

1. Introduction

Pluripotent stem cells (PSCs) are derived from the inner cell mass of the blastocyst [1,2]. Expansion of these cells during embryonic development or in vitro through self-renewal requires coordinated changes in cellular metabolism [3]. Like other rapidly dividing cells, PSCs must amplify their macromolecular contents such as nucleic acids, carbohydrates, proteins, lipopolysaccharides, and lipids, by generating precursor molecules to meet the metabolic requirements of cell proliferation. However, increasing evidence indicates that cellular metabolism not only plays an important role in regulating proliferative capacity but also self-renewal versus the differentiation of PSCs [4,5]. For example, lipid metabolites can act as signaling molecules and activate signaling pathways that converge on a unique network of genes controlled by stem cell-enriched transcription factors OCT4 and SOX2 [6]. OCT4 and SOX2 co-regulate a large number of genes to sustain stem cell pluripotency [7–10]. Intrinsic and extrinsic signals that perturb this transcriptional network impair PSC self-renewal and promote differentiation [11]. Therefore, regulating the availability and distribution of lipids and other macromolecules in PSCs could modulate cell signaling and influence the cell fate decision. Metabolite homeostasis reflects a balance between synthesis and degradation or export [12]. While the biosynthetic pathways of essential macromolecules are well-understood, the role of transporters in regulating their concentration and distribution remains underexplored.

The plasticity of PSCs is in part facilitated by the prevalence of open chromatin and elevated global transcriptional activities [13]. However, the permissive chromatin structure and the act of transcription itself are sources of genome instability, exposing DNA to DNA-modifying enzymes and genotoxic agents such as reactive oxygen species (ROS) [14,15]. In addition, unlike somatic cells, PSCs display a "compressed" cell cycle with a shortened G1, resulting in increased replicative stress [16]. Furthermore, PSCs do not undergo DNA damage-induced G1 cell cycle arrest, which in somatic cells is thought to provide time to repair critical damage before DNA replication occurs [17,18]. Therefore, ESCs are presumably at higher risk of acquiring mutations. Paradoxically, it has been found that the apparent mutation frequency in PSCs is about 100-fold lower than that in somatic cells [19], suggesting that there are additional mechanisms in PSCs that suppress mutagenesis and/or purge damaged cells. PSCs respond to DNA damage by undergoing rapid differentiation and apoptosis [20,21]. It is thought that hypersensitivity to DNA damage prevents deleterious mutations in PSCs from becoming amplified and propagated to progenitor cells [22]. Therefore, a regulated transcriptional switch from self-renewal to differentiation is not only important for embryonic development but also for genome maintenance in PSCs.

The seminal discovery that the PSC fate can be induced in somatic cells via the ectopic expression of a cadre of transcription factors opens the possibility of generating patient-specific induced pluripotent stem cells (iPSCs) for regenerative medicine [23,24]. While iPSCs are highly similar to bona fide ESCs [25], studies indicated that iPSC lines display altered gene expression patterns [26] and recurrent genetic abnormalities [26–28] that have been shown to increase the risk of tumorigenicity [29–31], thus posing serious challenges to using iPSCs for regenerative medicine due to significant safety concerns [31–34]. In order to fully realize the therapeutic potential of iPSCs, we suggest that a more complete understanding of the molecular underpinnings of stem cell pluripotency is required.

In this review, we focus on the "canonical" roles of membrane-bound ATP-binding cassette (ABC) transporters in the translocation of lipids, cholesterol, and ROS-scavenging glutathione peptides in PSCs, and the implications for modulating cellular signaling and homeostasis critical for stem cell pluripotency. We also discuss the unexpectedly diverse functions of non-membrane-bound ABC proteins in translation and in coordinating stem cell-specific transcription with genome surveillance, to maintain a pristine proteome and genome for proper stem cell function and regenerative medicine.

2. ABC Expression in PSCs

Ubiquitous from bacteria to humans, the ABC superfamily is one of the largest classes of transmembrane (TM) proteins [35]. In mammals, membrane-bound ABC proteins are efflux transporters that translocate essential substrates ranging from ions to macromolecules across membranes at the cost of ATP hydrolysis (Figure 1). It is perhaps not surprising that defects in these transporters are associated with human disorders, including metabolic diseases (Table 1) [36,37]. Of the 49 *ABC* genes in the human genome, 4 lack TM domains and thus are not transporters [38]. Transcriptomic and proteomic studies indicated that 26 *ABC* genes are expressed in PSCs [39–42] (Table 1), and that their expression levels change when PSCs exit from pluripotency and undergo differentiation [39,42,43]. However, the lack of specific antibodies against some of these ABC proteins precludes a confirmation of their expression at the protein level. Nonetheless, drawing on observations in PSCs and other cell systems, we suggest that cell type-specific expression patterns of ABC proteins not only reflect differences in metabolic requirements but may also contribute to cell fate regulation.

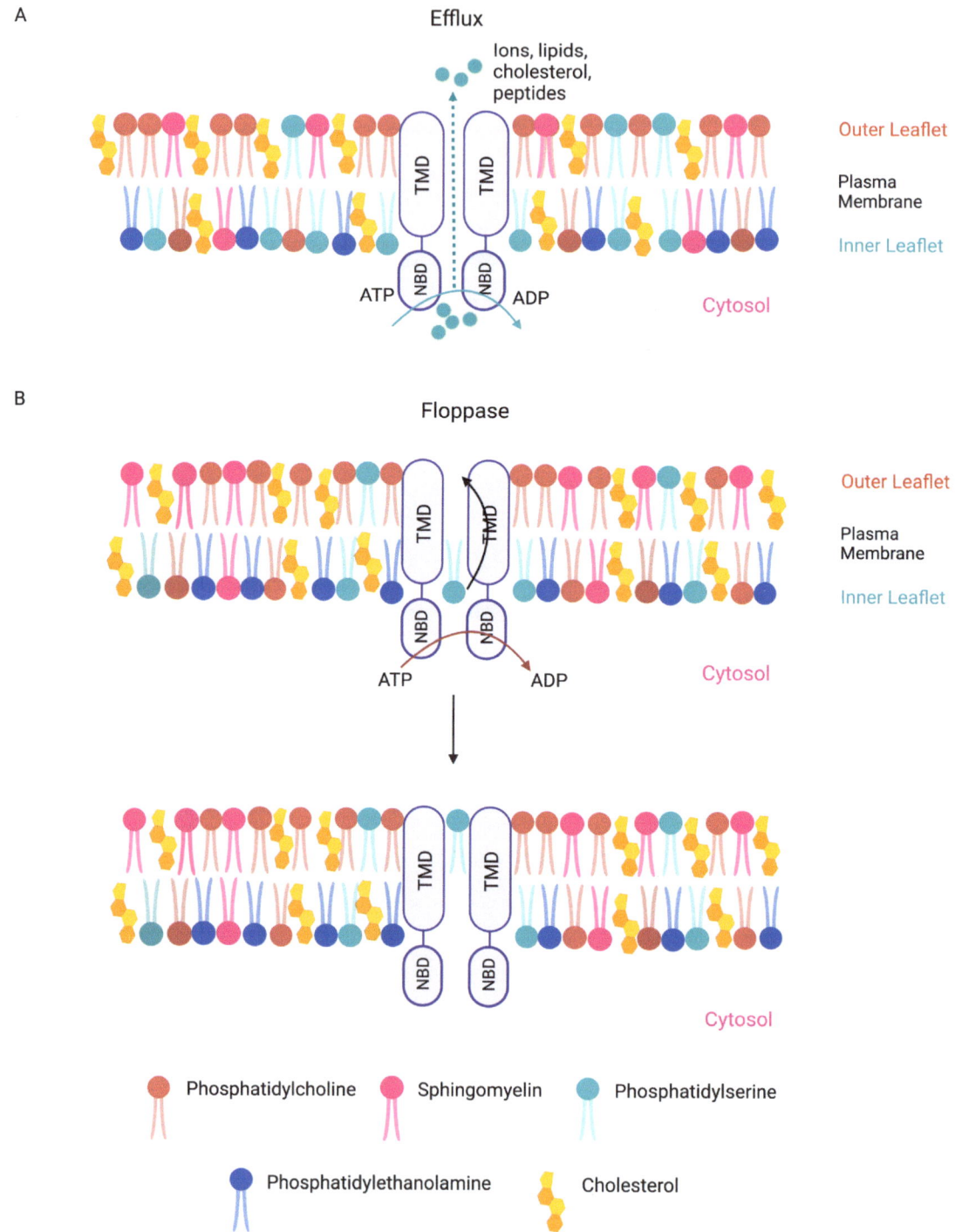

Figure 1. Membrane-bound mammalian ABC transporters are efflux pumps and/or floppases. (**A**) ABC proteins are essential membrane-bound transporters. ABC transporters are anchored at cell

membranes through their transmembrane domains (TMDs). ABC transporters can efflux ions and macromolecules (e.g., lipids, cholesterol, and peptides) across cell membranes. (**B**) ABC transporters are also lipid floppases. They are critical for maintaining the asymmetric distribution of phospholipids in the membrane. Phosphatidylcholine (beige) and sphingomyelin (pink) reside predominantly in the outer leaflet of the plasma membrane, whereas anionic lipids such as phosphatidylserine (cyan) and phosphatidylethanolamine (blue) are more prevalent in the inner leaflet. Membrane cholesterols are depicted (yellow). Phospholipids such as phosphatidylserine from the inner membrane leaflet are "flopped" to the outer leaflet. Efflux and floppase activities require ATP hydrolysis by the nucleotide-binding domains (NBDs).

Table 1. Summary of Human ABC proteins and their functions, involvement in diseases and expression in pluripotent stem cells. Abbreviations: PC, phosphatidylcholine; PS, phosphatidylserine; SM, Sphingomyelin; HDL, high-density lipoprotein.

Symbol	Alias	Subcellular Location	Function	Disease Associated	Expression at mRNA/Protein Level in PSCs
ABCA1	ABC1	Plasma membrane, endoplasmic reticulum	Cholesterol efflux onto HDL/phospholipids	Tangier disease	mRNA [39], Protein [43]
ABCA2	ABC2	Endosome, lysosome	Cholesterol, drug resistance	Alzheimer's disease	mRNA [39]
ABCA3	ABC3	Endosome, lysosome	Surfactant secretion	Surfactant metabolism dysfunction 3	mRNA [39]
ABCA5		Plasma membrane	Cholesterol efflux transporter		mRNA [39]
ABCA7		Plasma membrane, endoplasmic reticulum	Transport PC, PS, and SM from the cytoplasmic to the exocytoplasmic side of membranes,	Alzheimer's disease	mRNA [39]
ABCB1	PGY1, MDR	Plasma membrane	Glucosylceramides, multidrug resistance	Inflammatory bowel disease	mRNA [44]
ABCB2	TAP1	Endoplasmic reticulum	Peptide transport	Bare lymphocyte syndrome type I	mRNA [39]
ABCB3	TAP2	Endoplasmic reticulum	Peptide transport	Bare lymphocyte syndrome, type I due to TAP2 deficiency	mRNA [39]
ABCB4	PGY3	Plasma membrane	PC transport	Cholestasis 3 (PFIC3)	mRNA [45]
ABCB6	MTABC3	Plasma membrane, endosome, endoplasmic reticulum, Golgi, mitochondria, lysosome	Iron transport/heavy metal importer subfamily and role in porphyrin transport	Dyschromatosis universalis hereditaria 3, Lan blood group	mRNA [39,40], Protein [40,43]
ABCB7	ABC7	Mitochondria	Fe/S cluster transport	X-linked sideroblastic anemia with ataxia	mRNA [39,40,45], Protein [41]
ABCB8	MABC1	Mitochondria	Mitochondrial iron export; organic and inorganic molecules out of the mitochondria		mRNA [39], Protein [40]

Table 1. Cont.

Symbol	Alias	Subcellular Location	Function	Disease Associated	Expression at mRNA/Protein Level in PSCs
ABCB9		Lysosome	ATP-dependent low-affinity peptide transporter		mRNA [39]
ABCB10	MTABC2	Mitochondria	Enhances heme biosynthesis in developing red blood cells		mRNA [39,45,46]
ABCC1	MRP1	Plasma membrane, lysosome	Glutathione and other organic anions, drug resistance		mRNA [39,47], Protein [41,43]
ABCC4	MRP4	Plasma membrane	Cyclic nucleotides, bile acids, and eicosanoids/nucleoside transport/ glutathione		mRNA [39,40], Protein [40]
ABCC5	MRP5	Plasma membrane, endosome Golgi,	Nucleoside transport/glutamate conjugate and analog transporter/cAMP and cGMP, folic acid and N-lactoyl-amino acids		mRNA [39,40]
ABCC10	MRP7	Plasma membrane	Transport of glucuronide conjugates such as estradiol-17-beta-o-glucuronide and GSH conjugates such as leukotriene C4		mRNA [39]
ABCD1	ALD	Peroxisome	Peroxisomal transport of very long fatty acid/adrenoleukodystrophy	X-linked adrenoleuko-dystrophy	mRNA [39], Protein [40]
ABCD3	PXMP1, PMP70	Peroxisome	Peroxisomal transport of very long fatty acid/long-chain fatty acids (LCFA)-CoA, dicarboxylic acids-CoA, long-branched-chain fatty acids-CoA and bile acids from the cytosol to the peroxisome lumen for beta-oxidation		mRNA [39,40,45], Protein [41]
ABCD4	PMP69, P70R	Peroxisome, lysosome, endoplasmic reticulum	Cobalamin transporter	Methylmalonic aciduria and homocystinuria, cblJ type, inborn error of vitamin B12 metabolism	mRNA [39,45,46], Protein [40]
ABCE1	OABP, RNS4I	Cytoplasm, mitochondria	Oligoadenylate binding protein, Translation		mRNA [39,40,45], Protein [41]
ABCF1	ABC50	Ribosome, nucleus, cytoplasm	Transcription, translation, innate immune responses		mRNA [39,40,45], Protein [41,48]

Table 1. Cont.

Symbol	Alias	Subcellular Location	Function	Disease Associated	Expression at mRNA/Protein Level in PSCs
ABCF2					mRNA [39,40,45], Protein [41]
ABCF3					mRNA [39,40,46]
ABCG2	ABCP, MXR, BCRP	Mitochondria, Plasma membrane	Multidrug resistance,	Junior blood group system, gout	mRNA [39], Protein [49,50]

3. The Roles of ABC Transporters in PSCs

3.1. Lipid Transporters (ABCA1 and ABCC1)

Lipids are a diverse class of biomolecules. Glycerophospholipids, specifically phosphatidylcholine (PC), phosphatidylethanolamine (PE), phosphatidylserine (PS), and phosphatidylinositol (PI), as well as sphingolipids and cholesterol, serve as building blocks for membranes and organelles [51]. Some ABC transporters (ABCC1 [52,53]) act as "floppases" by catalyzing the movement of specific phospholipid species from the cytosolic leaflet to the extracellular leaflet of the plasma membrane (PM) [54], while others (ABCA1 [55]) function as extracellular phospholipid translocases (Figure 1). Indeed, ABC transporters have been shown to contribute to the asymmetric distribution of different phospholipids in the lipid bilayer, with PC and sphingolipids such as sphingomyelin (SM) residing predominantly in the outer leaflet of the PM, whereas anionic lipids such as PE, PS, and PI accumulate in the inner leaflet [56,57]. Increasing evidence indicates that changes in the composition and distribution of these phospholipids in the lipid bilayer can regulate signal transduction pathways that are known to regulate PSC cell fates [58,59].

Stem cell maintenance in human PSCs requires basic fibroblast growth factor (bFGF), which activates the RAS-RAF-MEK-ERK signal transduction cascade [60–63]. The association of RAS with the inner leaflet of the PM is an important step in the recruitment and activation of its effectors such as RAF and phosphatidylinositol 3-kinase (PI3K) [64]. Interestingly, it has been shown that RAS can adopt a distinct orientation at the PM, depending on the types of phospholipids (PC, PS, or phosphatidylinositol 4,5-bisphosphate [PIP2]) that interact with RAS [65]. As a result, the catalytic domain of membrane-bound RAS is predicted to become more exposed or partially obscured. Therefore, how RAS is anchored in the PM could modulate its ability to interact with its effectors (e.g., RAF versus PI3K) and regulate RAS-mediated downstream signaling choices. It appears that electrostatic interactions between RAS and lipids dictate interaction affinity and orientation preferences. Given that ABC transporters can translocate PC, PS, and PIP2 to the cell membrane outer leaflet [66–68], we propose that changes in the local distribution of phospholipids in the lipid bilayer by specific ABC transporters could influence the spatial arrangement of RAS. Future studies will be required to address the expression patterns of ABC transporters and their function in regulating the distribution of membrane phospholipids and RAS signal transduction, thereby controlling stem cell self-renewal versus differentiation. In a similar manner, it will be prudent to examine whether or not other signaling pathways (e.g., TGF-β [69] and EGFR [70]) that are known to contribute to stem cell pluripotency can also be modulated by PM phospholipid organization.

3.2. Cholesterol Transporters (ABCA1 and ABCG1)

Cholesterol is an important constituent of cell membranes. The bulk of cellular cholesterol (~90%) is localized at the PM [71]. Cholesterol homeostasis is determined by the biosynthesis, uptake, and efflux of cholesterol. ABCA1 and ABCG1 play crucial roles in the efflux of cellular cholesterol and thus are important regulators of membrane cholesterol level [72–74].

Cholesterol is a key modulator of membrane fluidity [75,76], which in turn regulates cell behaviors such as adhesion, proliferation, and migration [77]. However, recent evidence indicates that changes in PM stiffness may also regulate cell fate changes in PSCs [78]. It has been shown that the rigidification of the PM precedes or coincides with downregulation of gene expression programs that stabilize the pluripotent state in PSCs, suggesting that a decrease in membrane fluidity may prime PSCs to exit from pluripotency. Consistent with the notion that maintenance of membrane fluidity contributes to stem cell maintenance, enzymes in the cholesterol biosynthesis pathways have been shown to be expressed at higher levels in PSCs, thereby increasing membrane cholesterol content and fluidity [78,79]. Importantly, the inhibition of cholesterol production in PSCs accelerates their exit from pluripotency, as indicated by the rapid downregulation of stem cell marker alkaline phosphatase [78]. These observations underscore the importance of cholesterol homeostasis in stem cell maintenance. We propose that dissecting the mechanisms by which the expression and activities of ABCA1 and ABCG1 are controlled in PSCs will advance our understanding of the role of cholesterol efflux in regulating membrane fluidity and stem cell pluripotency.

In addition to regulating membrane fluidity, cholesterol, together with SM, has been shown to assemble dynamic, cholesterol-rich microdomains in the outer leaflet of the PM [80]. These compartmentalized domains, known as lipid rafts, have been shown to enrich specific receptors and their effectors to promote receptor–effector interactions, thereby lowering activation barriers. The ability of lipid rafts to partition and concentrate select signaling machineries depends on the intrinsic affinity of these signaling proteins to lipid rafts, which has been shown to be influenced by amino acid sequences in the TM domains of membrane receptors and protein palmitoylation [81,82]. Oligomerization of receptors has also been reported to increase their affinity to lipid rafts and residence time in these lipid subdomains [83], hinting at a potential mechanism by which lipid rafts amplify signaling. We suggest that a small change in the concentration of signaling components in lipid rafts may be sufficient, through amplification, to initiate signaling cascades. Therefore, lipid rafts may play an important role in increasing the responsiveness of signal transduction machineries to cellular stimuli.

It has been shown that ABCA1 and ABCG1 deficiency in macrophages leads to an increase in the number of lipid rafts and enhanced signaling responses [84]. This is likely due to the propensity of lipid rafts to cluster, resulting in the amplification of signals [85,86]. These observations suggest an inhibitory function of ABCA1 and ABCG1 in lipid raft formation, via the mobilization of cholesterol from lipid rafts to non-raft domains. It will be of interest to determine the mechanisms by which ABC transporters are recruited to lipid rafts. This is because the active efflux of membrane cholesterol by ABC transporters could facilitate the fine-tuning and dissolution of signal transduction hubs in lipid rafts and signal termination.

Lipid rafts are also detected in PSCs, but their roles in stem cell maintenance are less well-understood [87]. The self-renewal of mouse PSCs requires leukemia inhibitory factor (LIF) signaling [88]. It has been shown that depletion of membrane cholesterol in mouse PSCs by methyl-β-cyclodextrin (Mβ-CD), which has been shown to disrupt lipid rafts, compromises the recruitment of LIF receptor and its co-receptor gp130 to rafts and blunts LIF receptor-JAK-STAT3 signaling [87]. The observed reduction in expression levels of key pluripotency-associated transcription factors OCT4 and SOX2 in Mβ-CD-treated PSCs indicates a destabilized pluripotent state when lipid raft formation is impaired. These observations are consistent with the role of lipid rafts in enriching specific receptors and facilitating their activation. Lipid rafts have also been implicated in other signaling pathways that are known to promote stem cell self-renewal and pluripotency, such as EGFR [70] and RAS [89], and those that destabilize the stem cell state, including insulin receptor [90] and hedgehog [91]. An outstanding question is how ABC transporters may control lipid raft formation and dynamics to partition competing signaling in PSCs to favor self-renewal over differentiation.

3.3. Redox Regulation and Oxidative Stress (ABCC1 and ABCC4)

ROS are natural byproducts of cellular metabolism. ROS can cause damage to the basic building blocks of cells including DNA, protein, and lipids. Therefore, ROS pose significant threats to the ability of PSCs to maintain genome and proteome integrity as they self-renew. In addition to cellular damages inflicted by ROS build-up, an imbalance in ROS levels can also lead to the misregulation of redox sensor molecules via the oxidation of cysteine residues. Some of these redox sensors are key signaling effectors such as AKT and MAPK [92,93]. Therefore, it is conceivable that an increase in ROS concentration destabilizes the pluripotent cell state in part by interfering with signaling pathways essential for stem cell maintenance [94]. ROS levels in cells are determined by the rate of ROS generation and the rate of ROS scavenging by antioxidants. PSCs are able to maintain relatively low ROS levels compared to those of differentiated cells, in part due to their reliance on glycolysis rather than oxidative phosphorylation for energy production, which is known to generate less ROS [95,96]. Nevertheless, the neutralization of ROS species by antioxidants remains a critical mechanism in regulating ROS homeostasis in PSCs as it is essential for stem cell maintenance [97,98].

Glutathione (GSH) is a major antioxidant in cells [99,100]. GSH levels are balanced by its synthesis, transport, efflux, and degradation. Studies have shown that ABCC1 is a major GSH exporter and can regulate intracellular GSH levels. The overexpression of ABCC1 reduces intracellular GSH levels, while ABCC1 deficiency increases GSH concentrations [101,102]. Importantly, ABCC1 can export both GSH and various oxidized glutathione derivatives (e.g., glutathione disulfide (GSSG)), although with distinct substrate affinity [103–105]. Therefore, in addition to cellular enzymes that can degrade GSH (e.g., CHAC1 [106,107]) or regenerate GSH from GSSG (e.g., GSH reductase [108]), ABCC1 likely plays an integral role in maintaining the redox equilibrium in PSCs. It has been shown that oxidative stress downregulates key PSC-specific transcription factors OCT4 and SOX2, and compromises AKT signaling [97]. While the precise mechanism is unclear, the destabilization of OCT4 proteins and inactivation of AKT via the oxidation of critical cysteines residues could compromise the gene transcription and cellular signaling required for stem cell maintenance [92,109,110].

Like oxidative stress, reductive stress induced by excessive levels of GSH can also impair PSC functions. Physiological levels of ROS have been shown to promote PSC proliferation and accurate DNA synthesis [111]. High concentrations of antioxidants interfere with cell cycle progression and lead to the accumulation of DNA breaks [112], likely due to the toxic effects of high antioxidant levels on the stability of cell cycle regulators and proteins involved in the DNA damage response and DNA repair [111]. The balance between ROS and antioxidants must be optimal, as both extremes, oxidative and reductive stress, are damaging to PSCs. Functional studies on the role of ABCC1 and ABCC4 in PSCs will address the precise role of GSH/GSSG efflux in establishing a cellular redox state favorable for stem cell self-renewal and genome maintenance.

4. Non-Canonical Functions of ABCs in PSCs

While most ABC proteins are membrane-bound transporters, ABCE1 and the ABCF subfamily proteins (ABCF1, ABCF2, and ABCF3) lack TM domains [38]. Although their precise functions remain somewhat enigmatic, recent studies highlight the multifaceted function of ABCF1 in regulating translation, innate immune response, and transcription, thus expanding the functional repertoire of ABC proteins.

4.1. ABCF1 in mRNA Translation

The initiation of mRNA translation can occur via cap-dependent and independent mechanisms [113,114]. In addition to internal ribosome entry site (IRES) elements in mRNAs, RNA methylation at adenosines (m^6A) by m^6A methyltransferases such as METTL3 has been shown to also facilitate cap-independent translation initiation [115,116]. m^6A is the most abundant modification on mRNAs [117]. m^6A modifications have been shown to influence mRNA splicing and nuclear export [118], and regulate mRNA stability by targeting transcripts for degradation in RNA decay bodies [119,120]. In PSCs, mRNAs encoding core pluripotency transcription factors such as *Nanog* and *Klf4* are also marked by m^{6}As. However, it is less clear how PSCs overcome the destabilization effect of m^{6}A modification on core pluripotency gene transcripts to ensure their robust expression, which is necessary for self-renewal. A recent study suggested a potential active mechanism to translate m^{6}A-modified mRNAs [121]. It has been shown that ABCF1 promotes the cap-independent translation of m^{6}A-modified mRNAs, likely by facilitating the recruitment of the eukaryotic initiation factor 2 (eIF2) ternary complex in the absence of cap recognition machinery (Figure 2A). We speculate that ABCF1 may function to stabilize the pluripotent state during cellular stress, by ensuring the efficient translation of these pluripotency-associated transcripts when global cap-dependent translation is inhibited [122].

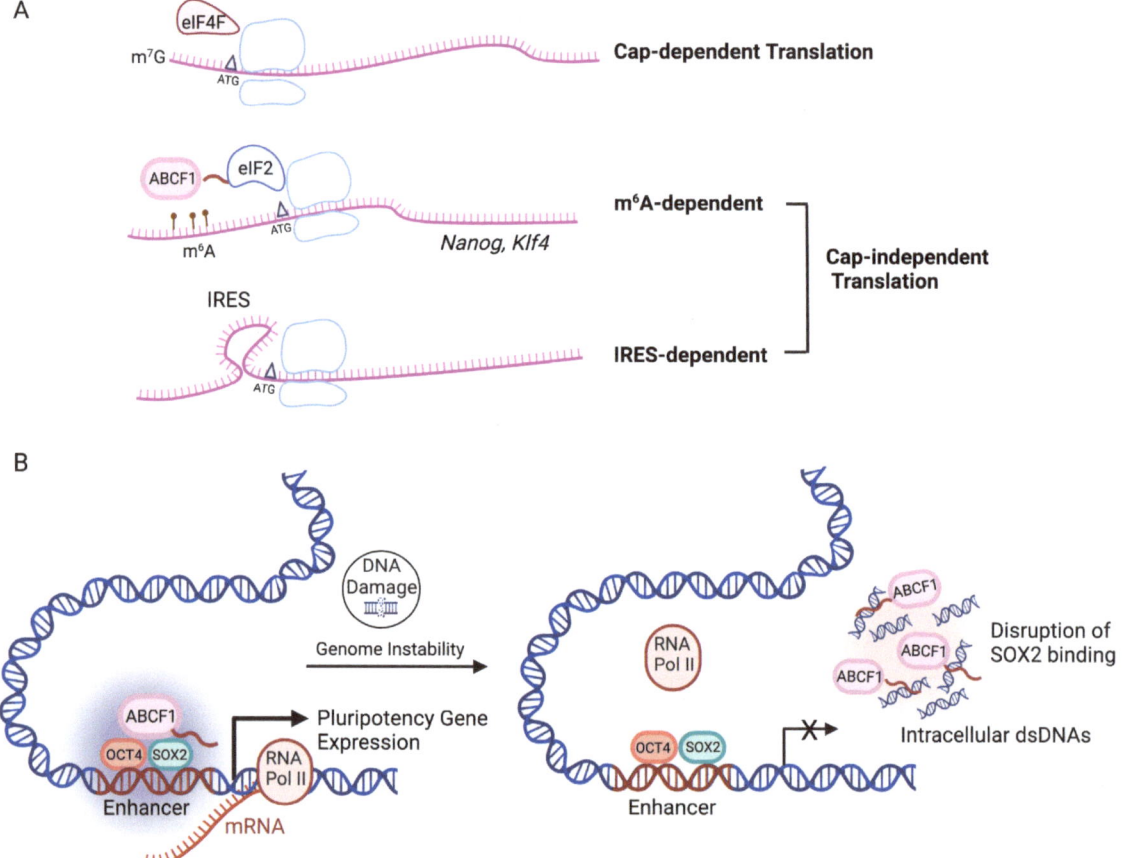

Figure 2. Multifaceted roles of ABCF1 in translation and transcription in PSCs. ABCF1 lacks TMD but contains a low-complexity domain (LCD) in the N-terminus critical for ABCF1 functions in PSCs. (**A**) Diagram showing that cap-dependent translation of m^{7}G capped mRNAs requires binding of translation initiating factor eIF4 to the cap structure. ABCF1 may promote the cap-independent translation of m^{6}A-modified pluripotency-associated mRNAs (e.g., *Nanog* and *Klf4*) in mouse PSCs,

via an interaction with eIF2 through its LCD. Internal ribosome entry site (IRES)-mediated cap-independent translation is not dependent on ABCF1. (**B**) A diagram showing that ABCF1 acts as transcriptional coactivator for SOX2 in PSCs. The LCD in ABCF1 directly interacts with SOX2 and assembles transcriptional complexes at pluripotency gene enhancers essential for gene activation. Upon DNA damage in PSCs, the LCD-dependent interaction of ABCF1 with SOX2 is disrupted due to competitive binding between ABCF1 and aberrant intracellular DNAs that accumulate in damaged PSCs. This leads to the downregulation of pluripotency gene expression and exit of damaged PSCs from self-renewal.

ABCF1 displays some sequence similarity to the yeast eEF3 subfamily ABC proteins including general control non-derepressible-20 (GCN20), which have been implicated in translational control [123,124]. However, the homology is restricted to the nucleotide-binding domains (NBDs). The residues outside of NBDs in ABCF1 are highly divergent from GCN20. Nonetheless, studies have shown that both ABCF1 and GCN20 employ their unique N-terminal regions to interact with eIF2 [124,125]. While the reported ABCF1-dependent translation has only been studied in mouse embryonic fibroblasts (MEFs), it is likely that this mechanism is also conserved in PSCs. Because ABCF1 expression is significantly higher in PSCs compared to that in somatic cells [48,126], we surmise that ABCF1 may play a more prominent role in the efficient translation of m^6A-modified mRNAs critical for stem cell pluripotency.

4.2. ABCF1 as an Intracellular DNA Sensor

Studies on differentiated mouse cells allowed researchers to identify ABCF1 as a sensor for aberrant intracellular DNAs [127,128]. ABCF1 interacts with critical regulators of the innate immune response and activates a pro-inflammatory response to intracellular DNAs resulting from infection or DNA damage [103,127], thereby promoting apoptosis and clearance of the affected cells [129]. While PSCs express ABCF1 and other known DNA sensors (e.g., cGAS and STING [130]), downstream signaling pathways required to stimulate the production of pro-inflammatory cytokines are absent or highly attenuated, in part due to active suppression by stem cell-specific transcription factors including OCT4 and SOX2 [131,132]. Whether or not ABCF1 also recognizes intracellular DNAs in PSCs and the biological consequences is unknown. Our recent work indicates that PSCs co-opt ABCF1's ability to detect intracellular DNAs to modulate stem cell-specific transcription in response to genome instability (discussed in the next sections) [48,133].

4.3. ABCF1 as a Stem Cell-Specific Transcriptional Coactivator

The unique transcriptional signatures that define the PSC state require cooperation between PSC-specific transcription factors and their coactivators [134,135]. Transcription factors OCT4 and SOX2 co-regulate a large number of genes that determine whether or not PSCs undergo self-renewal as they expand in the inner cell mass or commit to differentiation during embryonic development [7,8,136]. Therefore, the transcriptional activities of OCT4 and SOX2 are tightly regulated. Previous studies implicated the MED1 subunit of cell-ubiquitous coactivator complex Mediator in regulating OCT4 activity via a direct interaction [137,138]. However, other studies suggested the requirement of PSC-specific coactivators [139]. To this end, our laboratory developed an in vitro transcription assay and in an unbiased manner screened for factors in PSC nuclear extracts that can stimulate transcriptional activation by OCT4 and SOX2 [140]. We identified ABCF1 as a critical coactivator for OCT4 and SOX2 in PSCs. ABCF1 contains an unusual N-terminal region that is composed primarily of lysine and glutamic acid residues (40%). ABCF1 potentiates transcription by utilizing this low-complexity sequence domain (LCD) to interact directly with SOX2 and assemble PSC-specific transcriptional complexes at pluripotency-associated gene promoters (Figure 2B). Importantly, the yeast homologue GCN20 cannot be substituted for ABCF1 in transcriptional activation because the N-terminal region in GCN20 is highly divergent from the LCD of ABCF1. These observations suggest the acquisition of a mammalian-specific function of ABCF1 in transcriptional control. *Abcf1* knockout mouse embryos die at 3.5 days post coitus, a developmental stage that coincides with the emergence of pluripotent cells in the inner cell mass of the blastocyst [126]. Thus, genetic evidence indicates that ABCF1 is an essential transcriptional regulator of stem cell pluripotency.

The structural flexibility of the LCD in ABCF1 likely allows the rapid remodeling of transcriptional complexes to induce dynamic changes in gene expression to regulate stem cell self-renewal versus differentiation. LCDs are prevalent in transactivation domains in transcription factors [141]. The unique ability of LCDs to establish transient and multivalent interactions has been shown to allow transcription factors and coactivators to coalesce and overcome activation barriers [142]. The flexible nature of LCDs is also thought to facilitate the dynamic interaction with multiple protein partners, by virtue of their ability to rapidly adopt an ensemble of conformations [143].

4.4. ABCF1 Couples Transcription and Genome Surveillance in PSCs

PSCs appear to have developed several mechanisms to reduce the mutational load caused by elevated replicative and transcriptional stress [22]. As discussed in Section 1, damaged PSCs are efficiently eliminated through enforced exit from self-renewal via differentiation, thereby preserving the genome integrity of the self-renewing PSC population. DNA damage-induced PSC differentiation first requires the dismantling of the pluripotency gene transcriptional network that supports self-renewal, followed by the activation of differentiation programs. The tumor suppressor p53 has been proposed to regulate this transcriptional switch [144,145]. However, other studies indicated that the downregulation of the pluripotency gene network still occurs in ESCs lacking p53 [20,146]. The global shutdown of transcription upon DNA damage also cannot fully account for the transcriptional switch observed in damaged ESCs [147–149]. These observations suggest additional regulators that can relay signals from DNA damage to selectively modulate pluripotency gene transcription.

Our recent studies on the transcriptional function of ABCF1 revealed a new link between transcription and genome surveillance in PSCs [48]. Upon DNA damage, we found that ABCF1 binds intracellular DNAs that accumulate in damaged PSCs at the expense of its interaction with SOX2 (Figure 2B). The observed competition is likely due to the fact that both SOX2 and DNAs compete for the same LCD for binding. The disruption of an ABCF1-SOX2 complex by intracellular DNAs results in the dissociation of ABCF1 from its target pluripotency gene promoters, the downregulation of pluripotency gene expression, and differentiation of compromised PSCs. While DNA sensing by ABCF1 does not activate a canonical innate immune response in PSCs, PSCs appear to take advantage of ABCF1's intrinsic affinity to intracellular DNAs to modulate ABCF1-SOX2 interactions in the nucleus. We propose that the ABCF1–SOX2 complex represents an important regulatory nexus, wherein the constant tug of war between transcriptional activation and intracellular DNA sensing by ABCF1 could drive a PSC to self-renew under steady-state conditions, or alternatively to commit to differentiation and apoptosis when genome integrity is compromised. This switching of cell fates critically depends on whether or not intracellular DNA rises above a certain threshold that irreversibly tilts the balance toward the rapid exit of pluripotency.

5. Conclusions and Perspective

Although changes in metabolism have traditionally been viewed as a byproduct of cell fate changes and growth demands, there is growing evidence that metabolic regulation drives stem cell fate decisions. We have presented in this review evidence that the ABC family proteins contribute to pluripotent cell fate by coordinating an interconnected network of biological processes, from metabolism and signaling cascades involving macromolecule interactions at the cell membrane, to gene transcription and translation. In order for PSCs to dynamically respond to changing cellular cues, activities of ABC proteins must be coordinated and tuned. In this regard, stem cell-enriched transcription factors have been shown to bind the promoters of several *ABC* genes as discussed in this review, suggesting that their expression could be coupled to the pluripotent cell state [150]. Furthermore, activities of ABC transporters can be regulated by protein–protein interactions and post-translational modifications such as phosphorylation [151]. It is noteworthy that the efficient reprogramming of somatic cells to pluripotency also requires ABCF1, lipid and cholesterol metabolism, and an optimal redox status [48,152–154]. It is worth noting that the precise role of ABC proteins in stem cell pluripotency remains unclear, in large part because they have not been rigorously profiled and studied in PSCs. In this review, we synthesized observations from non-PSC types and proposed how cellular pathways controlled by ABC proteins may also contribute to stem cell maintenance. Future efforts on unraveling the biological impacts of ABC proteins on cell fate regulation in PSCs will be required. The knowledge gained is expected to significantly impact our understanding of embryonic development and the ability to manipulate PSCs for regenerative medicine.

Author Contributions: Conceptualization, P.S., S.A. and Y.W.F.; writing—original draft preparation, P.S. and Y.W.F.; writing—review and editing, P.S., S.A. and Y.W.F.; visualization, P.S. and Y.W.F.; supervision, Y.W.F. All authors have read and agreed to the published version of the manuscript.

Funding: We acknowledge the following funding sources: NIH grant R01HL125527, Harvard Stem Cell Institute, Boston Biomedical Innovation Center, Charles H. Hood Foundation, Brigham Research Institute, and Brigham and Women's Hospital HVC Junior Faculty Research Awards to Y.W.F.

Acknowledgments: We thank S. Agarwal and Z. Zhang for valuable discussion. Graphics were generated using Biorender.com.

Conflicts of Interest: Y.W.F. is a consultant to Rejuveron Life Sciences.

References

1. Evans, M.J.; Kaufman, M.H. Establishment in culture of pluripotential cells from mouse embryos. *Nature* **1981**, *292*, 154–156. [CrossRef] [PubMed]
2. Martin, G.R. Isolation of a pluripotent cell line from early mouse embryos cultured in medium conditioned by teratocarcinoma stem cells. *Proc. Natl. Acad. Sci. USA* **1981**, *78*, 7634–7638. [CrossRef]
3. Diamante, L.; Martello, G. Metabolic regulation in pluripotent stem cells. *Curr. Opin. Genet. Dev.* **2022**, *75*, 101923. [CrossRef] [PubMed]
4. Wu, J.; Ocampo, A.; Belmonte, J.C.I. Cellular Metabolism and Induced Pluripotency. *Cell* **2016**, *166*, 1371–1385. [CrossRef]
5. Gu, W.; Gaeta, X.; Sahakyan, A.; Chan, A.B.; Hong, C.S.; Kim, R.; Braas, D.; Plath, K.; Lowry, W.E.; Christofk, H.R. Glycolytic Metabolism Plays a Functional Role in Regulating Human Pluripotent Stem Cell State. *Cell Stem Cell* **2016**, *19*, 476–490. [CrossRef]
6. Chen, H.; Guo, R.; Zhang, Q.; Guo, H.; Yang, M.; Wu, Z.; Gao, S.; Liu, L.; Chen, L. Erk signaling is indispensable for genomic stability and self-renewal of mouse embryonic stem cells. *Proc. Natl. Acad. Sci. USA* **2015**, *112*, E5936–E5943. [CrossRef]
7. Boyer, L.A.; Lee, T.I.; Cole, M.F.; Johnstone, S.E.; Levine, S.S.; Zucker, J.P.; Guenther, M.G.; Kumar, R.M.; Murray, H.L.; Jenner, R.G.; et al. Core transcriptional regulatory circuitry in human embryonic stem cells. *Cell* **2005**, *122*, 947–956. [CrossRef]
8. Hainer, S.J.; Bošković, A.; McCannell, K.N.; Rando, O.J.; Fazzio, T.G. Profiling of Pluripotency Factors in Single Cells and Early Embryos. *Cell* **2019**, *177*, 1319–1329.e11. [CrossRef]
9. Dunn, S.-J.; Martello, G.; Yordanov, B.; Emmott, S.; Smith, A.G. Defining an essential transcription factor program for naïve pluripotency. *Science* **2014**, *344*, 1156–1160. [CrossRef]
10. Chen, X.; Xu, H.; Yuan, P.; Fang, F.; Huss, M.; Vega, V.B.; Wong, E.; Orlov, Y.L.; Zhang, W.; Jiang, J.; et al. Integration of external signaling pathways with the core transcriptional network in embryonic stem cells. *Cell* **2008**, *133*, 1106–1117. [CrossRef]
11. Young, R.A. Control of the embryonic stem cell state. *Cell* **2011**, *144*, 940–954. [CrossRef] [PubMed]
12. Li, X.; Hui, S.; Mirek, E.T.; Jonsson, W.O.; Anthony, T.G.; Lee, W.D.; Zeng, X.; Jang, C.; Rabinowitz, J.D. Circulating metabolite homeostasis achieved through mass action. *Nat. Metab.* **2022**, *4*, 141–152. [CrossRef]
13. Efroni, S.; Duttagupta, R.; Cheng, J.; Dehghani, H.; Hoeppner, D.J.; Dash, C.; Bazett-Jones, D.P.; Le Grice, S.; McKay, R.D.G.; Buetow, K.H.; et al. Global Transcription in Pluripotent Embryonic Stem Cells. *Cell Stem Cell* **2008**, *2*, 437–447. [CrossRef]
14. Fong, Y.W.; Cattoglio, C.; Tjian, R. The Intertwined Roles of Transcription and Repair Proteins. *Mol. Cell* **2013**, *52*, 291–302. [CrossRef]
15. Aguilera, A.; García-Muse, T. R loops: From transcription byproducts to threats to genome stability. *Mol. Cell* **2012**, *46*, 115–124. [CrossRef]
16. White, J.; Dalton, S. Cell cycle control of embryonic stem cells. *Stem Cell Rev.* **2005**, *1*, 131–138. [CrossRef]
17. Filion, T.M.; Qiao, M.; Ghule, P.N.; Mandeville, M.; van Wijnen, A.J.; Stein, J.L.; Lian, J.B.; Altieri, D.C.; Stein, G.S. Survival responses of human embryonic stem cells to DNA damage. *J. Cell. Physiol.* **2009**, *220*, 586–592. [CrossRef]

18. Suvorova, I.I.; Grigorash, B.B.; Chuykin, I.A.; Pospelova, T.V.; Pospelov, V.A. G1 checkpoint is compromised in mouse ESCs due to functional uncoupling of p53-p21Waf1 signaling. *Cell Cycle* **2016**, *15*, 52–63. [CrossRef]
19. Cervantes, R.B.; Stringer, J.R.; Shao, C.; Tischfield, J.A.; Stambrook, P.J. Embryonic stem cells and somatic cells differ in mutation frequency and type. *Proc. Natl. Acad. Sci. USA* **2002**, *99*, 3586–3590. [CrossRef]
20. Aladjem, M.I.; Spike, B.T.; Rodewald, L.W.; Hope, T.J.; Klemm, M.; Jaenisch, R.; Wahl, G.M. ES cells do not activate p53-dependent stress responses and undergo p53-independent apoptosis in response to DNA damage. *Curr. Biol.* **1998**, *8*, 145–155. [CrossRef]
21. Heyer, B.S.; MacAuley, A.; Behrendtsen, O.; Werb, Z. Hypersensitivity to DNA damage leads to increased apoptosis during early mouse development. *Genes Dev.* **2000**, *14*, 2072–2084. [CrossRef] [PubMed]
22. Vitale, I.; Manic, G.; De Maria, R.; Kroemer, G.; Galluzzi, L. DNA Damage in Stem Cells. *Mol. Cell* **2017**, *66*, 306–319. [CrossRef] [PubMed]
23. Yu, J.; Vodyanik, M.A.; Smuga-Otto, K.; Antosiewicz-Bourget, J.; Frane, J.L.; Tian, S.; Nie, J.; Jonsdottir, G.A.; Ruotti, V.; Stewart, R.; et al. Induced pluripotent stem cell lines derived from human somatic cells. *Science* **2007**, *318*, 1917–1920. [CrossRef]
24. Takahashi, K.; Yamanaka, S. Induction of Pluripotent Stem Cells from Mouse Embryonic and Adult Fibroblast Cultures by Defined Factors. *Cell* **2006**, *126*, 663–676. [CrossRef]
25. Yamanaka, S. Induced Pluripotent Stem Cells: Past, Present, and Future. *Cell Stem Cell* **2012**, *10*, 678–684. [CrossRef]
26. Ma, H.; Morey, R.; O'Neil, R.C.; He, Y.; Daughtry, B.; Schultz, M.D.; Hariharan, M.; Nery, J.R.; Castanon, R.; Sabatini, K.; et al. Abnormalities in human pluripotent cells due to reprogramming mechanisms. *Nature* **2014**, *511*, 177–183. [CrossRef]
27. Merkle, F.T.; Ghosh, S.; Kamitaki, N.; Mitchell, J.; Avior, Y.; Mello, C.; Kashin, S.; Mekhoubad, S.; Ilic, D.; Charlton, M.; et al. Human pluripotent stem cells recurrently acquire and expand dominant negative P53 mutations. *Nature* **2017**, *545*, 229–233. [CrossRef]
28. Kyriakides, O.; Halliwell, J.A.; Andrews, P.W. Acquired Genetic and Epigenetic Variation in Human Pluripotent Stem Cells. *Adv. Biochem. Eng. Biotechnol.* **2018**, *163*, 187–206. [CrossRef]
29. Assou, S.; Bouckenheimer, J.; De Vos, J. Concise Review: Assessing the Genome Integrity of Human Induced Pluripotent Stem Cells: What Quality Control Metrics? *Stem Cells* **2018**, *36*, 814–821. [CrossRef]
30. Yamamoto, T.; Sato, Y.; Yasuda, S.; Shikamura, M.; Tamura, T.; Takenaka, C.; Takasu, N.; Nomura, M.; Dohi, H.; Takahashi, M.; et al. Correlation Between Genetic Abnormalities in Induced Pluripotent Stem Cell-Derivatives and Abnormal Tissue Formation in Tumorigenicity Tests. *Stem Cells Transl. Med.* **2022**, *11*, 527–538. [CrossRef]
31. Lee, A.S.; Tang, C.; Rao, M.S.; Weissman, I.L.; Wu, J.C. Tumorigenicity as a clinical hurdle for pluripotent stem cell therapies. *Nat. Med.* **2013**, *19*, 998–1004. [CrossRef]
32. Yamanaka, S. Pluripotent Stem Cell-Based Cell Therapy-Promise and Challenges. *Cell Stem Cell* **2020**, *27*, 523–531. [CrossRef]
33. Martin, R.M.; Fowler, J.L.; Cromer, M.K.; Lesch, B.J.; Ponce, E.; Uchida, N.; Nishimura, T.; Porteus, M.H.; Loh, K.M. Improving the safety of human pluripotent stem cell therapies using genome-edited orthogonal safeguards. *Nat. Commun.* **2020**, *11*, 2713. [CrossRef]
34. Colter, J.; Murari, K.; Biernaskie, J.; Kallos, M.S. Induced pluripotency in the context of stem cell expansion bioprocess development, optimization, and manufacturing: A roadmap to the clinic. *NPJ Regen. Med.* **2021**, *6*, 72. [CrossRef]
35. Higgins, C.F. ABC transporters: From microorganisms to man. *Annu. Rev. Cell Biol.* **1992**, *8*, 67–113. [CrossRef]
36. Moore, J.M.; Bell, E.L.; Hughes, R.O.; Garfield, A.S. ABC transporters: Human disease and pharmacotherapeutic potential. *Trends Mol. Med.* **2023**, *29*, 152–172. [CrossRef]
37. Borst, P.; Elferink, R.O. Mammalian ABC Transporters in Health and Disease. *Annu. Rev. Biochem.* **2002**, *71*, 537–592. [CrossRef]
38. Vasiliou, V.; Vasiliou, K.; Nebert, D.W. Human ATP-binding cassette (ABC) transporter family. *Hum. Genom.* **2009**, *3*, 281–290. [CrossRef]
39. Barbet, R.; Peiffer, I.; Hutchins, J.R.A.; Hatzfeld, A.; Garrido, E.; Hatzfeld, J.A. Expression of the 49 human ATP binding cassette (ABC) genes in pluripotent embryonic stem cells and in early- and late-stage multipotent mesenchymal stem cells: Possible role of ABC plasma membrane transporters in maintaining human stem cell pluripotency. *Cell Cycle* **2012**, *11*, 1611–1620. [CrossRef]
40. Phanstiel, D.H.; Brumbaugh, J.; Wenger, C.D.; Tian, S.; Probasco, M.D.; Bailey, D.J.; Swaney, D.L.; Tervo, M.A.; Bolin, J.M.; Ruotti, V.; et al. Proteomic and phosphoproteomic comparison of human ES and iPS cells. *Nat. Methods* **2011**, *8*, 821–827. [CrossRef]
41. Chaerkady, R.; Kerr, C.L.; Kandasamy, K.; Marimuthu, A.; Gearhart, J.D.; Pandey, A. Comparative proteomics of human embryonic stem cells and embryonal carcinoma cells. *Proteomics* **2010**, *10*, 1359–1373. [CrossRef] [PubMed]
42. Apáti, Á.; Szebényi, K.; Erdei, Z.; Várady, G.; Orbán, T.I.; Sarkadi, B. The importance of drug transporters in human pluripotent stem cells and in early tissue differentiation. *Expert Opin. Drug Metab. Toxicol.* **2016**, *12*, 77–92. [CrossRef] [PubMed]
43. Erdei, Z.; Lőrincz, R.; Szebényi, K.; Péntek, A.; Varga, N.; Likó, I.; Várady, G.; Szakács, G.; Orbán, T.I.; Sarkadi, B.; et al. Expression pattern of the human ABC transporters in pluripotent embryonic stem cells and in their derivatives. *Cytom. B. Clin. Cytom.* **2014**, *86*, 299–310. [CrossRef]
44. Hirata, N.; Nakagawa, M.; Fujibayashi, Y.; Yamauchi, K.; Murata, A.; Minami, I.; Tomioka, M.; Kondo, T.; Kuo, T.F.; Endo, H.; et al. A Chemical Probe that Labels Human Pluripotent Stem Cells. *Cell Rep.* **2014**, *6*, 1165–1174. [CrossRef]
45. Fort, A.; Hashimoto, K.; Yamada, D.; Salimullah, M.; Keya, C.A.; Saxena, A.; Bonetti, A.; Voineagu, I.; Bertin, N.; Kratz, A.; et al. Deep transcriptome profiling of mammalian stem cells supports a regulatory role for retrotransposons in pluripotency maintenance. *Nat. Genet.* **2014**, *46*, 558–566. [CrossRef]

46. Yan, L.; Yang, M.; Guo, H.; Yang, L.; Wu, J.; Li, R.; Liu, P.; Lian, Y.; Zheng, X.; Yan, J.; et al. Single-cell RNA-Seq profiling of human preimplantation embryos and embryonic stem cells. *Nat. Struct. Mol. Biol.* **2013**, *20*, 1131–1139. [CrossRef]
47. Brandenberger, R.; Wei, H.; Zhang, S.; Lei, S.; Murage, J.; Fisk, G.J.; Li, Y.; Xu, C.; Fang, R.; Guegler, K.; et al. Transcriptome characterization elucidates signaling networks that control human ES cell growth and differentiation. *Nat. Biotechnol.* **2004**, *22*, 707–716. [CrossRef]
48. Choi, E.B.; Vodnala, M.; Zerbato, M.; Wang, J.; Ho, J.J.; Inouye, C.; Ding, L.; Fong, Y.W. ATP-binding cassette protein ABCF1 couples transcription and genome surveillance in embryonic stem cells through low-complexity domain. *Sci. Adv.* **2021**, *7*, eabk2775. [CrossRef]
49. Apáti, Á.; Orbán, T.I.; Varga, N.; Németh, A.; Schamberger, A.; Krizsik, V.; Erdélyi-Belle, B.; Homolya, L.; Várady, G.; Padányi, R.; et al. High level functional expression of the ABCG2 multidrug transporter in undifferentiated human embryonic stem cells. *Biochim. Biophys. Acta Biomembr.* **2008**, *1778*, 2700–2709. [CrossRef]
50. Erdei, Z.; Sarkadi, B.; Brózik, A.; Szebényi, K.; Várady, G.; Makó, V.; Péntek, A.; Orbán, T.I.; Apáti, Á. Dynamic ABCG2 expression in human embryonic stem cells provides the basis for stress response. *Eur. Biophys. J.* **2013**, *42*, 169–179. [CrossRef]
51. van Meer, G.; de Kroon, A.I.P.M. Lipid map of the mammalian cell. *J. Cell Sci.* **2011**, *124*, 5–8. [CrossRef]
52. Kamp, D.; Haest, C.W. Evidence for a role of the multidrug resistance protein (MRP) in the outward translocation of NBD-phospholipids in the erythrocyte membrane. *Biochim. Biophys. Acta* **1998**, *1372*, 91–101. [CrossRef]
53. Dekkers, D.W.; Comfurius, P.; Schroit, A.J.; Bevers, E.M.; Zwaal, R.F. Transbilayer movement of NBD-labeled phospholipids in red blood cell membranes: Outward-directed transport by the multidrug resistance protein 1 (MRP1). *Biochemistry* **1998**, *37*, 14833–14837. [CrossRef]
54. Daleke, D.L. Phospholipid flippases. *J. Biol. Chem.* **2007**, *282*, 821–825. [CrossRef]
55. Segrest, J.P.; Tang, C.; Song, H.D.; Jones, M.K.; Davidson, W.S.; Aller, S.G.; Heinecke, J.W. ABCA1 is an extracellular phospholipid translocase. *Nat. Commun.* **2022**, *13*, 4812. [CrossRef]
56. Fadeel, B.; Xue, D. The ins and outs of phospholipid asymmetry in the plasma membrane: Roles in health and disease. *Crit. Rev. Biochem. Mol. Biol.* **2009**, *44*, 264–277. [CrossRef]
57. Oude Elferink, R.P.J.; Paulusma, C.C. Function and pathophysiological importance of ABCB4 (MDR3 P-glycoprotein). *Pflugers Arch.* **2007**, *453*, 601–610. [CrossRef]
58. Grecco, H.E.; Schmick, M.; Bastiaens, P.I.H. Signaling from the living plasma membrane. *Cell* **2011**, *144*, 897–909. [CrossRef]
59. Castanieto, A.; Johnston, M.J.; Nystul, T.G. EGFR signaling promotes self-renewal through the establishment of cell polarity in Drosophila follicle stem cells. *Elife* **2014**, *3*, e04437. [CrossRef]
60. Lanner, F.; Rossant, J. The role of FGF/Erk signaling in pluripotent cells. *Development* **2010**, *137*, 3351–3360. [CrossRef]
61. Levenstein, M.E.; Ludwig, T.E.; Xu, R.-H.; Llanas, R.A.; Van Den Heuvel-Kramer, K.; Manning, D.; Thomson, J.A. Basic fibroblast growth factor support of human embryonic stem cell self-renewal. *Stem Cells* **2006**, *24*, 568–574. [CrossRef] [PubMed]
62. Haghighi, F.; Dahlmann, J.; Nakhaei-Rad, S.; Lang, A.; Kutschka, I.; Zenker, M.; Kensah, G.; Piekorz, R.P.; Ahmadian, M.R. bFGF-mediated pluripotency maintenance in human induced pluripotent stem cells is associated with NRAS-MAPK signaling. *Cell Commun. Signal.* **2018**, *16*, 96. [CrossRef] [PubMed]
63. Kubara, K.; Yamazaki, K.; Ishihara, Y.; Naruto, T.; Lin, H.-T.; Nishimura, K.; Ohtaka, M.; Nakanishi, M.; Ito, M.; Tsukahara, K.; et al. Status of KRAS in iPSCs Impacts upon Self-Renewal and Differentiation Propensity. *Stem Cell Rep.* **2018**, *11*, 380–394. [CrossRef] [PubMed]
64. Chavan, T.S.; Muratcioglu, S.; Marszalek, R.; Jang, H.; Keskin, O.; Gursoy, A.; Nussinov, R.; Gaponenko, V. Plasma membrane regulates Ras signaling networks. *Cell. Logist.* **2015**, *5*, e1136374. [CrossRef] [PubMed]
65. Li, Z.-L.; Buck, M. Computational Modeling Reveals that Signaling Lipids Modulate the Orientation of K-Ras4A at the Membrane Reflecting Protein Topology. *Structure* **2017**, *25*, 679–689.e2. [CrossRef]
66. Gulshan, K.; Brubaker, G.; Conger, H.; Wang, S.; Zhang, R.; Hazen, S.L.; Smith, J.D. PI(4,5)P2 Is Translocated by ABCA1 to the Cell Surface Where It Mediates Apolipoprotein A1 Binding and Nascent HDL Assembly. *Circ. Res.* **2016**, *119*, 827–838. [CrossRef]
67. Hamon, Y.; Broccardo, C.; Chambenoit, O.; Luciani, M.F.; Toti, F.; Chaslin, S.; Freyssinet, J.M.; Devaux, P.F.; McNeish, J.; Marguet, D.; et al. ABC1 promotes engulfment of apoptotic cells and transbilayer redistribution of phosphatidylserine. *Nat. Cell Biol.* **2000**, *2*, 399–406. [CrossRef]
68. Takahashi, K.; Kimura, Y.; Kioka, N.; Matsuo, M.; Ueda, K. Purification and ATPase activity of human ABCA1. *J. Biol. Chem.* **2006**, *281*, 10760–10768. [CrossRef]
69. Watabe, T.; Miyazono, K. Roles of TGF-β family signaling in stem cell renewal and differentiation. *Cell Res.* **2009**, *19*, 103–115. [CrossRef]
70. Yu, M.; Wei, Y.; Xu, K.; Liu, S.; Ma, L.; Pei, Y.; Hu, Y.; Liu, Z.; Zhang, X.; Wang, B.; et al. EGFR deficiency leads to impaired self-renewal and pluripotency of mouse embryonic stem cells. *PeerJ* **2019**, *7*, e6314. [CrossRef]
71. Lange, Y.; Ye, J.; Steck, T.L. How cholesterol homeostasis is regulated by plasma membrane cholesterol in excess of phospholipids. *Proc. Natl. Acad. Sci. USA* **2004**, *101*, 11664–11667. [CrossRef]
72. Kennedy, M.A.; Barrera, G.C.; Nakamura, K.; Baldán, A.; Tarr, P.; Fishbein, M.C.; Frank, J.; Francone, O.L.; Edwards, P.A. ABCG1 has a critical role in mediating cholesterol efflux to HDL and preventing cellular lipid accumulation. *Cell Metab.* **2005**, *1*, 121–131. [CrossRef]

73. Duong, M.; Collins, H.L.; Jin, W.; Zanotti, I.; Favari, E.; Rothblat, G.H. Relative contributions of ABCA1 and SR-BI to cholesterol efflux to serum from fibroblasts and macrophages. *Arterioscler. Thromb. Vasc. Biol.* **2006**, *26*, 541–547. [CrossRef]
74. Yvan-Charvet, L.; Wang, N.; Tall, A.R. Role of HDL, ABCA1, and ABCG1 transporters in cholesterol efflux and immune responses. *Arterioscler. Thromb. Vasc. Biol.* **2010**, *30*, 139–143. [CrossRef]
75. Szabo, G. Dual mechanism for the action of cholesterol on membrane permeability. *Nature* **1974**, *252*, 47–49. [CrossRef]
76. Subczynski, W.K.; Pasenkiewicz-Gierula, M.; Widomska, J.; Mainali, L.; Raguz, M. High Cholesterol/Low Cholesterol: Effects in Biological Membranes: A Review. *Cell Biochem. Biophys.* **2017**, *75*, 369–385. [CrossRef]
77. Reiss, K.; Cornelsen, I.; Husmann, M.; Gimpl, G.; Bhakdi, S. Unsaturated Fatty Acids Drive Disintegrin and Metalloproteinase (ADAM)-dependent Cell Adhesion, Proliferation, and Migration by Modulating Membrane Fluidity. *J. Biol. Chem.* **2011**, *286*, 26931–26942. [CrossRef]
78. Matsuzaki, T.; Matsumoto, S.; Kasai, T.; Yoshizawa, E.; Okamoto, S.; Yoshikawa, H.Y.; Taniguchi, H.; Takebe, T. Defining Lineage-Specific Membrane Fluidity Signatures that Regulate Adhesion Kinetics. *Stem Cell Rep.* **2018**, *11*, 852–860. [CrossRef]
79. Chen, W.-J.; Huang, W.-K.; Pather, S.R.; Chang, W.-F.; Sung, L.-Y.; Wu, H.-C.; Liao, M.-Y.; Lee, C.-C.; Wu, H.-H.; Wu, C.-Y.; et al. Podocalyxin-Like Protein 1 Regulates Pluripotency through the Cholesterol Biosynthesis Pathway. *Adv. Sci.* **2022**, *10*, e2205451. [CrossRef]
80. Jacobson, K.; Mouritsen, O.G.; Anderson, R.G.W. Lipid rafts: At a crossroad between cell biology and physics. *Nat. Cell Biol.* **2007**, *9*, 7–14. [CrossRef]
81. Scheiffele, P.; Roth, M.G.; Simons, K. Interaction of influenza virus haemagglutinin with sphingolipid-cholesterol membrane domains via its transmembrane domain. *EMBO J.* **1997**, *16*, 5501–5508. [CrossRef] [PubMed]
82. Melkonian, K.A.; Ostermeyer, A.G.; Chen, J.Z.; Roth, M.G.; Brown, D.A. Role of lipid modifications in targeting proteins to detergent-resistant membrane rafts. Many raft proteins are acylated, while few are prenylated. *J. Biol. Chem.* **1999**, *274*, 3910–3917. [CrossRef] [PubMed]
83. Harder, T.; Scheiffele, P.; Verkade, P.; Simons, K. Lipid domain structure of the plasma membrane revealed by patching of membrane components. *J. Cell Biol.* **1998**, *141*, 929–942. [CrossRef] [PubMed]
84. Yvan-Charvet, L.; Welch, C.; Pagler, T.A.; Ranalletta, M.; Lamkanfi, M.; Han, S.; Ishibashi, M.; Li, R.; Wang, N.; Tall, A.R. Increased inflammatory gene expression in ABC transporter-deficient macrophages: Free cholesterol accumulation, increased signaling via toll-like receptors, and neutrophil infiltration of atherosclerotic lesions. *Circulation* **2008**, *118*, 1837–1847. [CrossRef] [PubMed]
85. Janes, P.W.; Ley, S.C.; Magee, A.I.; Kabouridis, P.S. The role of lipid rafts in T cell antigen receptor (TCR) signalling. *Semin. Immunol.* **2000**, *12*, 23–34. [CrossRef]
86. Langlet, C.; Bernard, A.M.; Devrot, P.; He, H.T. Membrane rafts and signaling by the multichain immune recognition receptors. *Curr. Opin. Immunol.* **2000**, *12*, 250–255. [CrossRef]
87. Lee, M.Y.; Ryu, J.M.; Lee, S.H.; Park, J.H.; Han, H.J. Lipid rafts play an important role for maintenance of embryonic stem cell self-renewal. *J. Lipid Res.* **2010**, *51*, 2082–2089. [CrossRef]
88. Williams, R.L.; Hilton, D.J.; Pease, S.; Willson, T.A.; Stewart, C.L.; Gearing, D.P.; Wagner, E.F.; Metcalf, D.; Nicola, N.A.; Gough, N.M. Myeloid leukaemia inhibitory factor maintains the developmental potential of embryonic stem cells. *Nature* **1988**, *336*, 684–687. [CrossRef]
89. Simons, K.; Toomre, D. Lipid rafts and signal transduction. *Nat. Rev. Mol. Cell Biol.* **2000**, *1*, 31–39. [CrossRef]
90. Teo, A.K.K.; Nguyen, L.; Gupta, M.K.; Lau, H.H.; Loo, L.S.W.; Jackson, N.; Lim, C.S.; Mallard, W.; Gritsenko, M.A.; Rinn, J.L.; et al. Defective insulin receptor signaling in hPSCs skews pluripotency and negatively perturbs neural differentiation. *J. Biol. Chem.* **2021**, *296*, 100495. [CrossRef]
91. Li, Q.; Lex, R.K.; Chung, H.; Giovanetti, S.M.; Ji, Z.; Ji, H.; Person, M.D.; Kim, J.; Vokes, S.A. The Pluripotency Factor NANOG Binds to GLI Proteins and Represses Hedgehog-mediated Transcription. *J. Biol. Chem.* **2016**, *291*, 7171–7182. [CrossRef]
92. Murata, H.; Ihara, Y.; Nakamura, H.; Yodoi, J.; Sumikawa, K.; Kondo, T. Glutaredoxin exerts an antiapoptotic effect by regulating the redox state of Akt. *J. Biol. Chem.* **2003**, *278*, 50226–50233. [CrossRef]
93. Ito, K.; Hirao, A.; Arai, F.; Takubo, K.; Matsuoka, S.; Miyamoto, K.; Ohmura, M.; Naka, K.; Hosokawa, K.; Ikeda, Y.; et al. Reactive oxygen species act through p38 MAPK to limit the lifespan of hematopoietic stem cells. *Nat. Med.* **2006**, *12*, 446–451. [CrossRef]
94. Ji, A.-R.; Ku, S.-Y.; Cho, M.S.; Kim, Y.Y.; Kim, Y.J.; Oh, S.K.; Kim, S.H.; Moon, S.Y.; Choi, Y.M. Reactive oxygen species enhance differentiation of human embryonic stem cells into mesendodermal lineage. *Exp. Mol. Med.* **2010**, *42*, 175–186. [CrossRef]
95. Varum, S.; Rodrigues, A.S.; Moura, M.B.; Momcilovic, O.; Easley, C.A., 4th; Ramalho-Santos, J.; Van Houten, B.; Schatten, G. Energy metabolism in human pluripotent stem cells and their differentiated counterparts. *PLoS ONE* **2011**, *6*, e20914. [CrossRef]
96. Zhang, C.; Skamagki, M.; Liu, Z.; Ananthanarayanan, A.; Zhao, R.; Li, H.; Kim, K. Biological Significance of the Suppression of Oxidative Phosphorylation in Induced Pluripotent Stem Cells. *Cell Rep.* **2017**, *21*, 2058–2065. [CrossRef]
97. Wang, C.-K.; Yang, S.-C.; Hsu, S.-C.; Chang, F.-P.; Lin, Y.-T.; Chen, S.-F.; Cheng, C.-L.; Hsiao, M.; Lu, F.L.; Lu, J. CHAC2 is essential for self-renewal and glutathione maintenance in human embryonic stem cells. *Free Radic. Biol. Med.* **2017**, *113*, 439–451. [CrossRef]
98. Guo, Y.-L.; Chakraborty, S.; Rajan, S.S.; Wang, R.; Huang, F. Effects of oxidative stress on mouse embryonic stem cell proliferation, apoptosis, senescence, and self-renewal. *Stem Cells Dev.* **2010**, *19*, 1321–1331. [CrossRef]
99. Meister, A.; Anderson, M.E. Glutathione. *Annu. Rev. Biochem.* **1983**, *52*, 711–760. [CrossRef]
100. Schafer, F.Q.; Buettner, G.R. Redox environment of the cell as viewed through the redox state of the glutathione disulfide/glutathione couple. *Free Radic. Biol. Med.* **2001**, *30*, 1191–1212. [CrossRef] [PubMed]

101. Marchan, R.; Hammond, C.L.; Ballatori, N. Multidrug resistance-associated protein 1 as a major mediator of basal and apoptotic glutathione release. *Biochim. Biophys. Acta* **2008**, *1778*, 2413–2420. [CrossRef] [PubMed]
102. Cole, S.P.C.; Deeley, R.G. Transport of glutathione and glutathione conjugates by MRP1. *Trends Pharmacol. Sci.* **2006**, *27*, 438–446. [CrossRef] [PubMed]
103. Diner, B.A.; Li, T.; Greco, T.M.; Crow, M.S.; Fuesler, J.A.; Wang, J.; Cristea, I.M. The functional interactome of PYHIN immune regulators reveals IFIX is a sensor of viral DNA. *Mol. Syst. Biol.* **2015**, *11*, 787. [CrossRef]
104. Mueller, C.F.H.; Widder, J.D.; McNally, J.S.; McCann, L.; Jones, D.P.; Harrison, D.G. The role of the multidrug resistance protein-1 in modulation of endothelial cell oxidative stress. *Circ. Res.* **2005**, *97*, 637–644. [CrossRef]
105. Ballatori, N.; Krance, S.M.; Marchan, R.; Hammond, C.L. Plasma membrane glutathione transporters and their roles in cell physiology and pathophysiology. *Mol. Aspects Med.* **2009**, *30*, 13–28. [CrossRef]
106. Crawford, R.R.; Prescott, E.T.; Sylvester, C.F.; Higdon, A.N.; Shan, J.; Kilberg, M.S.; Mungrue, I.N. Human CHAC1 Protein Degrades Glutathione, and mRNA Induction Is Regulated by the Transcription Factors ATF4 and ATF3 and a Bipartite ATF/CRE Regulatory Element. *J. Biol. Chem.* **2015**, *290*, 15878–15891. [CrossRef]
107. Crawford, R.; Higdon, A.; Prescott, E.; Mungrue, I. CHAC1 degrades glutathione, sensitizing cells to oxidative injury (663.10). *FASEB J.* **2014**, *28*, 663-10. [CrossRef]
108. Hissin, P.J.; Hilf, R. A fluorometric method for determination of oxidized and reduced glutathione in tissues. *Anal. Biochem.* **1976**, *74*, 214–226. [CrossRef]
109. Marsboom, G.; Zhang, G.-F.; Pohl-Avila, N.; Zhang, Y.; Yuan, Y.; Kang, H.; Hao, B.; Brunengraber, H.; Malik, A.B.; Rehman, J. Glutamine Metabolism Regulates the Pluripotency Transcription Factor OCT4. *Cell Rep.* **2016**, *16*, 323–332. [CrossRef]
110. Watanabe, S.; Umehara, H.; Murayama, K.; Okabe, M.; Kimura, T.; Nakano, T. Activation of Akt signaling is sufficient to maintain pluripotency in mouse and primate embryonic stem cells. *Oncogene* **2006**, *25*, 2697–2707. [CrossRef]
111. Ivanova, J.S.; Pugovkina, N.A.; Neganova, I.E.; Kozhukharova, I.V.; Nikolsky, N.N.; Lyublinskaya, O.G. Cell cycle-coupled changes in the level of reactive oxygen species support the proliferation of human pluripotent stem cells. *Stem Cells* **2021**, *39*, 1671–1687. [CrossRef] [PubMed]
112. Li, T.-S.; Marbán, E. Physiological levels of reactive oxygen species are required to maintain genomic stability in stem cells. *Stem Cells* **2010**, *28*, 1178–1185. [CrossRef] [PubMed]
113. Hinnebusch, A.G.; Lorsch, J.R. The mechanism of eukaryotic translation initiation: New insights and challenges. *Cold Spring Harb. Perspect. Biol.* **2012**, *4*, a011544. [CrossRef] [PubMed]
114. Lacerda, R.; Menezes, J.; Romão, L. More than just scanning: The importance of cap-independent mRNA translation initiation for cellular stress response and cancer. *Cell. Mol. Life Sci.* **2017**, *74*, 1659–1680. [CrossRef] [PubMed]
115. Meyer, K.D.; Patil, D.P.; Zhou, J.; Zinoviev, A.; Skabkin, M.A.; Elemento, O.; Pestova, T.V.; Qian, S.B.; Jaffrey, S.R. 5′ UTR m6A Promotes Cap-Independent Translation. *Cell* **2015**, *163*, 999–1010. [CrossRef]
116. Zhou, J.; Wan, J.; Gao, X.; Zhang, X.; Jaffrey, S.R.; Qian, S.-B. Dynamic m(6)A mRNA methylation directs translational control of heat shock response. *Nature* **2015**, *526*, 591–594. [CrossRef]
117. Liu, N.; Pan, T. N6-methyladenosine–encoded epitranscriptomics. *Nat. Struct. Mol. Biol.* **2016**, *23*, 98–102. [CrossRef]
118. Meyer, K.D.; Jaffrey, S.R. The dynamic epitranscriptome: N6-methyladenosine and gene expression control. *Nat. Rev. Mol. Cell Biol.* **2014**, *15*, 313–326. [CrossRef]
119. Wang, X.; Lu, Z.; Gomez, A.; Hon, G.C.; Yue, Y.; Han, D.; Fu, Y.; Parisien, M.; Dai, Q.; Jia, G.; et al. N6-methyladenosine-dependent regulation of messenger RNA stability. *Nature* **2014**, *505*, 117–120. [CrossRef]
120. Kang, H.-J.; Jeong, S.-J.; Kim, K.-N.; Baek, I.-J.; Chang, M.; Kang, C.-M.; Park, Y.-S.; Yun, C.-W. A novel protein, Pho92, has a conserved YTH domain and regulates phosphate metabolism by decreasing the mRNA stability of PHO4 in Saccharomyces cerevisiae. *Biochem. J.* **2014**, *457*, 391–400. [CrossRef]
121. Coots, R.A.; Liu, X.-M.; Mao, Y.; Dong, L.; Zhou, J.; Wan, J.; Zhang, X.; Qian, S.-B. m(6)A Facilitates eIF4F-Independent mRNA Translation. *Mol. Cell* **2017**, *68*, 504–514.e7. [CrossRef]
122. Saba, J.A.; Liakath-Ali, K.; Green, R.; Watt, F.M. Translational control of stem cell function. *Nat. Rev. Mol. Cell Biol.* **2021**, *22*, 671–690. [CrossRef]
123. Vazquez de Aldana, C.R.; Marton, M.J.; Hinnebusch, A.G. GCN20, a novel ATP binding cassette protein, and GCN1 reside in a complex that mediates activation of the eIF-2 alpha kinase GCN2 in amino acid-starved cells. *EMBO J.* **1995**, *14*, 3184–3199. [CrossRef]
124. Marton, M.J.; Vazquez de Aldana, C.R.; Qiu, H.; Chakraburtty, K.; Hinnebusch, A.G. Evidence that GCN1 and GCN20, translational regulators of GCN4, function on elongating ribosomes in activation of eIF2alpha kinase GCN2. *Mol. Cell. Biol.* **1997**, *17*, 4474–4489. [CrossRef]
125. Paytubi, S.; Morrice, N.A.; Boudeau, J.; Proud, C.G. The N-terminal region of ABC50 interacts with eukaryotic initiation factor eIF2 and is a target for regulatory phosphorylation by CK2. *Biochem. J.* **2008**, *409*, 223–231. [CrossRef]
126. Wilcox, S.M.; Arora, H.; Munro, L.; Xin, J.; Fenninger, F.; Johnson, L.A.; Pfeifer, C.G.; Choi, K.B.; Hou, J.; Hoodless, P.A.; et al. The role of the innate immune response regulatory gene ABCF1 in mammalian embryogenesis and development. *PLoS ONE* **2017**, *12*, e0175918. [CrossRef]

127. Lee, M.N.; Roy, M.; Ong, S.-E.; Mertins, P.; Villani, A.-C.; Li, W.; Dotiwala, F.; Sen, J.; Doench, J.G.; Orzalli, M.H.; et al. Identification of regulators of the innate immune response to cytosolic DNA and retroviral infection by an integrative approach. *Nat. Immunol.* **2013**, *14*, 179–185. [CrossRef]
128. Cao, Q.T.; Aguiar, J.A.; Tremblay, B.J.-M.; Abbas, N.; Tiessen, N.; Revill, S.; Makhdami, N.; Ayoub, A.; Cox, G.; Ask, K.; et al. ABCF1 Regulates dsDNA-induced Immune Responses in Human Airway Epithelial Cells. *Front. Cell. Infect. Microbiol.* **2020**, *10*, 487. [CrossRef]
129. Jorgensen, I.; Rayamajhi, M.; Miao, E.A. Programmed cell death as a defence against infection. *Nat. Rev. Immunol.* **2017**, *17*, 151–164. [CrossRef]
130. Hopfner, K.-P.; Hornung, V. Molecular mechanisms and cellular functions of cGAS-STING signalling. *Nat. Rev. Mol. Cell Biol.* **2020**, *21*, 501–521. [CrossRef]
131. Eggenberger, J.; Blanco-Melo, D.; Panis, M.; Brennand, K.J.; TenOever, B.R. Type I interferon response impairs differentiation potential of pluripotent stem cells. *Proc. Natl. Acad. Sci. USA* **2019**, *116*, 1384–1393. [CrossRef]
132. Guo, Y.-L. The underdeveloped innate immunity in embryonic stem cells: The molecular basis and biological perspectives from early embryogenesis. *Am. J. Reprod. Immunol.* **2019**, *81*, e13089. [CrossRef]
133. Vodnala, M.; Choi, E.B.; Fong, Y.W. Low Complexity Domains, Condensates, and Stem Cell Pluripotency. *World J. Stem Cells* **2021**, *13*, 416–438. [CrossRef]
134. Fong, Y.W.; Cattoglio, C.; Yamaguchi, T.; Tjian, R. Transcriptional regulation by coactivators in embryonic stem cells. *Trends Cell Biol.* **2012**, *22*, 292–298. [CrossRef] [PubMed]
135. Pijnappel, W.W.M.P.; Esch, D.; Baltissen, M.P.A.; Wu, G.; Mischerikow, N.; Bergsma, A.J.; van der Wal, E.; Han, D.W.; vom Bruch, H.; Moritz, S.; et al. A central role for TFIID in the pluripotent transcription circuitry. *Nature* **2013**, *495*, 516–519. [CrossRef] [PubMed]
136. Marson, A.; Levine, S.S.; Cole, M.F.; Frampton, G.M.; Brambrink, T.; Johnstone, S.; Guenther, M.G.; Johnston, W.K.; Wernig, M.; Newman, J.; et al. Connecting microRNA Genes to the Core Transcriptional Regulatory Circuitry of Embryonic Stem Cells. *Cell* **2008**, *134*, 521–533. [CrossRef]
137. Boija, A.; Klein, I.A.; Sabari, B.R.; Dall'Agnese, A.; Coffey, E.L.; Zamudio, A.V.; Li, C.H.; Shrinivas, K.; Manteiga, J.C.; Hannett, N.M.; et al. Transcription Factors Activate Genes through the Phase-Separation Capacity of Their Activation Domains. *Cell* **2018**, *175*, 1842–1855.e16. [CrossRef]
138. Sabari, B.R.; Dall'Agnese, A.; Boija, A.; Klein, I.A.; Coffey, E.L.; Shrinivas, K.; Abraham, B.J.; Hannett, N.M.; Zamudio, A.V.; Manteiga, J.C.; et al. Coactivator condensation at super-enhancers links phase separation and gene control. *Science* **2018**, *361*, eaar3958. [CrossRef]
139. Rodda, D.J.; Chew, J.L.; Lim, L.H.; Loh, Y.H.; Wang, B.; Ng, H.H.; Robson, P. Transcriptional regulation of Nanog by OCT4 and SOX2. *J. Biol. Chem.* **2005**, *280*, 24731–24737. [CrossRef]
140. Fong, Y.W.; Inouye, C.; Yamaguchi, T.; Cattoglio, C.; Grubisic, I.; Tjian, R. A DNA repair complex functions as an Oct4/Sox2 coactivator in embryonic stem cells. *Cell* **2011**, *147*, 120–131. [CrossRef]
141. Zhang, Z.; Tjian, R. Measuring dynamics of eukaryotic transcription initiation: Challenges, insights and opportunities. *Transcription* **2018**, *9*, 159–165. [CrossRef]
142. Chong, S.; Mir, M. Towards Decoding the Sequence-Based Grammar Governing the Functions of Intrinsically Disordered Protein Regions. *J. Mol. Biol.* **2021**, *433*, 166724. [CrossRef]
143. Choi, U.B.; Sanabria, H.; Smirnova, T.; Bowen, M.E.; Weninger, K.R. Spontaneous switching among conformational ensembles in intrinsically disordered proteins. *Biomolecules* **2019**, *9*, 114. [CrossRef]
144. Li, M.; He, Y.; Dubois, W.; Wu, X.; Shi, J.; Huang, J. Distinct Regulatory Mechanisms and Functions for p53-Activated and p53-Repressed DNA Damage Response Genes in Embryonic Stem Cells. *Mol. Cell* **2012**, *46*, 30–42. [CrossRef]
145. Lin, T.; Chao, C.; Saito, S.; Mazur, S.J.; Murphy, M.E.; Appella, E.; Xu, Y. p53 induces differentiation of mouse embryonic stem cells by suppressing Nanog expression. *Nat. Cell Biol.* **2005**, *7*, 165–171. [CrossRef]
146. Jaiswal, S.K.; Oh, J.J.; DePamphilis, M.L. Cell cycle arrest and apoptosis are not dependent on p53 prior to p53-dependent embryonic stem cell differentiation. *Stem Cells* **2020**, *38*, 1091–1106. [CrossRef]
147. Fu, H.; Liu, R.; Jia, Z.; Li, R.; Zhu, F.; Zhu, W.; Shao, Y.; Jin, Y.; Xue, Y.; Huang, J.; et al. Poly(ADP-ribosylation) of P-TEFb by PARP1 disrupts phase separation to inhibit global transcription after DNA damage. *Nat. Cell Biol.* **2022**, *24*, 513–525. [CrossRef]
148. Nakazawa, Y.; Hara, Y.; Oka, Y.; Komine, O.; van den Heuvel, D.; Guo, C.; Daigaku, Y.; Isono, M.; He, Y.; Shimada, M.; et al. Ubiquitination of DNA Damage-Stalled RNAPII Promotes Transcription-Coupled Repair. *Cell* **2020**, *180*, 1228–1244.e24. [CrossRef]
149. Tufegdžić Vidaković, A.; Mitter, R.; Kelly, G.P.; Neumann, M.; Harreman, M.; Rodríguez-Martínez, M.; Herlihy, A.; Weems, J.C.; Boeing, S.; Encheva, V.; et al. Regulation of the RNAPII Pool Is Integral to the DNA Damage Response. *Cell* **2020**, *180*, 1245–1261.e21. [CrossRef]
150. Marques, D.S.; Sandrini, J.Z.; Boyle, R.T.; Marins, L.F.; Trindade, G.S. Relationships between multidrug resistance (MDR) and stem cell markers in human chronic myeloid leukemia cell lines. *Leuk. Res.* **2010**, *34*, 757–762. [CrossRef]
151. Crawford, R.R.; Potukuchi, P.K.; Schuetz, E.G.; Schuetz, J.D. Beyond Competitive Inhibition: Regulation of ABC Transporters by Kinases and Protein-Protein Interactions as Potential Mechanisms of Drug-Drug Interactions. *Drug Metab. Dispos.* **2018**, *46*, 567–580. [CrossRef] [PubMed]

152. Wu, Y.; Chen, K.; Xing, G.; Li, L.; Ma, B.; Hu, Z.; Duan, L.; Liu, X. Phospholipid remodeling is critical for stem cell pluripotency by facilitating mesenchymal-to-epithelial transition. *Sci. Adv.* **2019**, *5*, eaax7525. [CrossRef] [PubMed]
153. Wu, Y.; Chen, K.; Liu, X.; Huang, L.; Zhao, D.; Li, L.; Gao, M.; Pei, D.; Wang, C.; Liu, X. Srebp-1 Interacts with c-Myc to Enhance Somatic Cell Reprogramming. *Stem Cells* **2016**, *34*, 83–92. [CrossRef]
154. Zhou, G.; Meng, S.; Li, Y.; Ghebre, Y.T.; Cooke, J.P. Optimal ROS Signaling Is Critical for Nuclear Reprogramming. *Cell Rep.* **2016**, *15*, 919–925. [CrossRef]

Disclaimer/Publisher's Note: The statements, opinions and data contained in all publications are solely those of the individual author(s) and contributor(s) and not of MDPI and/or the editor(s). MDPI and/or the editor(s) disclaim responsibility for any injury to people or property resulting from any ideas, methods, instructions or products referred to in the content.

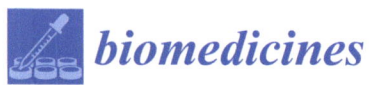

Article

Exogenous OCT4 and SOX2 Contribution to In Vitro Reprogramming in Cattle

Lucas Simões Machado [1,†], Camila Martins Borges [1], Marina Amaro de Lima [1], Juliano Rodrigues Sangalli [2], Jacinthe Therrien [3], Laís Vicari de Figueiredo Pessôa [2], Paulo Fantinato Neto [2], Felipe Perecin [2], Lawrence Charles Smith [1,3], Flavio Vieira Meirelles [1,2] and Fabiana Fernandes Bressan [1,*]

[1] Post-Graduate Program of Anatomy of Domestic and Wild Animals, Faculty of Veterinary Medicine and Animal Sciences, University of São Paulo, São Paulo 05508-270, SP, Brazil; lucas.machado@unifesp.br (L.S.M.); camila.martins.borges@usp.br (C.M.B.); marina.amaro.lima@usp.br (M.A.d.L.); lawrence.c.smith@umontreal.ca (L.C.S.); meirellf@usp.br (F.V.M.)

[2] Department of Veterinary Medicine, Faculty of Animal Sciences and Food Engineering, University of São Paulo, Pirassununga 13635-900, SP, Brazil; julianors@usp.br (J.R.S.); laisvpessoa@usp.br (L.V.d.F.P.); fantinato@usp.br (P.F.N.); fperecin@usp.br (F.P.)

[3] Centre de Recherche en Reproduction et Fertilité, Faculté de Médecine Vétérinaire, Université de Montréal, Saint-Hyacinthe, QC J2S 7C6, Canada; jacinthe.therrien@umontreal.ca

* Correspondence: fabianabressan@usp.br

† Current address: Department of Biochemistry, Paulista School of Medicine, Federal University of São Paulo (UNIFESP), São Paulo 04021-001, SP, Brazil.

Abstract: Mechanisms of cell reprogramming by pluripotency-related transcription factors or nuclear transfer seem to be mediated by similar pathways, and the study of the contribution of OCT4 and SOX2 in both processes may help elucidate the mechanisms responsible for pluripotency. Bovine fibroblasts expressing exogenous *OCT4* or *SOX2*, or both, were analyzed regarding the expression of pluripotency factors and imprinted genes *H19* and *IGF2R*, and used for in vitro reprogramming. The expression of the *H19* gene was increased in the control sorted group, and putative iPSC-like cells were obtained when cells were not submitted to cell sorting. When sorted cells expressing OCT4, SOX2, or none (control) were used as donor cells for somatic cell nuclear transfer, fusion rates were 60.0% vs. 64.95% and 70.53% vs. 67.24% for SOX2 vs. control and OCT4 vs. control groups, respectively; cleavage rates were 66.66% vs. 81.68% and 86.47% vs. 85.18%, respectively; blastocyst rates were 33.05% vs. 44.15% and 52.06% vs. 44.78%, respectively. These results show that the production of embryos by NT resulted in similar rates of in vitro developmental competence compared to control cells regardless of different profiles of pluripotency-related gene expression presented by donor cells; however, induced reprogramming was compromised after cell sorting.

Keywords: bovine; epigenetics; pluripotency; cellular reprogramming; OCT4; SOX2

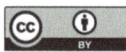

1. Introduction

Assisted reproductive biotechniques (ARTs) such as in vitro embryo production (IVP), intracytoplasmic sperm injection (ICSI), and mechanisms of in vitro induced reprogramming by either nuclear transfer (NT) or exogenous expression of pluripotency-related transcription factors (iPSCs generation) have important applications in regenerative medicine, and they may also greatly contribute to enhance animal production. In particular, in vitro reprogramming is a promising tool to overcome challenges in acquired infertilities or conservation of endangered species, and they may also lead to a better understanding of the underlying mechanism involved in initial embryonic development [1,2].

Nonetheless, ARTs are often performed in an environment that differs from the "in vivo" conditions, concerning, for example, the gaseous atmosphere and the nutrient supply in the culture. It has been shown that in vitro manipulations of gametes and embryos at the beginning of an organism's development may lead to changes in epigenetic regulation, particularly due to the possible disruption of the gene expression pattern during the reprogramming cycles [3–8], which can lead to the occurrence of abnormalities in the development and even after birth of individuals derived from these techniques [3–6]. Indeed, a high incidence of epigenetic syndromes has been reported more frequently in ART-derived offspring than when natural reproduction occurs, particularly due to an abnormal epigenetic reprogramming leading to altered gene expression and dysfunctions in embryonic development and in the embryonic annexes in imprinted genes after in vitro reprogramming [7,9].

Several human epigenetic syndromes have been associated with disrupted imprinted genes, including Beckwith–Wiedemann or BWS [10], Silver–Russel or SRS [11], Angelman [12], and Prader–Willi [13] syndromes. In particular, BWS and SRS are reported to be closely related to the *H19* and *IGF2* imprinted status. Usually, patients affected with syndromes resulting from disorders in the *H19/IGF2* locus present growth disorders, body asymmetry, intellectual disability, and the appearance of tumors [14]. A common condition in ruminants derived from ARTs is large offspring syndrome or LOS), with causes and phenotypes very similar to the BWS in humans [15–17].

Mechanisms of pluripotency acquaintance, in vivo or in vitro, seem to be mediated by the same pathways, eliciting nuclear remodeling and modulating gene expression. Two transcription factors, OCT4 and NANOG, were the first to be identified as essential for early embryonic development and for maintaining stem-cell pluripotency [18,19]. It was also shown that SOX2, another transcription factor, heterodimerizes with OCT4, regulating several genes in pluripotent cells [18–22]. Hence, not only are these transcription factors bound to their target DNA sites, the proteins are known to interact with each other and with chromatin remodeling agents, modulating the chromatin conformation and, therefore, the gene expression [23,24]. Interestingly, more recently, both OCT4 and SOX2 factors have been reported to have a considerable influence on the regulation of some imprinted genes, especially at locus *H19/IGF2*, known to be essential for normal embryo and placenta development [25–27].

In mouse embryos, Zimmerman et al. reported that the binding of OCT/SOX pluripotency factors to the *H19/IGF2* locus ICR contributed to hypomethylation in post-compaction embryos, thus relating the methylation status of these genes to the main factors of pluripotency [28]. Habib et al. (2014), through a study with 57 patients with BWS, demonstrated that some patients who present methylation gain in the *H19/IGF2* locus also present mutations in the binding site of the OCT4/SOX2 factors, showing that the SOX/OCT motifs within *H19/IGF2* ICR also participate in maintaining hypomethylation of the maternal allele [29].

It is, therefore, important to investigate possible factors involved in the induction and regulation of pluripotency acquisition, imprinting maintenance, and gene expression of the genes relevant to the development in cattle, possibly one of the livestock species where in vitro technologies are currently used in favor of animal production. Herein, we present an experimental in vitro model where pluripotency factors were studied together or separately regarding their influence on cellular genomic imprinting regulation and pluripotency acquisition in vitro.

2. Materials and Methods

All procedures were performed in accordance with the Guide for the Care and Use of Laboratory Animals of the National Institutes of Health and The ARRIVE Guidelines, as well as with the rules issued by the National Council for Control of Animal Experimentation (CONCEA, Ministry of Science, Technology, and Innovations and Communications, and in accordance with Law 11.794 of 8 October 2008, Decree 6899 of 15 July 2009) and in accordance with the provisions of the Resolution 466/12 of the National Health Council. Protocols were then approved by the Ethics Committee on Animal Use of the School of Veterinary Medicine and Animal Science University of São Paulo, Brazil (protocol number 8077020516) and by the Ethics Committee on the Use of Animals of the Faculty of

Animal Science and Food Engineering, University of São Paulo, Brazil (protocol number 3526250717).

2.1. Bovine Fetal Fibroblast (bFF) Isolation and Experimental Design

The cell lines were obtained from three *Bos indicus* (maternal) × *Bos taurus* (paternal) fetuses at approximately 50 days of gestational age conceived after artificial insemination. The crossbred (F1) model was used to study allele-specific imprinted genes expression as previously described by our group and others, detailed below. After the removal of the head and organs, tissue was washed with PBS (phosphate-buffered saline) and minced into small fragments, followed by a 3 h incubation in collagenase IV (0.040 g/mL, Sigma-Aldrich Corp., St. Louis, MO, USA) at 38.5 °C. Next, the dissociated tissue was plated and cells were cultured in Iscove's modified Dulbecco's medium (IMDM, Thermo Fisher Scientific; Carlsbad, CA, USA) supplemented with 10% fetal bovine serum (FBS, Hyclone) and antibiotics (penicillin/streptomycin, Thermo Fisher Scientific; Carlsbad, CA, USA) [30]. All lineages were cryopreserved at low passages (p2–3) and thawed for experiments.

All three bovine fetal fibroblast (bFF) lineages were used for exogenous expression of OCT4, SOX2, or both, and then submitted to fluorescence analysis and cellular sorting. A previously validated bicistronic vector system for iPSC induction that allows for simultaneous real-time tracking of expression of the individual transgenes in single cells was used [31].

After cell recovery, bFF1 (male) was characterized regarding epigenetic maintenance at the *H19/IGF2* imprinted locus, and further reprogrammed by nuclear transfer (cells expressing OCT4, SOX2, and control) or induced reprogramming (cells named non-sorted control, sorted control, OCT4+, SOX2+, and OCT4 + SOX2).

The experimental design is briefly shown in Figure 1.

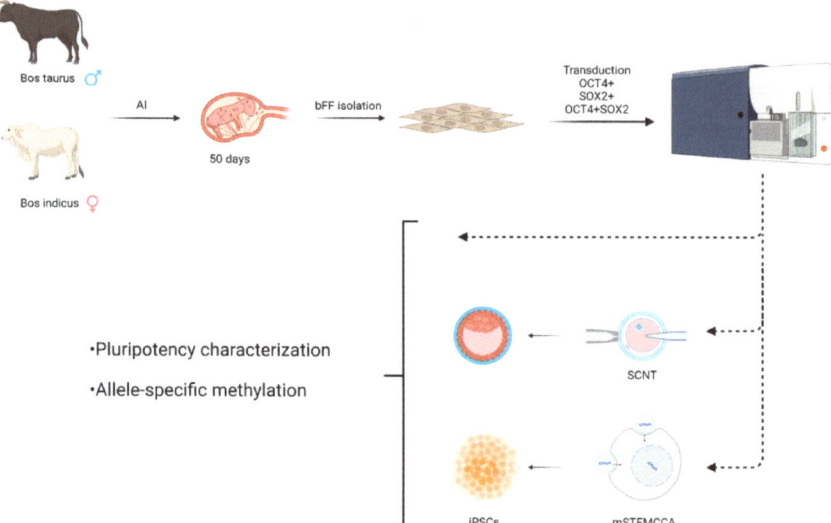

Figure 1. Experimental design showing the cell isolation from *Bos taurus* × *Bos indicus* animals, transduction, sorting, and cellular reprogramming through nuclear transfer or induced in vitro reprogramming.

2.2. Generation of Fibroblasts Expressing Exogenous OCT4 and SOX2

For the production of the cells with exogenous expression of OCT4 and SOX2 and the association of both OCT4 and SOX2, the pLM-vexGFP-Oct4 and pLM-mCitrine-Sox2 vectors were used for lentivirus production as previously described [31]. The first contained human OCT4 (hOCT4) and a fluorescent reporter protein coding sequence for the vexGFP (excitable at 407 nm and emission at 535 nm, Addgene #22240); the second contained hSOX2 and the mCitrine (excitable at 516 nm and emission at 529 nm, Addgene #23242) fluorescent reporter. The use of bicistronic lentiviral vectors encoding the reprogramming factors being co-expressed with discernable fluorescent proteins guarantees the monitoring of expression of each individual reprogramming factor in cells during the course of reprogramming, in a stoichiometric and temporal manner.

Lentiviral particles of OCT4-vexGFP and SOX2-mCitrine were produced by lipofection of 293FT cells (Thermo Fisher Scientific; Carlsbad, CA, USA) with Lipofectamine 2000 (Thermo Fisher Scientific; Carlsbad, CA, USA), using 5 µg of pLM-vexGFP-Oct4 and pLM-mCitrine-Sox2 vectors, 1.2 µg of PLP1 and PLP2 and 2.4 µg of PLP/VSVG (ViraPower kit, Thermo Fisher Scientific; Carlsbad, CA, USA), following the manufacturer's protocol. The supernatant (culture medium) was collected and refreshed at 48 h and 72 h after transfection, filtered, and used for transduction. Pluripotency was induced as previously described, using mouse OCT4, SOX2, c-MYC, and KLF4 transcription factors (mOSKM, mSTEMCCA) [32,33].

2.3. Flow Cytometry Analysis

After 72 h of transduction, protein expression was analyzed by flow cytometry. The gating strategy comprised using non-transduced cells as controls. Positive cells were sorted (BD FACSDiva software and BD FACSAria II SORP equipment—excitation laser 405 nm and detection filter 510/30 for the vexGFP protein and excitation laser 488 nm and 530/30 detection filter for the mCitrine protein). The recovered cells were re-cultured and induced to pluripotency; some were cryopreserved (experimental group pre-induction), and others were used in the subsequent analyses. On the basis of a higher transduction efficiency detected by flow cytometry, one cellular lineage was used for in vitro reprogramming.

2.4. Gene Expression of Imprinted and Pluripotency Genes

RNA was extracted with the RNeasy mini kit (Qiagen, Hilden, Germany) according to the manufacturer's recommendations, and its quality and quantity were assessed by spectrophotometer (Nanodrop 2000). cDNA was synthesized with the High-Capacity cDNA reverse transcription kit (Thermo Fisher Scientific; Carlsbad, CA, USA) according to the manufacturer's recommendations. Experimental groups were quantified regarding their transcripts of imprinted genes *H19* and *IGF2R* and genes related to pluripotency OCT4 and SOX2. Beta-actin (ACTB) and CCR4-NOT transcription complex subunit 11 (ACTB and C2ORF29 or CNOT11) were used as housekeeping genes.

Relative analysis of transcripts was performed by RT-qPCR (7500 Fast Real-Time PCR System, Thermo Fisher Scientific; Carlsbad, CA, USA) using a commercial assay in duplicate (Power SYBR®Green PCR Master Mix, Thermo Fisher Scientific; Carlsbad, CA, USA), where 5 µL of the sample cDNA was added to a 20 µL final volume reaction. The primers' (Table 1) final concentration was 200 nM, and standard curves were performed to evaluate the efficiency of each gene. The qPCR reaction consisted of a denaturation step of 95 °C for 5 s, and an annealing temperature of 60 °C, for 40 cycles. Data were analyzed using the delta–delta CT method [34].

2.5. Allele-Specific Methylation Analyses of the DMR at the H19/IGF2 Locus

DNA extraction was performed with the DNeasy Blood and Tissue Kit (Qiagen, Hilden, Germany) according to the manufacturer's recommendations, and quality and quantity were determined by a spectrophotometer (Nanodrop 2000). The EpiTect Bisulfite Kit (#59104 Qiagen, Hilden, Germany) was used according to the manufacturer's recommendations in a thermocycler for 5 min at 99 °C, 25 min at 60 °C, then 5 more min at 99 °C, 85 min at 60 °C, back to 5 min at 99 °C, 175 min at 60 °C, and finally, 20 °C overnight.

Table 1. Primer sequences for the quantitative analysis of transcripts and methylation analysis at the IGF2/H19 locus.

Name	5'–3' Sequence
ACTB_FWD	GCGGACAGGATGCAGAAA
ACTB_REV	ACGGAGTACTTGCGCTCAG
C2ORF29_FWD	ACTGAGCCTGACCATGCGATC
C2ORF29_REV	GGCTGGAGTGAGGCCAATATG
H19_FWD	AGTGGGAGGGGCATTGGACT
H19_REV	GACCATATCATATCCCTCTGTGC
SOX2_FWD	ATGGGCTCGGTGGTGAAGT
SOX2_REV	TGGTAGTGCTGGGACATGTGA
OCT4_FWD	GCAAACGATCAAGCAGTGACTAC
OCT4_REV	GGCGCCAGAGGAGAGGATACG

Amplification of fragments from the H19/IGF2 DMR (proximally −3327 to −2675 base pairs away from exon 1 was performed using the primers U-H19 F1 and U-H19 R4 (Table 1). The PCR reaction contained 38.5 µL of ultrapure H_2Od, 5 µL of Buffer TPN 10× (Invitrogen), 1.5 µL of dNTP (Invitrogen), 1.5 µL of $MgCl_2$, 1 µL of primer (one for each, forward and reverse), and 0.5 µL of Platinum Taq (Invitrogen, #10966) for each sample, before adding 1 µL of DNA. Each PCR reaction was performed in triplicates. The protocol used was 1 min of plate pre-heating, 50 cycles of 30 s at 94 °C, 30 s at 53 °C and 30 s at 72 °C, and one final 7 min step at 72 °C. Amplified samples were run in a 1.2% agarose gel alongside a 1 Kb ladder, and the master mix lacking DNA as control was purified from the agarose gel and sequenced.

Global and allelic expression analysis of imprinted genes was realized as described by Suzuki and collaborators [35]. A single-nucleotide polymorphism (SNP) at the IGF2/H19 locus between *Bos indicus* and *Bos taurus* allowed for allele-specific DNA methylation analysis after sequencing and allele-specific gene expression analysis. The nucleotide guanine at the sequence TTTATGTATTA indicates *Bos indicus* origin; therefore, the allele is of maternal origin. If the nucleotide adenine were present in its place, that would indicate an allele of paternal origin.

2.6. In Vitro Induced Reprogramming into Pluripotency

Three repetitions (R1, R2, and R3) were submitted to the pluripotency induction. The lentiviral particles containing mouse OSKM (mSTEMCCA) were produced by lipofection of 293FT cells, as previously described [32,33]. At 5 or 6 days after transduction, the cells were transferred to culture plates containing a monolayer of mitotically inactivated (mitomycin C, M4287 Sigma-Aldrich) mouse embryonic fibroblasts (MEFs).

During the cellular reprogramming, the cells were cultured in iPSC medium consisting of DMEM/F12 Knockout (Thermo Fisher Scientific), supplemented with 20% knockout serum replacement (KSR, Thermo Fisher Scientific), 1% glutamine (Thermo Fisher Scientific), 3.85 µM β-mercaptoethanol (Thermo Fisher Scientific), 1% non-essential amino acids (Thermo Fisher Scientific), 10 ng/mL bFGF (Peprotech) and antibiotics (penicillin/streptomycin, Thermo Fisher Scientific). Morphologically typical colonies were manually picked at the first passage, and clonal lines were further dissociated for passaging with TrypLE Express (Life Technologies).

2.7. Somatic Cell Nuclear Transfer

Fetal fibroblasts expressing either OCT4-vexGFP or SOX2-mCitrine were analyzed for OCT4 and SOX2 gene expression through qPCR and flow cytometry analysis, which enabled the sorting of positive cells used as donor cells for somatic cell nuclear transfer procedures as previously described [36,37]. Briefly, bovine oocytes obtained from slaughterhouses were in vitro matured for 18 h, enucleated, and reconstructed with fibroblasts expressing OCT4-vexGFP (n = 182, in four replicates), SOX2-mCitrine (n = 203, in four replicates), or control cells (non-transduced, n = 178 and n = 149, in four replicates as control of OCT4 or SOX2 expressing cells each). After reconstruction, embryos were activated with ionomycin (5 µM, 5 min) and 6-DMAP (2 mM, 3 h) and in vitro cultured until blastocyst stage (7 days) in SOF medium supplemented with 2.5% FBS and 3mg/mL BSA.

2.8. Statistical Analysis

Data obtained from the experimental procedures were analyzed using the statistical program Statistical Analysis System (SAS University Edition), with previous verification of the normality of the residues by the Shapiro–Wilk test (PROC UNIVARIATE) and submitted to analysis of variance. Gene expression data were then submitted to the Bonferroni test. A significance level of 5% was considered for all statistical analyses.

3. Results

3.1. bFF Expressing Exogenous OCT4 and SOX2

The exogenous expression of OCT4 and SOX2 was confirmed by flow cytometry (Figure 2), where the positive populations were sorted out and recovered for in vitro culture and reprogramming procedures. The percentage of positive cells in each cell line and treatment group is presented in Table 2. The post-sorting purity percentage was 90% or greater.

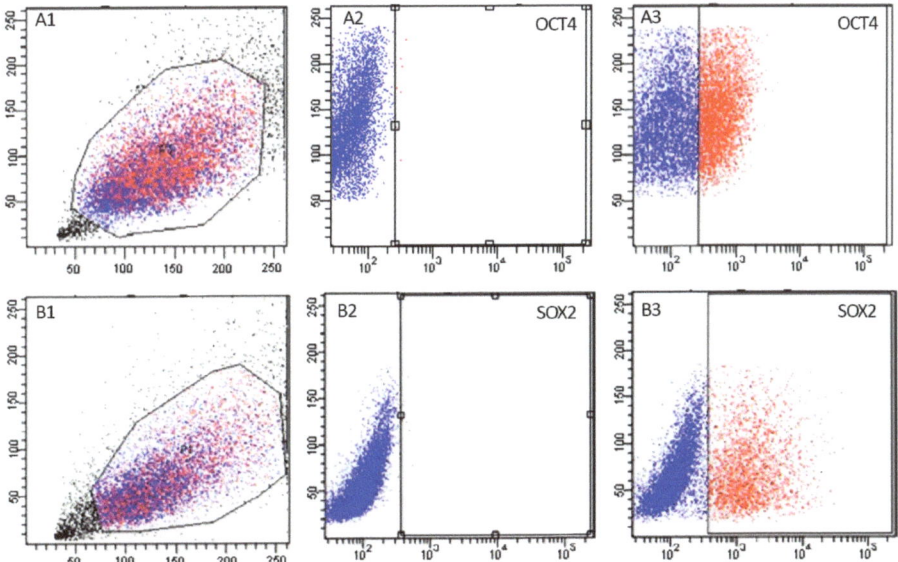

Figure 2. Representative scatter plots of flow cytometric analysis of stable lines expressing OCT4-vexGFP (**A1–A3**) and SOX2-mCitrine (**B1–B3**) used for sorting nuclear donor cells. Blue dots represent negative cells (non-fluorescent) and red dots present positive cells (fluorescent cells). In (**A1,B1**), the Y-axis represents side scatter (SSC) and X-axis represents forward scatter (FSC). (**A2,B2**) represent the control groups, where the Y-axis represents the cell count and X-axis represents the fluorescence in arbitrary units. (**A3,B3**) represent the hOCT4 and the hSOX2 groups, where the Y-axis represents the cell count and X-axis represents the fluorescence in arbitrary units.

Due to higher fluorescence detection of bFF1, the post-sorting recovery was more efficient, enabling its utilization for the subsequent experiments. Cells expressing both OCT4 and SOX2 presented very high proliferation levels, followed by early senescence. Such behavior was observed over three repetitions; therefore, they were used for induced pluripotency, and nuclear transfer was not conducted.

Table 2. Percentage of fluorescent cells by flow cytometry in three bovine fetal fibroblast cell lines.

	hOCT4%	hSOX2%	hOCT4 + hSOX2%
bFF1	79.8	10.2	1.3
bFF2	22.7	4.2	0.4
bFF3	18.7	3.9	0.2
Average	40.4	6.1	0.63

3.2. Quantitative Gene Expression Analyzes of Imprinted Genes or Genes Related to Pluripotency

The experimental groups from the three repetitions were induced to pluripotency (R1, R2, and R3) and evaluated regarding the expression of pluripotency factors OCT4 and SOX2 and imprinted genes H19 and IGF2R. OCT4+ cells showed higher OCT4 expression, and SOX2+ cells had greater SOX2 expression, as expected. This analysis enabled us to detect the high exogenous expression of the target genes.

Double-positive cells (OCT4+/SOX2+) OCT4 + SOX2 cells showed an increase in both OCT4 and SOX2 expression, albeit not statistically significant, probably because the expression was similar to groups expressing only OCT4 and SOX2, and there is apparently an interaction between exogenous OCT4 expression and endogenous SOX2 expression. It is noteworthy that SOX2+ cells had an approximately 10-fold OCT4 level increase when compared to the control (Figure 3).

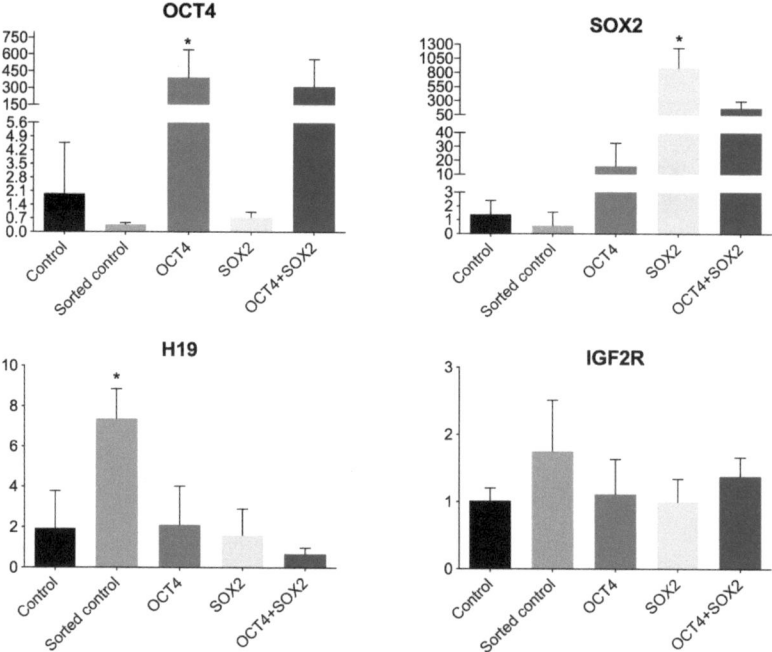

Figure 3. Quantitative gene expression of OCT4, SOX2 (pluripotency-related genes), H19, and IGF2R (imprinted genes) in bovine cells from experimental groups: control, sorted control, expressing exogenous OCT4, expressing exogenous SOX2, or expressing both (OCT4 + SOX2), in arbitrary units. The X-axis represents arbitrary units and the Y-axis represents the experimental groups. Bars presenting an asterisk (*) showed a statistical difference ($p < 0.05$).

The analysis of the imprinted gene H19 expression showed an increased expression in control sorted group, which was not expected. It is speculated herein that the pluripotency factors somehow protect the locus against possible deregulation caused by the sorting procedure, and such possibility must be further investigated with analyses of more repetitions and the methylation pattern of this specific locus.

No differences among the groups were observed when the imprinted gene IGF2R was analyzed; however, there was an approximately 50% increase in expression levels in the sorted control group when compared to the non-sorted control, indicating, once more, a possible effect caused by the flow cytometry analysis and sorting on the regulation of imprinted genes. More repetitions are needed to further understand this possibility.

The analysis of each repetition showed that, even though the gene expression pattern seemed very similar in the groups, the non-sorted R1 had a unique pattern (Figure 4). R1 had a higher expression of OCT4 and a lower expression of H19 in relation to R2 and R3, indicating a possible relationship between them, and R1 was the group able to produce iPSCs colonies more efficiently. The existence of more reprogrammable populations has already been described in the literature [38,39], and more studies are necessary to reveal if such pre-disposition may be related to the regulation between imprinted and pluripotency genes.

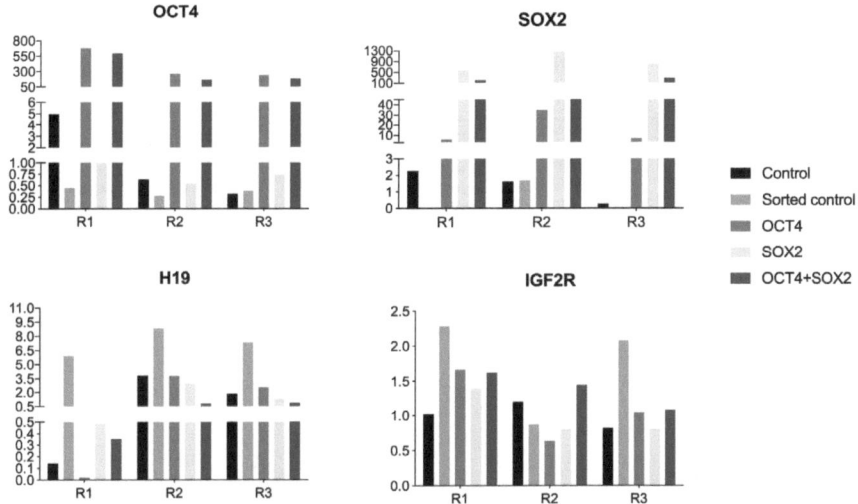

Figure 4. Quantitative gene expression of OCT4, SOX2 (pluripotency-related genes), H19, and IGF2R (imprinted genes) in bovine cells from experimental groups: control, sorted control, expressing exogenous OCT4, expressing exogenous SOX2, or expressing both (OCT4 + SOX2), in arbitrary units. R1, R2, and R3 are representative bars for each lineage (repetition).

3.3. Allele-Specific Methylation Analyses of the DMR at the H19/IGF2 Locus

The methylation was analyzed, and the bisulfite conversion rate (number of non-converted cytosines in relation to all convertible cytosines) was considered appropriate when superior to 90% (Table 3).

Table 3. Bisulfite conversion efficiency rate.

	Non-Sorted Control	Sorted Control	OCT4+	SOX2+	OCT4 + SOX2
Conversion rate	98.03%	98.23%	95.09%	98.89%	98.32%

The percentage of total methylation, as well as the methylation at the CTCF region, was calculated using the number of methylated and not methylated CpG islands. In general, the paternal allele (taurus) was methylated, and the maternal allele (indicus) was not methylated (Table 4).

Table 4. Methylation percentage in the DMR at the H19/IGF2 locus in the experimental groups.

	Non-Sorted Control (%DMR; %CTCF)	Sorted Control (%DMR, %CTCF)	OCT4+ (%DMR, %CTCF)	SOX2+ (%DMR, %CTCF)	OCT4 + SOX2 (%DMR, %CTCF)
Maternal allele	21.42; 33.33	0; 0	21.24; 6.67	2.4; 5.55	5.95; 11.11
Paternal allele	100; 100	92.85; 100	100; 100	96.42; 100	92.3

3.4. Pluripotency Induction (iPSC Production)

bFF1 was used for pluripotency induction. Interestingly, non-sorted cells generated biPS colonies, whereas sorted cells (control non-transgenic, OCT4-, SOX2-, and OCT4- + SOX2-expressing cells) did not generate biPS cells.

The percentage of colonies formed is described in Table 5 (the number of colonies formed divided by the number of plated transduced cells). The groups transduced with hOSKM did not produce iPSC colonies.

Table 5. Percentage of iPSC colonies formed in each experimental group in all three repetitions (percentage and number of colonies).

	Non-Sorted Control	Sorted Control	OCT4+	SOX2+	OCT4 + SOX2
R1	0.00035 (7)	0	0	0	0
R2	0.00005 (1)	0	0	0	0
R3	0	0	0	0	0

Cells showed typical colony morphology with approximately 15 to 20 days post transduction (Figure 5).

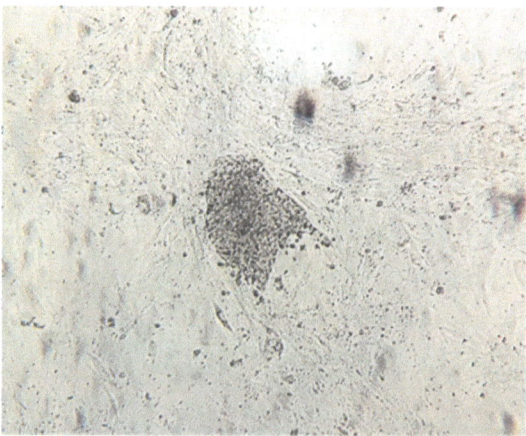

Figure 5. Representative image of a reprogrammed colony of cells from the non-sorted control before first picking (p0), 200×.

Colonies were manually picked at the first passage and later enzymatically passaged. Among the repetitions, different passages on bFF1 were used since the same cell line was cultured continuously while used on the repetitions. Therefore, R1 had the lowest number of passages in vitro.

3.5. Somatic Cell Nuclear Transfer Using hOCT4 and hSOX2 Overexpressing Donor Cells

Fusion rates were 60.0% vs. 64.95% and 70.53% vs. 67.24% for SOX2 vs. control and OCT4 vs. control groups, respectively; cleavage rates (48 h after activation) were 66.66% vs. 81.68% and 86.47% vs. 85.18%, respectively; blastocyst rates (192 h after activation) were 33.05% vs. 44.15% and 52.06% vs. 44.78%, respectively (Figure 6).

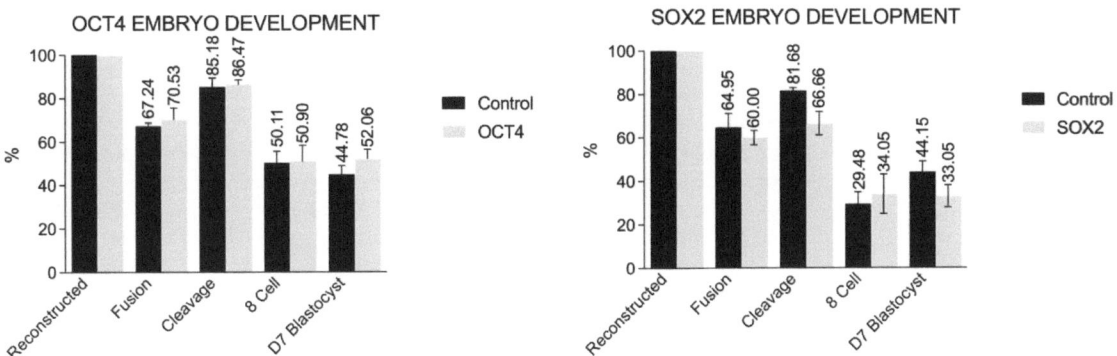

Figure 6. Development competence (percentage of reconstructed and fused embryos, cleavage, and development—8 cell and blastocyst rates) of nuclear transfer-derived embryos produced with donor cells expressing exogenous OCT4, SOX2, or none (control cells).

There were no differences in the rate of fusion, cleavage, percentage of embryos in eight cells, and capacity of development to blastocysts on the seventh day of in vitro culture between clone embryos reconstructed with modified or not cells.

4. Discussion

During development, a mammal's genome is epigenetically reprogrammed on two different and essential occasions: gametogenesis and early embryogenesis. The reprogramming processes occur in the primordial germ cells (PGCs), where epigenetic markers are erased, and new ones are established at specific moments, both before and after fertilization. After fertilization, a second wave of global demethylation occurs, except for imprinted genes, followed by de novo methylation, which sets a new epigenetic layout allowing totipotency and following cell line committed differentiation [40,41]. Epigenetic modifications may be inherited but also modified by the environment, thus explaining the more frequent and different phenotypical alterations observed in ART-generated individuals [42]. In this study, the creation of an in vitro experimental model that enables the study of OCT4 and SOX2 transcription factors, as well as their combination, in the regulation of the imprinting in the H19/IGF2 locus in bovine cells and cells reprogrammed in vitro was proposed.

In this study, bovine cell lines expressing pluripotency exogenous factors OCT4, SOX2, or both were produced. These lines are important to better understand the acquisition and maintenance of the pluripotency process in vitro. The sorting of positive cells for those factors allows us to use only those cells that have integrated the factors, increasing, in theory, reprogramming efficiency. The production of such factors was accomplished by the lentiviral approach, and the lentiviral production was confirmed through fluorescence analysis of the 293FT cells after transfection. After 5 or 6 days post transduction, the percentage of positive cells for the reporter genes was quantified by flow cytometry and used as a lentiviral transduction efficiency parameter. Such measurement is valid for the qualitative and quantitative analysis of the efficiency of integration of the transgene since the multiplicity of infection of these vectors results in a linear title of the average fluorescence intensity of each corresponding fluorescent protein [31]. The same group reported that a threefold increase of OCT4 in relation to the SOX2, KLF4, and c-MYC levels raised the reprogramming efficiency, and the opposite resulted in a drastic decrease in reprogramming efficiency [31]. In 2011, Yamaguchi and collaborators reported that decreased SOX2 levels increased efficiency in partially reprogrammed cells production [43], showing that both expression and interaction of OCT4 and SOX2 need to be finely regulated for acquiring and maintaining pluripotency in vitro.

The expression of the imprinted genes H19 and IGF2 was also analyzed on the cell lines produced, and the methylation of the DMR at the H19/IGF2 locus. Nevertheless, the hypothesis that the overexpression of OCT4 and SOX2 in bovine cell lines is not only possible but leads to modifications in expression and imprinting pattern in the H19/IGF2 locus, as well as in bovine reprogramming into pluripotency by TNCS or iPSC generation efficiency, was not confirmed in this study.

Even though further analyses are needed, it is possible to observe that the methylation pattern of the non-sorted group was slightly different from the others that were submitted to the same sorting process; the maternal allele was, herein, completely demethylated. To infer if the expression of the exogenous factors acts in a protective way toward the H19/IGF2 locus from external interferences, such as sorting or reprogramming, further analyses are still needed.

The generation of induced pluripotency models (induced pluripotent stem cells) made it possible to study the process of in vitro reprogramming more precisely. In this study, cell reprogramming after OSKM transduction was observed only in the control group, and the study of whether the imbalance between OCT4 and SOX2 expression may hamper induced reprogramming will be of great importance to better understand the role of these pluripotency factors in the acquisition and maintenance of the epigenetic patterns of reprogrammed cells.

Nonetheless, the results obtained herein (reprogrammed cells generated only from the non-sorted control group and, within that group, a higher number of colonies on the first repetition, fewer colonies on the second repetition, and none on the third), two effects can be inferred: (1) a sorting effect, and (2) an in vitro passage number effect. The environmental factor must also be considered, with possible effects caused by the laboratory routine itself as changes in the culture medium lot or supplements.

Moreover, the embryo production by NT from cells expressing hOCT4 or hSOX2 resulted in similar in vitro embryonic development rates regardless of the gene expression profiles of factors related to the pluripotency of the nucleus donor cells.

Lastly, in this study, we analyzed whether the overexpression of two important pluripotency-related genes could be related to the success of cellular reprogramming and to a specific imprinting deregulation, which is commonly reported (H19/IGF2 locus). There is limited research on the influence of specific genes in the in vitro reprogramming of animals other than rodents and primates. Herein, we showed that the overexpression of pluripotency-related factors, proven by a reporter gene and molecular analysis, is not able to completely impact the epigenetics and the efficiency of the in vitro reprogramming in cattle, and other strategies should be implemented in order to generate healthy cloned cattle or bona fide pluripotent stem cells in this species.

5. Conclusions

The results described in this study allow us to conclude that the production of cells expressing exogenous pluripotent factors was successful, as shown by the gene expression experiments. Cellular reprogramming to pluripotency by cloned embryo production was achieved in the present study when cells expressing OCT4 or SOX2 were used as donor cells; however, in our conditions, these cell lines did not result in iPSCs after induced reprogramming in vitro. There was interference from the flow cytometer analysis and sorting process in the expression of the imprinted gene H19 in at least one of the experimental groups.

The production of embryos by NT of hSOX2- or hOCT4-expressing donor cells resulted in similar rates of in vitro developmental competence compared to control cells regardless of different profiles of pluripotency-related gene expression presented by donor cells. A better understanding of the contribution of each reprogramming factor used in induced reprogramming will establish strategies to enhance in vitro reprogramming performance. Such knowledge will contribute to in vitro animal production by increasing the cloning efficiency at term and regenerative medicine through the derivation and adequate culture of reprogrammed pluripotent stem cells.

Author Contributions: Conceptualization, F.V.M. and F.F.B.; methodology, L.S.M., C.M.B., M.A.d.L., J.R.S., J.T., F.P., and F.F.B.; investigation, L.S.M., J.T., L.V.d.F.P., P.F.N., F.P., L.C.S., F.V.M., and F.F.B.; writing—original draft preparation, L.S.M. and C.M.B.; writing—review and editing, L.V.d.F.P. and F.F.B.; supervision, F.F.B. All authors have read and agreed to the published version of the manuscript.

Funding: This work was supported by grants #2009/11631-6, #2011/08376-4, #2012/24766-0, #2013/08135-2, #2013/13686-8, #2015/01407-2, #2015/26818-5, #2017/02159-8—Fundação de Amparo à Pesquisa do Estado de São Paulo (FAPESP); CNPq; and CAPES.

Institutional Review Board Statement: All procedures were performed in accordance with the Guide for the Care and Use of Laboratory Animals of the National Institutes of Health and the ARRIVE Guidelines, as well as with the rules issued by the National Council for Control of Animal Experimentation (CONCEA, Ministry of Science, Technology and Innovations and Communications, and in accordance with Law 11.794 of 8 October 2008, Decree 6899 of 15 July 2009), and in accordance with the provisions of the Resolution 466/12 of the National Health Council. Protocols were then approved by the Ethics Committee on Animal Use of the School of Veterinary Medicine and Animal Science University of São Paulo, Brazil (protocol number 8077020516) and by the Ethics Committee on the Use of Animals of the Faculty of Animal Science and Food Engineering, University of São Paulo, Brazil (protocol number 3526250717).

Informed Consent Statement: Not applicable.

Data Availability Statement: Data are contained within the article.

Acknowledgments: The authors would like to acknowledge the scientific and technical support received from Alexandre Basso and Daniela Teixeira (UNIFESP) for flow cytometry analysis, Eirini Papapetrou for providing the plasmids encoding for OCT4-vexGFP and SOX2-mCitrine, Jose Eduardo Krieger, Vinicius Bassaneze, and Chester Bitencourt Sacramento (INCOR, FMUSP) for lentivirus transduction and scientific support, and Kaiana Recchia for scientific discussion.

Conflicts of Interest: The authors declare no conflict of interest.

References

1. Brezina, P.R.; Ning, N.; Mitchell, E.; Zacur, H.A.; Baramki, T.A.; Zhao, Y. Recent Advances in Assisted Reproductive Technology. *Curr. Obstet. Gynecol. Rep.* **2012**, *1*, 166–173. [CrossRef]
2. Herrick, J.R. Assisted Reproductive Technologies for Endangered Species Conservation: Developing Sophisticated Protocols with Limited Access to Animals with Unique Reproductive Mechanisms. *Biol. Reprod.* **2019**, *100*, 1158–1170. [CrossRef]
3. Bird, A. DNA Methylation Patterns and Epigenetic Memory. *Genes Dev.* **2002**, *16*, 6–21. [CrossRef] [PubMed]
4. Bortvin, A.; Eggan, K.; Skaletsky, H.; Akutsu, H.; Berry, D.L.; Yanagimachi, R.; Page, D.C.; Jaenisch, R. Incomplete Reactivation of Oct4-Related Genes in Mouse Embryos Cloned from Somatic Nuclei. *Dev. Camb. Engl.* **2003**, *130*, 1673–1680.
5. Eilertsen, K.J.; Power, R.A.; Harkins, L.L.; Misica, P. Targeting Cellular Memory to Reprogram the Epigenome, Restore Potential, and Improve Somatic Cell Nuclear Transfer. *Anim. Reprod. Sci.* **2007**, *98*, 129–146. [CrossRef]
6. Santos, F.; Dean, W. Epigenetic Reprogramming during Early Development in Mammals. *Reprod. Camb. Engl.* **2004**, *127*, 643–651. [CrossRef]
7. Smith, L.C.; Therrien, J.; Filion, F.; Bressan, F.; Meirelles, F.V. Epigenetic Consequences of Artificial Reproductive Technologies to the Bovine Imprinted Genes SNRPN, H19/IGF2, and IGF2R. *Front. Genet.* **2015**, *6*, 58. [CrossRef]
8. Hansen, P.J. Implications of Assisted Reproductive Technologies for Pregnancy Outcomes in Mammals. *Annu. Rev. Anim. Biosci.* **2020**, *8*, 395–413. [CrossRef]
9. Smith, L.C.; Suzuki, J.; Goff, A.K.; Filion, F.; Therrien, J.; Murphy, B.D.; Kohan-Ghadr, H.R.; Lefebvre, R.; Brisville, A.C.; Buczinski, S.; et al. Developmental and Epigenetic Anomalies in Cloned Cattle. *Reprod. Domest. Anim. Zuchthyg.* **2012**, *47* (Suppl. S4), 107–114. [CrossRef]

10. Brown, K.W.; Villar, A.J.; Bickmore, W.; Clayton-Smith, J.; Catchpoole, D.; Maher, E.R.; Reik, W. Imprinting Mutation in the Beckwith-Wiedemann Syndrome Leads to Biallelic IGF2 Expression through an H19-Independent Pathway. *Hum. Mol. Genet.* **1996**, *5*, 2027–2032. [CrossRef]
11. Bartholdi, D.; Krajewska-Walasek, M.; Ounap, K.; Gaspar, H.; Chrzanowska, K.H.; Ilyana, H.; Kayserili, H.; Lurie, I.W.; Schinzel, A.; Baumer, A. Epigenetic Mutations of the Imprinted IGF2-H19 Domain in Silver-Russell Syndrome (SRS): Results from a Large Cohort of Patients with SRS and SRS-like Phenotypes. *J. Med. Genet.* **2009**, *46*, 192–197. [CrossRef]
12. Runte, M.; Kroisel, P.M.; Gillessen-Kaesbach, G.; Varon, R.; Horn, D.; Cohen, M.Y.; Wagstaff, J.; Horsthemke, B.; Buiting, K. SNURF-SNRPN and UBE3A Transcript Levels in Patients with Angelman Syndrome. *Hum. Genet.* **2004**, *114*, 553–561. [CrossRef] [PubMed]
13. Reed, M.L.; Leff, S.E. Maternal Imprinting of Human SNRPN, a Gene Deleted in Prader-Willi Syndrome. *Nat. Genet.* **1994**, *6*, 163–167. [CrossRef] [PubMed]
14. Amor, D.J.; Halliday, J. A Review of Known Imprinting Syndromes and Their Association with Assisted Reproduction Technologies. *Hum. Reprod. Oxf. Engl.* **2008**, *23*, 2826–2834. [CrossRef] [PubMed]
15. Young, L.E.; Sinclair, K.D.; Wilmut, I. Large Offspring Syndrome in Cattle and Sheep. *Rev. Reprod.* **1998**, *3*, 155–163. [CrossRef]
16. Ceelen, M.; Vermeiden, J.P. Health of Human and Livestock Conceived by Assisted Reproduction. *Twin Res. Off. J. Int. Soc. Twin Stud.* **2001**, *4*, 412–416. [CrossRef]
17. Chen, Z.; Robbins, K.M.; Wells, K.D.; Rivera, R.M. Large Offspring Syndrome: A Bovine Model for the Human Loss-of-Imprinting Overgrowth Syndrome Beckwith-Wiedemann. *Epigenetics Off. J. DNA Methylation Soc.* **2013**, *8*, 591–601. [CrossRef]
18. Nichols, J.; Zevnik, B.; Anastassiadis, K.; Niwa, H.; Klewe-Nebenius, D.; Chambers, I.; Schöler, H.; Smith, A. Formation of Pluripotent Stem Cells in the Mammalian Embryo Depends on the POU Transcription Factor Oct4. *Cell* **1998**, *95*, 379–391. [CrossRef]
19. Mitsui, K.; Tokuzawa, Y.; Itoh, H.; Segawa, K.; Murakami, M.; Takahashi, K.; Maruyama, M.; Maeda, M.; Yamanaka, S. The Homeoprotein Nanog Is Required for Maintenance of Pluripotency in Mouse Epiblast and ES Cells. *Cell* **2003**, *113*, 631–642. [CrossRef]
20. Boyer, L.A.; Lee, T.I.; Cole, M.F.; Johnstone, S.E.; Levine, S.S.; Zucker, J.P.; Guenther, M.G.; Kumar, R.M.; Murray, H.L.; Jenner, R.G.; et al. Core Transcriptional Regulatory Circuitry in Human Embryonic Stem Cells. *Cell* **2005**, *122*, 947–956. [CrossRef]
21. Hammachi, F.; Morrison, G.M.; Sharov, A.A.; Livigni, A.; Narayan, S.; Papapetrou, E.P.; O'Malley, J.; Kaji, K.; Ko, M.S.H.; Ptashne, M.; et al. Transcriptional Activation by Oct4 Is Sufficient for the Maintenance and Induction of Pluripotency. *Cell Rep.* **2012**, *1*, 99–109. [CrossRef] [PubMed]
22. Rizzino, A.; Wuebben, E.L. Sox2/Oct4: A Delicately Balanced Partnership in Pluripotent Stem Cells and Embryogenesis. *Biochim. Biophys. Acta* **2016**, *1859*, 780–791. [CrossRef] [PubMed]
23. Chen, L.; Daley, G.Q. Molecular Basis of Pluripotency. *Hum. Mol. Genet.* **2008**, *17*, R23–R27. [CrossRef] [PubMed]
24. Whitworth, K.M.; Prather, R.S. Somatic Cell Nuclear Transfer Efficiency: How Can It Be Improved through Nuclear Remodeling and Reprogramming? *Mol. Reprod. Dev.* **2010**, *77*, 1001–1015. [CrossRef]
25. Reik, W.; Constância, M.; Fowden, A.; Anderson, N.; Dean, W.; Ferguson-Smith, A.; Tycko, B.; Sibley, C. Regulation of Supply and Demand for Maternal Nutrients in Mammals by Imprinted Genes. *J. Physiol.* **2003**, *547*, 35–44. [CrossRef]
26. Nelissen, E.C.M.; Dumoulin, J.C.M.; Busato, F.; Ponger, L.; Eijssen, L.M.; Evers, J.L.H.; Tost, J.; van Montfoort, A.P.A. Altered Gene Expression in Human Placentas after IVF/ICSI. *Hum. Reprod. Oxf. Engl.* **2014**, *29*, 2821–2831. [CrossRef]
27. Constância, M.; Hemberger, M.; Hughes, J.; Dean, W.; Ferguson-Smith, A.; Fundele, R.; Stewart, F.; Kelsey, G.; Fowden, A.; Sibley, C.; et al. Placental-Specific IGF-II Is a Major Modulator of Placental and Fetal Growth. *Nature* **2002**, *417*, 945–948. [CrossRef]
28. Zimmerman, D.L.; Boddy, C.S.; Schoenherr, C.S. Oct4/Sox2 Binding Sites Contribute to Maintaining Hypomethylation of the Maternal Igf2/H19 Imprinting Control Region. *PLoS ONE* **2013**, *8*, e81962. [CrossRef]
29. Abi Habib, W.; Azzi, S.; Brioude, F.; Steunou, V.; Thibaud, N.; Das Neves, C.; Le Jule, M.; Chantot-Bastaraud, S.; Keren, B.; Lyonnet, S.; et al. Extensive Investigation of the IGF2/H19 Imprinting Control Region Reveals Novel OCT4/SOX2 Binding Site Defects Associated with Specific Methylation Patterns in Beckwith-Wiedemann Syndrome. *Hum. Mol. Genet.* **2014**, *23*, 5763–5773. [CrossRef]
30. Pessoa, L.V.F.; Bressan, F.F.; Chiaratti, M.R.; Pires, P.R.L.; Perecin, F.; Smith, L.C.; Meirelles, F.V. Mitochondrial DNA Dynamics during in Vitro Culture and Pluripotency Induction of a Bovine Rho0 Cell Line. *Genet. Mol. Res.* **2015**, *14*, 14093–14104. [CrossRef]
31. Papapetrou, E.P.; Tomishima, M.J.; Chambers, S.M.; Mica, Y.; Reed, E.; Menon, J.; Tabar, V.; Mo, Q.; Studer, L.; Sadelain, M. Stoichiometric and Temporal Requirements of Oct4, Sox2, Klf4, and c-Myc Expression for Efficient Human IPSC Induction and Differentiation. *Proc. Natl. Acad. Sci. USA* **2009**, *106*, 12759–12764. [CrossRef] [PubMed]
32. Pessoa, L.V.F.; Pires, P.R.L.; Collado, M.; Pieri, N.C.G.; Recchia, K.; Souza, A.F.; Perecin, F.; Da Silveira, J.C.; Andrade, A.F.C.; Ambrosio, C.E.; et al. Generation and MiRNA Characterization of Equine Induced Pluripotent Stem Cells Derived from Fetal and Adult Multipotent Tissues. *Stem Cells Int.* **2019**, *2019*, 1393791. [CrossRef] [PubMed]
33. Bressan, F.F.; Bassanezze, V.; de Figueiredo Pessôa, L.V.; Sacramento, C.B.; Malta, T.M.; Kashima, S.; Fantinato Neto, P.; Strefezzi, R.D.F.; Pieri, N.C.G.; Krieger, J.E.; et al. Generation of Induced Pluripotent Stem Cells from Large Domestic Animals. *Stem Cell Res. Ther.* **2020**, *11*, 247. [CrossRef]
34. Livak, K.J.; Schmittgen, T.D. Analysis of Relative Gene Expression Data Using Real-Time Quantitative PCR and the 2(-Delta Delta C(T)) Method. *Methods* **2001**, *25*, 402–408. [CrossRef] [PubMed]

35. Suzuki, J.; Therrien, J.; Filion, F.; Lefebvre, R.; Goff, A.K.; Perecin, F.; Meirelles, F.V.; Smith, L.C. Loss of Methylation at H19 DMD Is Associated with Biallelic Expression and Reduced Development in Cattle Derived by Somatic Cell Nuclear Transfer. *Biol. Reprod.* **2011**, *84*, 947–956. [CrossRef] [PubMed]
36. Miranda, M.D.S.; Bressan, F.F.; Zecchin, K.G.; Vercesi, A.E.; Mesquita, L.G.; Merighe, G.K.F.; King, W.A.; Ohashi, O.M.; Pimentel, J.R.V.; Perecin, F.; et al. Serum-starved apoptotic fibroblasts reduce blastocyst production but enable development to term after SCNT in cattle. *Cloning Stem Cells* **2009**, *11*, 565–573. [CrossRef]
37. Bressan, F.F.; dos Santos Miranda, M.; Perecin, F.; De Bem, T.H.; Pereira, F.T.V.; Russo-Carbolante, E.M.; Alves, D.; Strauss, B.; Bajgelman, M.; Krieger, J.E.; et al. Improved production of genetically modified fetuses with homogeneous transgene expression after transgene integration site analysis and recloning in cattle. *Cell. Reprogram.* **2011**, *13*, 29–36. [CrossRef]
38. Pan, S.; Chen, W.; Liu, X.; Xiao, J.; Wang, Y.; Liu, J.; Du, Y.; Wang, Y.; Zhang, Y. Application of a Novel Population of Multipotent Stem Cells Derived from Skin Fibroblasts as Donor Cells in Bovine SCNT. *PLoS ONE* **2015**, *10*, e0114423. [CrossRef]
39. Rodríguez-Alvarez, L.; Manriquez, J.; Velasquez, A.; Castro, F.O. Constitutive Expression of the Embryonic Stem Cell Marker OCT4 in Bovine Somatic Donor Cells Influences Blastocysts Rate and Quality after Nucleus Transfer. *Vitro Cell. Dev. Biol.-Anim.* **2013**, *49*, 657–667. [CrossRef]
40. Ruvinsky, A. Basics of Gametic Imprinting. *J. Anim. Sci.* **1999**, *77* (Suppl. S2), 228–237. [CrossRef]
41. Reik, W.; Dean, W.; Walter, J. Epigenetic Reprogramming in Mammalian Development. *Science* **2001**, *293*, 1089–1093. [CrossRef] [PubMed]
42. Urdinguio, R.G.; Sanchez-Mut, J.V.; Esteller, M. Epigenetic Mechanisms in Neurological Diseases: Genes, Syndromes, and Therapies. *Lancet Neurol.* **2009**, *8*, 1056–1072. [CrossRef] [PubMed]
43. Yamaguchi, S.; Hirano, K.; Nagata, S.; Tada, T. Sox2 Expression Effects on Direct Reprogramming Efficiency as Determined by Alternative Somatic Cell Fate. *Stem Cell Res.* **2011**, *6*, 177–186. [CrossRef] [PubMed]

Disclaimer/Publisher's Note: The statements, opinions and data contained in all publications are solely those of the individual author(s) and contributor(s) and not of MDPI and/or the editor(s). MDPI and/or the editor(s) disclaim responsibility for any injury to people or property resulting from any ideas, methods, instructions or products referred to in the content.

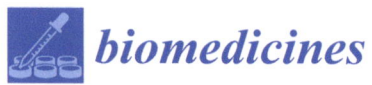

Review

Progress and Prospects of Gene Editing in Pluripotent Stem Cells

Zhenwu Zhang, Xinyu Bao and Chao-Po Lin *

School of Life Science and Technology, ShanghaiTech University, Shanghai 201210, China; zhangzhw2@shanghaitech.edu.cn (Z.Z.); baoxy2022@shanghaitech.edu.cn (X.B.)
* Correspondence: linzhb@shanghaitech.edu.cn

Abstract: Applying programmable nucleases in gene editing has greatly shaped current research in basic biology and clinical translation. Gene editing in human pluripotent stem cells (PSCs), including embryonic stem cells (ESCs) and induced pluripotent stem cells (iPSCs), is highly relevant to clinical cell therapy and thus should be examined with particular caution. First, since all mutations in PSCs will be carried to all their progenies, off-target edits of editors will be amplified. Second, due to the hypersensitivity of PSCs to DNA damage, double-strand breaks (DSBs) made by gene editing could lead to low editing efficiency and the enrichment of cell populations with defective genomic safeguards. In this regard, DSB-independent gene editing tools, such as base editors and prime editors, are favored due to their nature to avoid these consequences. With more understanding of the microbial world, new systems, such as Cas-related nucleases, transposons, and recombinases, are also expanding the toolbox for gene editing. In this review, we discuss current applications of programmable nucleases in PSCs for gene editing, the efforts researchers have made to optimize these systems, as well as new tools that can be potentially employed for differentiation modeling and therapeutic applications.

Keywords: pluripotent stem cell; induced pluripotent stem cell; CRISPR-Cas9; base editor; prime editor; gene editing

Citation: Zhang, Z.; Bao, X.; Lin, C.-P. Progress and Prospects of Gene Editing in Pluripotent Stem Cells. *Biomedicines* **2023**, *11*, 2168. https://doi.org/10.3390/biomedicines11082168

Academic Editor: Aline Yen Ling Wang

Received: 30 June 2023
Revised: 16 July 2023
Accepted: 18 July 2023
Published: 1 August 2023

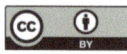

Copyright: © 2023 by the authors. Licensee MDPI, Basel, Switzerland. This article is an open access article distributed under the terms and conditions of the Creative Commons Attribution (CC BY) license (https://creativecommons.org/licenses/by/4.0/).

1. Introduction

Pluripotent stem cells (PSCs) possess two unique characteristics, indefinite self-renewal and the potential to differentiate into nearly all cell types of three germ layers, therefore holding great promise for regenerative medicine. The two major types of PSCs are embryonic stem cells (ESCs) derived from the inner cell mass of the preimplantation embryo [1] and induced pluripotent stem cells (iPSCs) generated by reprogramming of somatic cells [2,3]. With technical advances in the past decade, human iPSCs can now be generated by RNA viruses, episomal vectors, or chemical cocktails, avoiding genomic integrations [4–9]. Compared with human ESCs, iPSCs are generated from autologous cells and are easier to obtain, enabling iPSCs to be applied in cell-based therapies [10–12]. For example, mutations of patient-derived iPSCs can be corrected and differentiated towards specific cell types for therapeutic purposes [13,14]. For cancer immunotherapy, autologous or immune-compatible iPSCs can be modified (e.g., introducing chimeric antigen receptors) and serve as unlimited, "off-the-shelf" sources of engineered immune cells [15,16].

In addition to clinical purposes, PSCs also possess great value in basic research [17]. PSCs are long-standing models for investigating determinants or modulators of lineage specification or terminal differentiation. The advent of organoid cultures further expanded PSC applications [18,19]. Organoids are self-organized cell aggregates that recapitulate cellular compositions and organizations of corresponding tissues, and have been widely employed as in vitro models to study tissue development or diseases [20–24]. PSC-based in vitro differentiation models in 2D and 3D conditions are also platforms for high-throughput screening [25,26] or lineage tracing [27,28], serving as precious tools for studying human-specific development or diseases lacking appropriate mouse models (Figure 1).

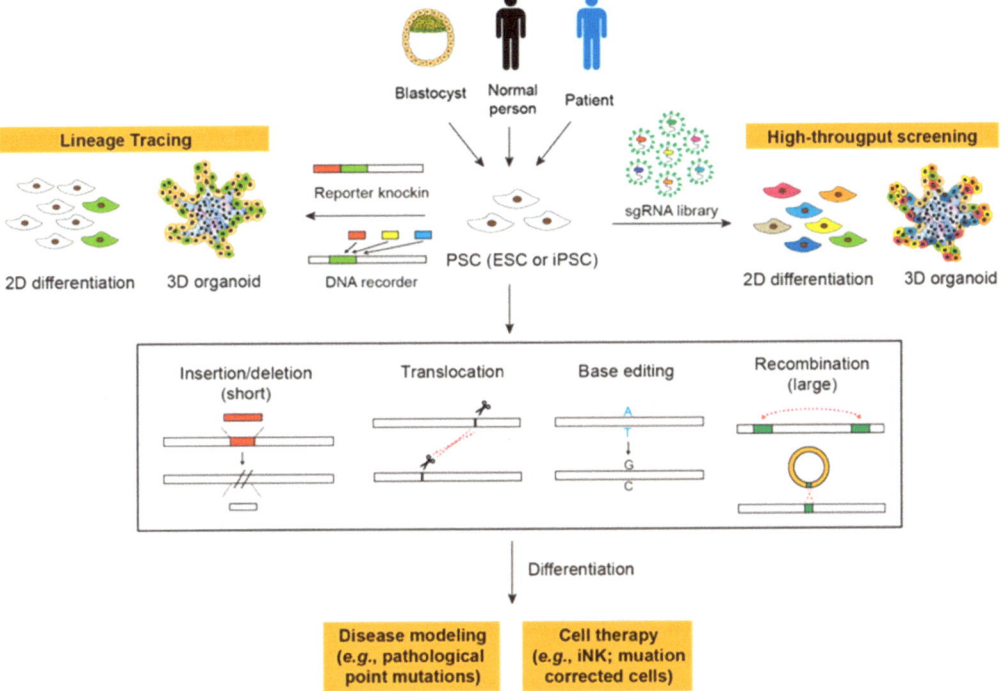

Figure 1. Gene editing in PSC-based basic research and clinical applications. ESC, embryonic stem cell; iPSC, induced pluripotent stem cell; iNK, iPSC-derived NK cells. See the text for details.

Many of those aforementioned applications require gene editing in PSCs. A major merit of performing gene editing in PSCs is the high stability in both the genome and the cell fate potential. Thus, the integrity of the genome of engineered PSCs can be thoroughly examined before any application. Recently, the ability to edit the genome of PSCs has been greatly elevated with the development of gene editing tools, especially programmable nucleases. The ease of use and the high editing efficiency of programmable nucleases greatly facilitate the applications of PSCs in basic research, such as knock-out/knock-in, disease modeling, and correction of genetic mutations [29–31]. Nonetheless, gene editing in PSCs also requires careful evaluation due to their spectacular properties: comparing with adult (stem) cells which have limited longevity, PSCs can propagate almost indefinitely and pass all mutations to their progenies, making the preciseness of gene editing in PSCs of great concern. This concern is further exacerbated with recent studies demonstrating that gene editing mediated by CRISPR associated protein 9 (Cas9)-induced DNA cleavage in human PSCs produces genome-wide mutations and rearrangements [32,33]. Moreover, the selection of successfully edited PSC clones also favors the accumulation of p53 mutations, hampering further utilization of this powerful technology in human PSCs [33,34]. Here, we review the current progress and prospects of gene editing, which we define as inducing permanent changes on DNA sequences, in PSCs and the efforts researchers have made to optimize those tools (Table 1).

Table 1. Multifaceted comparison of gene editing tools.

	DSB-Dependent Editor			Base Editor					Prime Editor
	ZFN	TALEN	SpCas9	CBE	ABE	CGBE	AXBE/AYBE		
Type of DNA damage	DSB	DSB	DSB	SSB	SSB	SSB	SSB		SSB (PE2) or DSB (PE3)
Type of editing	Indel; Knock-in; Base mutation /correction	Indel; Knock-in; Base mutation /correction	Indel; Knock-in; Translocation; Base mutation /correction	Base substitution	Base substitution	Base substitution	Base substitution;		Base substitution; Indel; Recombination
p53 activation?	Yes	Yes	Yes	No	No	N/A	N/A		No
On-target specificity	+	+	++	++	+++	++	+ (C/T mix)		+++
Off-target effects on DNA	++	++	++	++	Very low	++ (based on CBE)	Very low (based on ABE)		Low
Off-target effects on RNA	-	-	-	++	+	++ (based on CBE)	+ (based on ABE)		-
Applied in human PSCs?	Yes	Yes	Yes	Yes	Yes	No	No		Yes
Clinical trial?	Yes	Yes	Yes	Yes	Yes	No	No		No

2. DSB-Mediated Gene Editing by Programmable Nucleases

Since late 1980, homologous recombination (HR) has been widely employed for genome editing in mouse ESCs to create genetically modified mice, establishing a paradigm for studying gene functions, disease mechanisms, and lineage specifications [35]. In a general protocol, donor DNAs with homologous arms are electroporated to mouse ESCs, and the HR-mediated editing (knock-out or knock-in) occurs spontaneously at very low frequencies [36]. This laborious and time-consuming procedure was changed by groundbreaking works of the Haber and Jasin groups, demonstrating that the induction of double-strand breaks (DSBs) by endonucleases at sites aimed to be edited could trigger DNA repair pathways and dramatically increase the efficiencies of HR in yeasts and mammalian cells [37,38]. On the other hand, repair of DSBs by non-homologues end joining (NHEJ) can generate insertions/deletions (indels), ablating the protein expression or function. These findings inspired researchers to look for programmable nucleases that can induce DSBs at desired sites. To date, zinc finger nucleases (ZFNs), transcription activator-like effector nucleases (TALENs), and CRISPR-Cas systems are the most frequently employed methods.

Different cells exhibit distinct sensitivities to DSBs. PSCs, as derived from early embryos, have evolved at least two mechanisms to keep low DNA mutation rates compared to somatic cells, thus protecting the genome integrity from the accumulation of genetic mutations. First, PSCs possess a superior ability to repair DNA damages by expressing abundant mismatch repair proteins or avoiding error-prone repair pathways [39–42]. The high DNA repair capability also suggests the fast removal of the DSB marker γ-H2AX, thus antagonizing its association with apoptosis-inducing factor (AIF) for the formation of the "degradosome" that leads to chromatin remodeling and large-scale DNA fragmentation [43,44]. Second, once the level of DNA damage accumulates over a threshold, PSCs are highly prone to apoptosis, eliminating themselves from the whole population. Those self-protection mechanisms of PSCs are double-edged swords for applying those powerful DSB-dependent gene editing tools in PSCs, since the sensitivity of PSCs toward DNA damages could lead to the low editing efficiency or undesired loss/mutation of genomic safeguards [32,33].

Here, we briefly review those three DSB-dependent programmable nucleases and their off-target effects in the context of PSCs, as their development and mechanisms have been extensively reviewed [30,45–49].

2.1. Zinc-Finger Nuclease (ZFN)

Zinc-finger nucleases (ZFNs) are artificially engineered endonucleases that recognize specific DNA sequences by customized zinc-finger protein arrays [50,51]. The zinc finger domain of a ZFN, which binds to a specific DNA sequence, is fused with the FokI nuclease. With a pair of ZFNs binding to target sites of genome DNA in the opposite orientation, FokI will be dimerized and produce DNA DSBs that strongly activate the DNA repair pathway and greatly increase gene editing efficiencies compared with the natural recombination rate in the absence of DNA breaks. NHEJ or homology-directed repair (HDR) of these DSBs will lead to random indels or sequence replacement, which can be utilized for gene knock-out or knock-in, respectively [52]. Recently, new dimer architectures, made possible by different linkers between zinc finger proteins and FokI, were successfully developed and greatly increased the design flexibility [53]. Currently, several ZFN-based gene- and cell-therapies developed by Sangamo Therapeutics are under clinical trials.

ZFNs-mediated genetic manipulation in human PSCs was first reported in 2007. The ZFN and the donor DNA were delivered to human ESCs by lentiviruses to knock-in a green fluorescent protein (GFP)-expressing cassette to the end of the *CCR5* gene through HDR with a 5.3% efficiency [54]. ZFN was also used to disrupt the *PIG-A* gene in human ESCs and iPSCs [55]. Hockemeyer et al. used ZFNs to tag *EGFP* to *PITX3* or insert *EGFP* to the safe harbor locus, *AAVS1*, to generate reporter or drug-inducible cell lines in human ESCs [56]. These pioneer studies demonstrated the superior efficiencies of DSB-activated recombination in PSCs.

On- and Off-Targeting of ZFNs

With the high genome editing efficiency, the specificity of the programmable nucleases also came into view. The on-target efficiency of nucleases can be examined by Sanger/high-throughput sequencing or mismatch-sensitive enzymes such as T7 endonuclease I (T7E1) [57,58]. Nonetheless, the evaluation of off-target effects is not as trivial as it appears to be: high-throughput transcriptomic sequencing (RNA-seq) is able to detect mutations on coding and non-coding genes with good coverage, yet can neither determine whether mutations happen on DNA or RNA, nor reveal gene duplications, chromosome translocations, and mutations in regulatory regions [59]. The whole-genome/exome sequencing (WGS/WES) has been applied to examine the ZFN-mediated correction of a point mutation on the *A1AT* site in human iPSCs [60]. Nonetheless, although the WGS is a reliable way to measure off-target edits in single cell-derived colonies, it is not suitable for measuring the rate of off-target editing at the population level, as the mutation frequencies at off-target sites are too low to be detected by typical sequencing depth.

To resolve these issues, other methods have been developed to enhance the sensitivity of off-target measurement in an unbiased, genome-wide manner. For example, the in vitro selection and the integrase-deficient lentivirus (IDLV) capture were developed to examine the ZFN cleavage sites [61]. The former uses DNA substrate libraries to determine the specificity of nucleases in vitro [61], while the latter uses IDLV to integrate at cleavage sites and detect off-target edits in cells [62]. Both methods were employed to examine the off-target effects of a *CCR5*-targeting ZFN and uncovered a previously known off-target site, *CCR2* [61–64]. In addition to the *CCR2* site, in vitro selection also identified large numbers of off-targets from the substrate library, some of which can be identified in cells [61]. Together, these studies suggest that the off-target effects of ZFNs should be meticulously evaluated. As various methods have been developed for measuring CRISPR-Cas9 off-targets (see later), the specificity of ZFNs can be systematically addressed.

2.2. Transcription Activator-like Effector Nucleases (TALENs)

The transcription activator-like effector nuclease (TALEN) is composed of the DNA binding domain and the DNA cutting domain [65,66]. The DNA binding domain, derived from the transcription activator-like effector (TALE) protein in the *Flavobacterium*, contains multiple tandem repeats of 33–34 amino acids with divergent dual residues at positions 12 and 13 (repeat variable di-residue, or RVD), which determine TALE's binding specificity. The DNA cutting domain is the cleavage domain of FokI endonuclease. Thus, both ZFNs and TALENs can be viewed as FokI endonucleases targeted by engineered proteins that recognize specific DNA sequences. Similar to ZFNs, TALENs were also introduced into cells for genome editing, making knock-out, knock-in, and site-specific mutations [66,67]. One advantage of TALENs for researchers is that all the RVDs and their recognized sequences are open resources, while ZFNs are only available from Sangamo Therapeutics, Richmond, CA, USA. So far, there have been several TALEN-based gene- and cell-therapies under clinical trials [68,69].

In PSCs, TALENs have been used for genome editing in iPSCs generated from dermal fibroblasts in MELAS (myopathy, encephalopathy, lactic acidosis, and stroke-like episodes) patients with mitochondrial G13513A mutation [70]. Moreover, genes associated with human cardiovascular diseases, such as *TNNT2, LMNA/C, TBX5, MYH7, ANKRD1*, and *NKX2.5*, were also knocked-out by TALENs in human iPSCs to build cardiovascular disease models [71]. X-linked chronic granulomatous disease (X-CGD) is an inherited disorder of the immune system caused by mutations in the *GP91PHOX* (*NOX2*) gene that regulates reactive oxygen species (ROS) production [72]. Wild-type *NOX2* was knocked into the *AAVS1* site of X-CGD patient-derived iPSCs, which can be derived to granulocytes exhibiting restored ROS production [72]. TALEN was also used to correct the mutation of beta-globin alleles in sickle cell disease (SCD) patient-derived iPSCs [73]. Together, these results suggest the effectiveness of TALEN-mediated gene editing in PSCs.

The specificities of TALENs were also investigated. In a parallel comparison of the ZFN and TALEN targeting *CCR6*, the TALEN exhibits lower off-target activity at the *CCR2* site [74]. Further study revealed that the ZFN and TALEN have different mutation signatures, as the TALEN induces significantly fewer insertions [75]. Off-target effects of TALENs can be further avoided by carefully choosing target sequences [76]. In PSCs, two studies employed WGS to confirm the off-target effects of TALENs in single-cell derived colonies [77,78]. As aforementioned, off-target rates at the population level of TALENs still await systematic evaluation with the new techniques (see the Section 2.3.1).

2.3. CRISPR-Cas System

Clustered Regularly Interspaced Short Palindromic Repeats (CRISPR)-Cas are bacterial and archaeal adaptive immunity systems that integrate segments of foreign nucleic acids into CRISPR arrays in host genomes [79,80]. Transcripts of these inserted segments (spacers) are employed as guide RNAs (gRNAs) to recognize and interfere with cognate targets (protospacers) [81]. The most important components of CRISPR-Cas systems are CRISPR RNAs (crRNAs) and Cas effectors [46]. With the assistance of crRNAs that recognize protospacer sequences, Cas effectors exhibit nuclease activities toward target DNAs or RNAs [46]. In the CRISPR-Cas9 system, which has been employed extensively in gene editing, another small RNA, the trans-activating crRNA (tracrRNA), is required [58,81,82]. The crRNA and tracrRNA form a double-stranded RNA which recruits the Cas9 protein to form a ribonucleoprotein (RNP) complex for target recognition and cleavage [81,83]. For the application, the crRNA and tracrRNA are further combined to the single-guide RNA (sgRNA) for ease of use [81]. One essential determinant for target recognition is the adjacent protospacer motif (PAM), the short DNA sequence next to protospacers [84]. For example, the PAM sequence for *Streptococcus pyogenes* Cas9 (*Sp*Cas9) is NGG [81]. The DNA cleavage induced by Cas9, like ZFNs or TALENs, triggers NHEJ or HDR repair pathways depending on the absence or presence of DNA templates, respectively, and results in indels or HR products. Thus, different from ZFNs or TALENs which recognize DNA targets by the protein–DNA interaction, the CRISPR-Cas systems utilize the nucleic acid base pairing as the mechanism to recognize their targets (DNA or RNA), greatly simplifying their design and application.

There are two distinct nuclease domains, HNH and RuvC, in Cas9, which cleave the target and non-target stand, respectively [81,83]. Inactivation of either HNH or RuvC domain creates the Cas9 nickase (nCas9), which can cleave only one DNA strand. If both HNH and RuvC domains are inactivated, the enzymatically dead Cas9, dCas9, could serve as a scaffold for recruiting effectors to the desired site without making DNA breaks. Depending on the factors fused with, dCas9 can be used for activating (CRISPRa) or suppressing (CRISPRi) gene expression, epigenetic modification (e.g., DNA methylation or histone modifications), or molecular imaging [85–87]. Although epigenetic regulations play key roles in PSC functions, applications excellently reviewed elsewhere are omitted in the present review due to the space limitation and the absence of permanent alterations of DNA sequences induced by these variants.

Except for Cas9, other Cas proteins, such as Cas3, Cas10, Cas12, Cas13, and Cas14, are also employed for other purposes based on their properties and substrates. For example, Cas3 and Cas10 cleave ssDNAs [88,89], Cas12 (including *As*Cas12a and *Lb*Cas12b from *Acidaminococcus* and *Lachnospiraceae* bacterium, respectively) cleaves both dsDNAs and ssDNAs [90], and Cas13 (including Cas13a and Cas13b) cleaves ssRNAs [91]. The diversity of the CRISPR-Cas system greatly expands the application repertoire, which is reviewed elsewhere [92]. Here, we focus on the utilization and off-target effects of the CRISPR-Cas9 system in human PSCs.

The CRISPR-Cas9 system has been extensively applied in human PSCs, although its off-target and side effects on genome integrity have not been extensively investigated yet. In addition to knocking out and knocking in specific genes, CRISPR-Cas9 has been employed for high-throughput screening using sgRNA libraries, which is less feasible for ZFNs or TALENs [93–95] (Figure 1). To build PSC-derived disease models, CRISPR-Cas9 usually performs genome engineering at the pluripotent stage, followed by differentiating PSCs into the desired cells/organoids. For example, CRISPR-Cas9 was applied to introduce *RBM20* mutations in human iPSCs, which were differentiated into cardiomyocytes to establish an in vitro model of dilated cardiomyopathy (DCM) [96]. CRISPR-Cas9 can also introduce inter-chromosome translocations to model blood cancers [97] (Figure 1). In addition to modeling disease, CRISPR-Cas9 was used to reverse disease mutations as exemplified by the correction of a diabetes-causing pathogenic mutant of *Wolfram syndrome 1* (*WFS1*) gene in iPSCs derived from a Wolfram syndrome (WS) patient. After transplantation, the genetically-corrected WS iPSC-derived β cells can reverse severe diabetes in mice [98].

Apart from 2D differentiation, human PSCs are also employed to build disease models or perform lineage tracing in organoids (Figure 1). Multiple organoids, including the brain, liver, retina, lung, blood vessels, heart, and kidney, have been generated from human PSCs [99–104]. For example, CRISPR-Cas9-mediated knockout of *PKD1* or *PKD2* in human ESC-derived kidney organoids can model polycystic kidney disease [105]. CRISPR-Cas9-mediated introduction of oncogenic mutations in human ESCs, which are then differentiated to cerebral organoids, can serve as a model to recapitulate brain tumorigenesis [106]. The introduction of the E50K mutation in optineurin (*OPTN*) by CRISPR-Cas9 has also been used to model glaucoma in ESC-derived retinal organoids [107]. To track hair cell induction during human inner ear organogenesis, CRISPR-Cas9 was used to construct *ATOH1* reporters in human ESCs, which are differentiated into inner cell organoids [108]. Recently, CRISPR-Cas systems have also served as DNA recorders and writers to trace sequential events during differentiation (see Conclusion and Future Prospects). Together, these results indicate the versatility of the CRISPR-Cas system in PSC applications (Figure 1).

CRISPR-Cas9-mediated gene editing has also been proposed for clinical cell therapies using human PSCs. For instance, cytokine-inducible SH2-containing protein (CISH) is a key negative regulator of interleukin-15 (IL-15) signaling in natural killer (NK) cells. Knockout of *CISH* in human iPSC-derived NK (iNK) cells by CRISPR-Cas9 improves their expansion capability, cytotoxic activity, and in vivo persistence to inhibit tumor progression in the leukemia xenograft model [109]. Knocking out the ectoenzyme *CD38* by CRISPR-Cas9 also improves in vivo persistence and antitumor activity of iPSC-derived NK cells in the absence of exogenous cytokine and elicits superior antitumor activity [110]. Thus, human PSCs could be a potentially unlimited, stable source of engineered "off-the-shelf" immune cells for cancer therapy (Figure 1).

2.3.1. Evaluating Off-Target Effects of CRISPR-Cas9

As mentioned above, advanced methods have been developed to examine the off-target effects of programmable nucleases, especially CRISPR-Cas9. For example, Digenome-seq (digested genome sequencing), GUIDE-seq (genome-wide, unbiased identification of DSBs enabled by sequencing), HTGTS (the high-throughput genomic translocation sequencing), and BLESS (labeling, enrichments on streptavidin, and next-generation sequencing) can all identify DSBs generated by Cas9 in vitro or in vivo (reviewed in [111]). A parallel comparison between the ZFN, TALEN, and Cas9 targeting the same site demonstrated that Cas9 is more efficient and specific than the other two, although whether it is universal for other target sites remains to be determined [112]. Despite its superior specificity, genome-wide analyses have shown that Cas9, like other programmable nucleases, can recognize and cleave DNA at off-target sites with sequences resembling on-target sites [113–115]. Employing a pair of nCas9 to create two single-strand breaks instead of one DSB can reduce the off-target rates, although it also compromises the editing efficiency [116]. Compared with other programmable endonucleases, the specificity of CRISPR-Cas9 can be and has been further improved by engineering Cas9 proteins. Mutations of the residues in Cas9 which are involved in Cas9-DNA interaction can reduce the binding of Cas9 at off-target sites, while the binding and editing ability at on-target sites are largely retained [117–119]. Modifications on the sgRNA, such as adjusting the length of the spacer region or adding secondary structures onto the 5′ ends of a sgRNA, also reduce off-target effects [113,120,121].

3. Base Editors

Since DSB-mediated editing raises concerns for undesired mutations in PSCs, base editors, which make base substitutions without introducing DSBs, are reasonably favored for gene editing in PSCs. Theoretically, six base editors will be needed for "any base to any base" substitutions (please refer to Chen et al. [125] for the illustration). Yet, pathogenic point mutations in humans are not evenly distributed (also Chen et al. [125] for the statistics), making it possible to cover most human diseases with fewer editors. The first two base editors reported, the cytidine base editor (CBE) and the adenine base editor (ABE), were realized by David Liu's lab in 2016 and 2017, respectively [112,122]. CBE converts cytidines to thymines on one strand and thus can be used to create both C>T (C•T→T•A) and G>A (G•C→A•T) substitutions. Similarly, ABE substitutes adenines with guanines and thus can make both A>G (A•T→G•A) and T>C (T•A→C•G) substitutions. Those four types of editing cover ~60% of edits needed for correcting pathogenic mutations [125]. In 2020, two labs reported the glycosylase base editor that can make C>G and G>C conversions, which constitute ~10% of pathological mutations [123,124]. Recently, new editors were reported to be able to convert A to C or T [125,126], covering another ~25% of pathological mutations. In addition to these single-base editors, dual-base editors, which fuse two types of single-base editors, were also created to introduce multiple substitutions [127–130]. Together, these base editors constitute a tool collection for introducing or correcting point mutations in somatic or stem cells. In this section, we briefly review these single-base editors and discuss their strengths and remaining issues in PSC-based applications.

3.1. Cytidine Base Editor (CBE)

CBEs take advantage of the cytidine deaminase activity, which converts cytidines to uracils (U), equivalent to T in base pairing, for base substitution. The rat APOBEC1 (apolipoprotein B mRNA editing enzyme, catalytic polypeptide-like 1, or rAPOBEC1) and the sea lamprey AID (activation-induced cytidine deaminase) were first employed in the BE series [131] and Target-AID [132], respectively. Cytidine deaminases from different species, including the CDA, AID, and APOBEC3 family, are also employed to build CBEs with different editing efficiencies and sequence preferences [133]. BE3 and BE4 are the third and fourth generation of BE, containing nCas9, rAPOBEC1, as well as one (BE3) or two (BE4) copies of uracil DNA glycosylase inhibitor (UGI) from the *Bacillus subtilis* bacteriophage [131] (Figure 2a). UGI can suppress the repair of U by inhibiting the uracil DNA glycosylase (UNG), which excises uracil bases to form abasic sites for base excision repair (BER). To date, more than thirty CBE variants have been made by changing the editing window, expanding the PAM compatibility, or increasing/decreasing their on-target/off-target activities [134]. Notably, despite its successful application in multiple cell lines, BE3 exhibits lower editing efficiency in human PSCs [135] and may need further optimization for better efficiency [136] (see the Section 3.5.2).

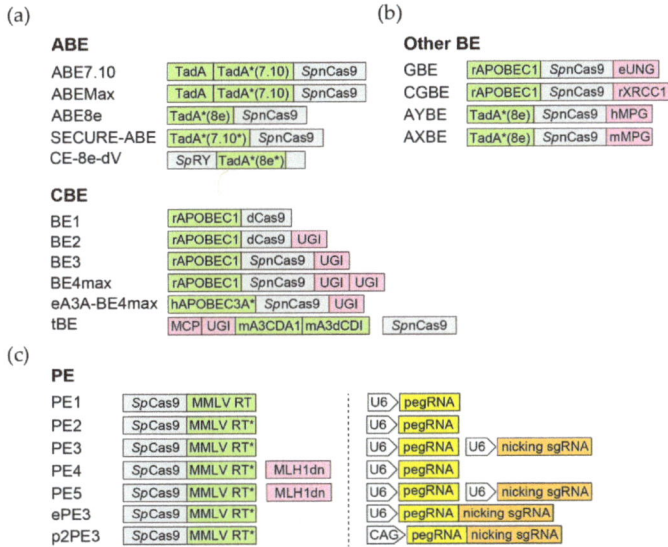

Figure 2. Base editors and prime editors. Representative versions of base editors and prime editors. The Cas9 derivatives are highlighted in grey, the key enzymatic components of BEs (**a**,**b**) and PEs (**c**) are highlighted in green, and the associated components are highlighted in pink. For PEs, the archi-tectures of promoters, pegRNAs (yellow), and nicking sgRNAs (orange) are also shown. The CAG promoter of p2PE3 can be replaced by other Pol II promoters.

3.2. Adenine Base Editor (ABE)

In 2017, David Liu's lab reported the first ABE, which realized the A>G and T>C substitutions [122]. Theoretically, deamination of adenosines results in inosines (I), which could complement with cytidines and be eventually converted to guanines by the mismatch repair. However, there are no known DNA adenine deaminases. To solve this issue, Gaudelli et al. subjected the *E. coli* tRNA adenine deaminase TadA to extensive evolution to alter its activity towards DNA [122]. ABE7.10, which contains a wild-type TadA and an evolved TadA* (contains 14 amino acid substitutions in the catalytic domain), was finally retrieved with the highest efficiency of converting A•T to G•C [122]. This breakthrough opens the gate for the subsequent derivation of ABE variants with improved nuclear localization/expression (ABEmax) [137] or smaller size and faster editing kinetics (ABE8e) [138]. Recently, several groups, including us, modified those ABEs to further reduce their off-targeting activities [139–141] or expand the PAM compatibility [142,143] (Figure 2a). Notably, compared with CBE, ABE exhibits high product purity and low rates of indels in mammalian cells, including human PSCs, possibly due to their lack of efficient glycosylase to initiate BER [122].

3.3. Glycosylase Base Editor (GBE) and C-to-G Base Editor (CGBE)

In 2020, three research groups reported base editors that can make C>G and G>C base transversions (purine > pyrimidine or pyrimidine > purine) in mammalian cells [123,124,135] (Figure 2b). All three base editors employ nCas9 and rAPOBEC1 (the same one CBE uses), while two of them (Kurt et al. [GBE] and Zhao et al. [CGBE]) replace the UGI with UNG and Chen et al. use XRCC1 protein instead of UGI. The UNG excises the U base created by the deaminase and generates the apurinic/apyrimidinic (AP) site that, in combination with the nick made by nCas9, initiates the DNA repair process (translesion synthesis) which favors insertion of G at the AP site. The C-to-G BE designed by Chen et al. uses XRCC1 to recruit BER proteins to repair the AP site created by endogenous UNG [135]. GBE and CGBE are further modified or optimized to relieve the PAM restriction, as well as to be more predictable and purer [144,145]. Recently, the Li lab reported a TadA-derived C-to-G base editor, Td-CGBE, which is based on an N46L variant of TadA-8e [146].

3.4. Adenine Transversion Editors (AYBE and AXBE)

As mentioned above, the A>C substitution is required to reverse ~25% pathological point mutations. Recently, two breakthrough studies reported base editors that can transverse A to C or T in mammalian cells [125,126] (Figure 2b). Both groups employ a strategy similar to GBE/CGBE, but aim at creating the AP site on A instead of C (in the GBE/CGBE case), which is expected to be mutagenized by the DNA repair pathway. To achieve this, Tong et al. constructed the adenine transverse base editor (AYBE, Y = C or T) by fusing the ABE8e with an engineered human hypoxanthine glycosylase enzyme, N-methylpurine DNA glycosylase (MPG, also called AAG). MPG excises the hypoxanthine group from the inosine produced by ABE, resulting in an AP site. The AP site will then be processed by the translesion synthesis pathway and replaced by C or T as the most common outcomes [126]. Chen et al. employed a similar strategy but used mouse AAG (MPG) instead of the human one, creating the AXBE. Importantly, by mutagenesis and Cas embedding strategies, Chen et al. further created the ACBE-Q editor, which exhibited high A>C activity and reduced A>G bystander substitutions [125]. Although the purity and efficiency of adenine transversion editors remain to be improved, these two editors have substantially expanded the potential of base editing.

3.5. Pros and Cons of Using Base Editors in PSCs

Although base editors cannot introduce indels or HR, they still possess wide applications in correcting point mutations, creating premature stop codons (knockout), and alternating splicing events. In contrast to DSB-dependent genome editing, base editors are considerably favored since most of them use nCas9, which only generates nicks. This advantage is particularly important for PSCs, in which the activation of p53-dependent DNA damage responses leads to detrimental consequences [33]. However, the deaminases may lead to undesired off-target edits on RNA or DNA in PSCs. Since off-target mutations on RNA could cause undesired phenotypes, and mutations on DNA will be transferred to all differentiated progenies, the off-target issue is one of the major concerns for applying base editors in PSCs. Here, we summarize the current knowledge on the off-target effects of base editors and the efforts researchers have made to resolve this issue.

3.5.1. Dealing with Off-Target Effects of CBE and ABE

The rAPOBEC1 used by the BE series has off-target activities towards both DNA and RNA. Expressing BE3 in mouse embryos resulted in substantial off-target DNA single-nucleotide variants (SNVs) with more than 20-fold higher frequencies compared to CRISPR-Cas9 or ABE [147]. Most of the appeared mutations are independent of sgRNAs, suggesting that these off-target edits are attributed to the random, Cas9-independent binding of rAPOBEC1 to DNA [147]. A cohort study of BE3 transgenic mice also revealed five times more SNVs in the muscle tissue compared with the GFP control [148]. In contrast, ABE transgenic mice show barely detectable off-target DNA SNVs. The higher genome-wide off-target mutation rate of CBE over ABE is also observed in plants [149]. Although the off-target activity of the cytidine deaminase employed by the Target-AID system, pmCDA1, has not been evaluated by WGS, the R-loop assay on specific sites also suggests a high off-target activity on DNA [150]. Together, these results draw the attention to off-target DNA mutations generated by cytidine deaminases.

The off-target DNA activities of CBE and ABE in PSCs were also evaluated. In a well-controlled experiment, BE4 was tested for its off-target activities using syngeneic human iPSC clones with doxycycline-inducible CBE [151]. The WGS revealed that BE4 induces 10 times more SNVs compared with the control in human iPSCs. We also examined the off-target effects of overexpressed enhanced ABE (CE-8e-dV) in human ESC clones with a similar approach and did not observe mutations beyond the background level [143]. These results confirm that early version CBEs exhibit higher off-target rates on DNA compared with ABE in PSCs. Notably, we only uncovered a few (<50) differentially expressed genes upon CE-8e-dV overexpression, and no activation of the p53 signaling pathway was observed, further indicating the safety of ABE in PSCs [143].

The off-target activity on RNA is an even more important issue for rAPOBEC1-based CBE. Grünewald et al. performed RNA-seq and WGS on BE3-overexpressed human cells. On the transcriptome-wide scale, they uncovered tens of thousands of C>U edits with frequencies ranging from 0.07–100% in 38–58% of expressed genes, which resulted in missense, nonsense, splice site, 5′ UTR, and 3′ UTR mutations [152]. The parallel WGS confirmed that most of those RNA mutations are not originated from DNA [152]. In contrast to the nature of rAPOBEC1 that targets both DNA and RNA, DNA is likely the only natural substrate for AID [153]. For ABE, despite its minimal off-target DNA editing activity, researchers also found ABE generates lower but evident A>I editing in cellular RNAs, possibly due to the deaminase activity of TadA/TadA* towards RNA [140]. Our study in human ESCs also revealed RNA off-target activity of ABE8e [143]. Together, these results suggest diverse influences on the transcriptome by CBE and ABE in PSCs.

Many efforts have been made to resolve the off-target issue of CBE and ABE. For CBE, mutations were introduced to cytidine deaminases to segregate its activity towards DNA and RNA. For example, the Joung group engineered two SECURE-bEs by introducing R33A or R33A/K34A to rAPOBEC1, which greatly reduces the C>U editing on RNA while maintaining the on-target efficiency on DNA [152]. They also replaced rAPOBEC1 with an engineered human APOBEC3A (hA3A) domain in the BE3 system, which can perform base editing in the CpG context with low off-target rates [154]. The Liu and Yang groups found that W90Y/R126E mutations in rAPOBEC1 (YE1) greatly reduce the off-target activity of BE3 on DNA and RNA [155–157]. Wang et al. constructed a transformer BE (tBE) system by fusing a cleavable deoxycytidine deaminase inhibitor (dCDI) domain to cytidine deaminases, resulting in efficient editing with only a background level of off-target mutations in the whole transcriptome and the genome [158] (Figure 2a). Recently, three groups reported TadCBE, CBE-T, and Td-CBE, all of which use engineered/evolved TadA (the ABE component) to perform cytidine deamination with the advantages of high on-target activities, smaller sizes, and substantially lower DNA and RNA off-target activities [146,159,160].

Similar to CBEs, ABEs were also engineered for better on- and off-target performance on both DNA and RNA. Liu and other groups employed different strategies to further reduce off-target mutations induced by adenosine deaminases, including the point mutation V106W [140,161], deletion of the key residue R153 [162], and embedding the editing enzymes into the middle of nCas9 to hamper their access to off-targets [139]. We combined those three strategies to make a new ABE, CE-8e-dV, and tested its performance in human ESCs [143]. By WGS and RNA-seq analyses, we confirmed that CE-8e-dV exhibits background-level DNA off-target effects and only ~1/3 off-target RNA edits compared with

ABE8e [139]. Chen et al. reported that introducing the L145T mutation to ABE8e (ABE9) could further decrease its editing window and bystander editing [163]. Finally, mutagenesis-based engineering also enables researchers to create ABE9e (R111T/N127K/Q154R), which has a significantly lower bystander mutation rate in human ESCs [164].

3.5.2. On- and Off-Targets of Other Base Editors in PSCs

GBE, CGBE, AYBE, and AXBE are newly developed base editors. The efficiency of CGBE has been examined in human H9 ESCs: both CGBE and BE3 exhibit low editing efficiency in H9 cells, which might be due to specific methylation profiles in stem cells that inhibit editing [135]. Although AXBE has been employed in mice and human cells [125], its activity in human PSCs remains to be evaluated since linking hAAG to ABEmax or ABE8e (same as the AYBE design) does not result in A>Y transversion in PSCs [165]. In the aggregate, the on-target efficiencies of C>G and A>Y editors in human PSCs still await examination by transcriptome- and genome-wide analysis. Finally, overexpression of some components of editors, such as XRCC1 or MPG, could also have unexpected influences on PSCs and needs to be addressed.

4. Prime Editor (PE)

In 2019, a versatile gene-editing tool, prime editor (PE), was developed by the Liu lab [166,167]. The two essential components of the PE system are the editor, a nCas9 fused with reverse transcriptase (RT), and a single engineered prime editing guide RNA (pegRNA) which consists of the sgRNA and the intended sequence to edit. After being guided to the target site by the sgRNA component of the pegRNA, the nCas9 generates a nick in the single-stranded R-loop of the target site. The pegRNA then hybridizes with the nicked target DNA strand and serves as the template for RT to polymerize the desired sequence onto the nicked target DNA. After resolving the flap of the edited DNA by DNA repair machinery, the desired sequence will be incorporated into the genome. Decided by the templates, PE can make all types of base substitutions or insertions/deletions of small DNA fragments in mammalian cells [166,167].

PEs have evolved through multiple versions (Figure 2c). The original version of prime editor (PE1) uses the wild-type RT from Moloney murine leukemia virus (MMLV) [166]. Although PE1 can make all gene edits in human cells, the gene editing efficiency is low, typically <5% [166]. In PE2, five mutations are introduced to MMLV-RT to enhance its thermostability, processivity, and binding affinity to the template. The gene editing efficiency of PE2 is increased 1.6- to 5.1-fold compared to PE1 in human cells [166]. On the basis of PE2, PE3 includes an additional sgRNA to direct the nCas9 component of the prime editor to also nick the non-edited strand, promoting the replacement of the non-edited strand with the sequence complementary to the edited DNA [166]. The gene editing efficiency of PE3 is further increased 1.5- to 4.2-fold compared to PE2 in HEK293T cells [166]. PE4 and PE5 prime editing systems are developed by the transient expression of an engineered mismatch repair (MMR)-inhibiting protein, MLH1dn, with PE2 and PE3, respectively. The rationale behind this design is that the MMR was found to strongly antagonize prime editing and promote the generation of undesired indel byproducts [168]. Compared with PE2 and PE3 systems, PE4 and PE5 prime editing systems enhance the editing efficiency by an average of 7.7- and 2.0-fold, respectively [168]. PEmax, which contains R221K/N394K mutations in Cas9, two NLS (nuclear localization signal) tags, and a codon-optimized MMLV-RT, exhibits further elevated editing efficacy [168]. Finally, replacing the nCas9 with the DSB-making Cas9 also significantly enhances the editing efficiency [169–172]. Notably, since DSBs are made by late versions of PE (since PE3), their side effects need to be determined, particularly in PSCs.

The PE system was also modified or optimized by researchers from the perspectives of editors or pegRNAs. The modification on editors is mostly by fusing with other proteins to enhance the editor's performance. In the hyPE2 design, the Rad51 DNA-binding domain is inserted between nCas9 and RT to facilitate reverse transcription [173]. Fusion of the chromatin-modulating peptide to PE3 (CMP-PE3) or a DNA repair-related peptide to PE2 (IN-PE2) can significantly increase the editing efficiency in mammalian cells [174,175]. On the other hand, the pegRNA design is optimized by various rationales. The pegRNA contains a primer binding site (PBS) sequence to trigger the reverse transcription, whose length greatly affects the editing efficiency [176]. Several algorithms or approaches were developed to optimize the PBS length or the pegRNA sequence [177–183]. Modifying the pegRNA by stabilizing its secondary structure or preventing its circularization also enhances the editing efficiency [176,183–186].

The efficiencies of PEs vary widely, depending on the genomic context, the pegRNA design, and the cell type. In our work, PE editing efficiencies on the same sites are consistently lower in PSCs compared with immortalized cells, such as HEK293T [187]. The causes of such differences remain unclear. One possibility of the low efficiency could be simply the level of PE/pegRNA expressed in cells (see Conclusion and Future Prospects). The high MMR repair capacity of PSCs could also result in this low editing efficiency, as overexpressing MLH1dn (PE4/5) enhanced the editing efficiency of PE in PSCs [187]. Interestingly, inhibition of p53 by SV40 large T antigen (SV40LT) further increases the editing efficiency, suggesting p53 plays a role in modulating PE-mediated edits [187]. Despite the involvement of p53, our and other researchers' results suggest that PE-editing, in the presence or absence of editing boosters (MLH1dn or SV40LT), does not lead to off-target mutations beyond the background level [187,188].

Although the efficiency remains to be improved, prime editing has been successfully applied for gene editing in human PSCs to induce nucleotide substitutions or small insertions/deletions. Habib et al. used PE to correct a liver disease-related mutation of *SERPINA1* in patient-derived human iPSCs. PE was also used to precisely delete the intronic splicing silencer-N1 (ISS-N1) within survival motor neuron 2 (*SMN2*) to rescue full-length SMN expression in human iPSCs derived from spinal muscular atrophy (SMA) patients [189]. Finally, Li. et al. reported that delivering PE and pegRNA in the mRNA form greatly enhances the editing efficiency on multiple sites, which greatly facilitates applying PEs in human PSCs [190]. However, whether this approach can generally increase the efficiencies of PEs on different target sites remains to be investigated. Finally, compared with the base editors (CBEs or ABEs), PEs exhibit lower efficiency but fewer bystander edits. Importantly, the WGS confirmed that PE does not lead to off-target mutations in the genome in PSCs [188]. Together, these results suggest that PEs are promising editing tools to for PSCs, although their caveats remain to be solved.

5. New Gene Editing Tools

Although DSB-independent editing tools currently used are favored in PSCs, one major restriction of those tools is the inability or low efficiency to insert large DNA fragments. PEs can insert short DNA fragments (<20 nt), yet their efficiencies drop dramatically with the increased length of insertion [187]. This property does not meet the need of many clinical applications (e.g., CAR-iNK), which call for much larger insertions. Currently, several new gene editing tools have been developed for knocking in larger DNA fragments (see Sections 5.1–5.3) or to enrich cell populations containing these insertions (see Section 5.4). Of note, some of these tools are still under development and need improvements for applying in mammalian cells or PSCs.

5.1. CRISPR-Associated Transposon (CAST)

As the name suggests, the CRISPR-associated transposon (CAST) is the transposon containing a specific subtype of CRISPR-Cas systems [191]. Compared with RNA-guided endonucleases that function in the defense against MGE (mobile genetic elements), this specific CRISPR-Cas subtype is employed for RNA-guided transposition [192]. The mechanisms of two types of CASTs, CAST I-F and CAST V-K, were elucidated in prokaryotes [193]. As the recognition–integration process is independent of HDR, transposon-based CRISPR systems hold great expectation for inserting large DNA fragments into specific sites in eukaryotic cells. Recently, a system based on CAST, the HE-assisted large-sequence integrating CAST-complex (HELIX), has been able to insert DNA fragments into exogenous plasmids in human cells [194]. Furthermore, Lampe et al. reported that with the help of bacterial ClpX, Type I-F CAST could reach single-digit efficiencies in human endogenous genes [195]. Despite this success, CAST is still ineffective in editing human endogenous genes, possibly due to the unidentified regulatory factors, components, or features of eukaryotic chromatin. More understanding of structures and mechanisms of CASTs could facilitate their application in eukaryotic cells, even PSCs.

5.2. CRISPR-Associated Serine Recombinases (twinPE and PASTE)

Another strategy to integrate large DNA fragments is using recombinases, which integrate MGE into bacterial genomes on attachment sites, the specific sequences into which the payloads will be inserted. Recently, thousands of large serine recombinases (LSRs) and DNA attachment sites were predicted using computational approaches, and over 60 new LSRs were experimentally validated in human cells [196]. In combination with TwinPE, which exhibits superior ability to insert the landing pad sequence into the desired site, large DNA fragment insertion can be mediated by the site-specific serine recombinase/integrase, Bxb1 [197]. Another approach with a similar concept, PASTE (programmable addition via site-specific targeting elements), uses the PE-Bxb1 fusion protein and the pegRNA containing the attachment sequence (atgRNA for attachment site-containing guide RNA) [198]. Both twinPE and PASTE can insert large DNA fragments ranging from 5.6~36 kb into human immortalized cells or cancer cells, sufficient for most purposes. It will be valuable to test the efficiencies of those tools in PSCs.

5.3. Retron

Retrons are non-transposable retroelements firstly identified in prokaryotes [199]. A typical retron contains a reverse transcriptase (RT) and a template sequence, on which the RT acts to create the multi-copy single-stranded DNA (msDNA) [200,201]. The msDNAs are then joined to their template RNAs by a $2'$–$5'$ phosphodiester bond, forming a special DNA–RNA hybrid structure [201]. Although the functions of retrons in their hosts remain poorly understood [202], the retron scaffold has been modified for the purpose of genome editing: a sgRNA can be added to the RNA component of the retron to guide it to the target site in the presence of Cas, while the desired donor sequence can be inserted into the retron scaffold and retro-transcribed into the msDNA [203]. As the consequence, those msDNAs containing desired sequences will be enriched in the proximity of the sgRNA-guided cleavage site and be used as the donor template for HR [203]. This system, named CRISPEY (Cas9 retron precise parallel editing via homology), has been employed in yeasts for massive parallel genome editing [203]. Recently, retrons have been successfully applied for gene editing in mammalian cells, although their efficiencies remain low [204,205]. Other concerns for the retron system are its DSB-dependent HDR mechanism and the limited fragment size (~700 bp) that can be inserted into the retron framework. Together, more mechanistic studies are required to apply retrons in mammalian cells.

5.4. SeLection by Essential-Gene Exon Knock-in (SLEEK)

Precise knock-in of genes at desired, endogenous sites is required for many clinical purposes. However, the desired knock-in mediated by CRISPR-Cas9-induced HDR is usually mixed or even overwhelmed by undesired indels generated by NHEJ. Recently, a simple but efficient approach to enrich cells with correct knock-in was developed. In SLEEK (selection by essential-gene exon knock-in), the donor DNA fragment is targeted to a site within an exon of an essential gene. The cargo template is designed in a way that the correct knock-in will retain the essential gene function, while all the cells containing undesired products get wiped out without the need for drug selection [206]. Importantly, this method has been applied in iPSCs to knock-in *CD16* and *mbIL-15*, which enhance the anti-tumor activity and persistence of iNK cells [206]. Although the WGS of those iPSC clones is still needed to evaluate the consequences of DSB-dependent HDR, this method provides a great advantage in saving the cost of generating clinical level PSCs.

6. Conclusions and Future Prospects

6.1. Improving Editing Efficiencies in Human PSCs

Considering the laborious process to isolate and characterize single-cell derived colonies, improving the gene editing efficiencies is crucial to apply gene editing tools in human PSCs. The Doudna and Church groups demonstrated that Cas9-mediated gene editing in PSCs is less efficient than in other somatic cells [82,207]. Previous studies also reported decreased editing efficiencies of CBE and PE in human PSCs [208]. However, it is over-simplistic to directly compare the editing efficiencies between somatic/immortal cells and PSCs. Human PSCs are notoriously hard to deliver exogenous genes with high copies. Thus, the low editing efficiencies of editors in PSCs could be simply due to their low expression levels compared to cell lines that can be easily transfected. In agreement with this notion, recent studies suggested that PE delivered in the mRNA form greatly enhances the editing efficiency compared to other forms, such as plasmids or RNP complexes [190]. Recent studies also showed that delivering Cas RNPs (Cas9 or Cas12) by cell-penetrating peptides greatly enhances editing efficiencies in human T cells or hematopoietic progenitor cells [209,210]. It is anticipated that the editing efficiencies of base editors or PEs in human PSCs can also be improved with these delivery techniques.

In addition to modifications on editors or gRNAs, small molecules were also found to be able to manipulate editing efficiencies. Small molecules that can enhance the HDR activity, such as L755507 and Brefeldin A, also increase CRISPR-mediated HDR efficiencies in mouse ESCs and human non-pluripotent cells [211]. Inhibitors targeting key components of NHEJ also increase the HDR rate in human non-pluripotent cells and mouse embryos [212–214]. In addition, inhibition of ATM or ATR could enhance both knockout and knock-in efficiencies of Cas12a (Cpf1) in human PSCs, although whether it is applicable for Cas9 remains to be determined [215]. Finally, histone deacetylase (HDAC) inhibitors can enhance Cas9-, CBE-, and ABE-mediated editing by increasing both the expression level of proteins and target accessibility in human non-pluripotent cells [215]. Investigating these boosters and their influences on off-target effects as well as genome integrity in the context of human PSCs will benefit future applications.

6.2. Conditional Gene Editing

The major concern of performing gene editing in PSCs is that off-target edits will be carried to their differentiated progenies. One potential solution of that is to construct inactive editing components in PSCs which will be activated upon differentiation to perform editing in somatic (stem) cells that have limited longevity. This design can be achieved by putting editors and/or gRNAs under the control of specific promoters. However, most RNA polymerase III promoters used to drive gRNA expression are constitutively active. We recently established a novel PE, p2PE3, using RNA polymerase II promoters to drive the expression of pegRNA and sgRNA [187] (Figure 2c). The p2PE3 displays 2.1-fold higher editing efficiency compared to PE3, and can be combined with SV40LT and/or MLH1dn to further increase its editing efficiency in human PSCs [187]. Using this system, the PE and pegRNA can be integrated as a cassette and put under the control of drug-inducible or lineage-specific promoters. This conditional editing strategy can also be employed by Cas9 or base editors to avoid undesired mutation in PSCs.

6.3. CRISPR-Cas as DNA Recorders of Cell Fates

PSCs are reliable in vitro models for differentiation, which involves progressive transitions of cellular states. General lineage tracing approaches only allow marking one or two states (e.g., the Cre or the Cre/Dre dual system). Recently, the CRISPR-Cas system has been employed to record signaling, cellular, or transcriptional events on DNA of eukaryotic cells (i.e., using DNA as the memory device) [216–219]. Among them, the "DNA typewriter" technique employs an elegant design, using sequential prime editing to capture different events in the happening order [219]. With this technique, different events, such as transcription activation or signal transduction, can be encoded by different pegRNAs driven by specific promoters (i.e., the p2PE3 system mentioned before) built in PSCs. Upon 2D or 3D differentiation, the order of happened events can be recorded on the "DNA tape" in each cell and decoded by single-cell sequencing. This system could be a unique tool to reveal complex event histories during cell fate specification.

6.4. New Systems to Be Explored

In nature, there are still broad varieties of RNA-guided nucleases, transposases, and recombinases that remain unexplored and can be potentially employed as gene editing tools. For example, the Doudna group identified the CIRSPR-CasΦ system from the Biggiephage [220], which is only half the size of Cas9 and has been employed for gene editing in plants [221]. A more thorough investigation identified ~6000 phage CRISPR-Cas systems covering all six known CRISPR-Cas types [222]. One of them, Casλ, was characterized and able to perform gene editing in HEK293T cells [222]. By tracing the ancestor of Cas proteins, the Zhang and Siksnys groups identified three IS200/IS605 transposon-encoded proteins, IscB, IsrB, and TnpB, which are also RNA-guided DNA nucleases [223,224]. Both IscB and TnpB exhibit gene editing activity and can be incorporated in base editors with high efficiencies in human cells [223–226]. Surprisingly, two very recent studies suggest that TnpB homologs are widespread in eukaryotes [227,228]. Saito et al. and Jiang et al. characterized the RNA-guided DNA nuclease activity of the eukaryotic transposon-encoded Fanzor proteins. Both studies demonstrated that Fanzor proteins from different species can be reprogrammed for human genome engineering in HEK293T cells [227,228]. Those eukaryotic RNA-guided endonucleases not only have hypercompact sizes but also exhibit low cleavage activity on collateral nucleic acids. Since they are originated from eukaryotic cells, Fanzor proteins are expected to have great application potential in the future.

In addition to novel nucleases, the Zhang group also elucidated the transposition mechanism of a non–long terminal repeat (non-LTR) retrotransposon, the R2 retrotransposon. Non-LTR transposons are inserted into genomes by a mechanism called target-primed reverse transcription (TPRT), during which the target DNA sequence is nicked, priming the reverse transcription of retrotransposon RNA. The Zhang group resolved the structure of the silk moth R2Bm (LINE type) TPRT complex and elucidated the mechanism of how R2Bm recognizes its native target to initiate TPRT [229]. Importantly, the Zhang group found that Cas9 can retarget R2 in vitro and initiate TPRT [229]. Although the integration events have not yet been observed in vitro or in vivo, this finding suggests its future use as a site-specific insertion tool.

6.5. Conclusions

With the optimization of current tools and the discovery of new tools, it is predictable that "safe" gene editing in PSCs will be easier to perform in the future. Notably, since the specificity of gene editing in PSCs has to meet the highest criteria, those gene editors validated in PSCs can also be potentially applied to other gene- or cell-therapies. Undeniably, current PSC-based therapies still face concerns, such as the removal of residual undifferentiated cells as well as the immunogenicity and under-performance of PSC-derived cells. Gene editing could also be employed to resolve those issues by engineering cells for lower immunogenicity (e.g., removal of HLA) or high efficacies/functions (e.g., expression of stimulatory or sustaining cytokines). Considering PSCs' unique merits of stability and unlimited quantity, it is worthy to further develop and validate gene editing tools for PSCs to facilitate their applications in both basic and translational research.

Funding: This work was funded by National Key R&D Program of China (2020YFA0710800), National Natural Science Foundation of China (31871487, 81703090), and the ShanghaiTech University start-up fund.

Acknowledgments: We thank Guanglei Li, Shisheng Huang, and Wanyu Tao for their critical reading. Due to space limitation, we apologize for important works that were not included.

Conflicts of Interest: The authors declare no conflict of interest.

References

1. Thomson, J.A.; Itskovitz-Eldor, J.; Shapiro, S.S.; Waknitz, M.A.; Swiergiel, J.J.; Marshall, V.S.; Jones, J.M. Embryonic stem cell lines derived from human blastocysts. *Science* **1998**, *282*, 1145–1147. [CrossRef] [PubMed]
2. Takahashi, K.; Tanabe, K.; Ohnuki, M.; Narita, M.; Ichisaka, T.; Tomoda, K.; Yamanaka, S. Induction of pluripotent stem cells from adult human fibroblasts by defined factors. *Cell* **2007**, *131*, 861–872. [CrossRef] [PubMed]
3. Yu, J.; Vodyanik, M.A.; Smuga-Otto, K.; Antosiewicz-Bourget, J.; Frane, J.L.; Tian, S.; Nie, J.; Jonsdottir, G.A.; Ruotti, V.; Stewart, R.; et al. Induced pluripotent stem cell lines derived from human somatic cells. *Science* **2007**, *318*, 1917–1920. [CrossRef] [PubMed]
4. Chen, G.; Gulbranson, D.R.; Hou, Z.; Bolin, J.M.; Ruotti, V.; Probasco, M.D.; Smuga-Otto, K.; Howden, S.E.; Diol, N.R.; Propson, N.E.; et al. Chemically defined conditions for human iPSC derivation and culture. *Nat. Methods* **2011**, *8*, 424–429. [CrossRef] [PubMed]
5. Okita, K.; Matsumura, Y.; Sato, Y.; Okada, A.; Morizane, A.; Okamoto, S.; Hong, H.; Nakagawa, M.; Tanabe, K.; Tezuka, K.; et al. A more efficient method to generate integration-free human iPS cells. *Nat. Methods* **2011**, *8*, 409–412. [CrossRef]
6. Fusaki, N.; Ban, H.; Nishiyama, A.; Saeki, K.; Hasegawa, M. Efficient induction of transgene-free human pluripotent stem cells using a vector based on Sendai virus, an RNA virus that does not integrate into the host genome. *Proc. Jpn. Acad. Ser. B Phys. Biol. Sci.* **2009**, *85*, 348–362. [CrossRef]
7. Yu, J.; Hu, K.; Smuga-Otto, K.; Tian, S.; Stewart, R.; Slukvin, I.I.; Thomson, J.A. Human induced pluripotent stem cells free of vector and transgene sequences. *Science* **2009**, *324*, 797–801. [CrossRef]
8. Guan, J.; Wang, G.; Wang, J.; Zhang, Z.; Fu, Y.; Cheng, L.; Meng, G.; Lyu, Y.; Zhu, J.; Li, Y.; et al. Chemical reprogramming of human somatic cells to pluripotent stem cells. *Nature* **2022**, *605*, 325–331. [CrossRef]
9. Liuyang, S.; Wang, G.; Wang, Y.; He, H.; Lyu, Y.; Cheng, L.; Yang, Z.; Guan, J.; Fu, Y.; Zhu, J.; et al. Highly efficient and rapid generation of human pluripotent stem cells by chemical reprogramming. *Cell Stem Cell* **2023**, *30*, 450–459.e9. [CrossRef]
10. Yamanaka, S. Pluripotent Stem Cell-Based Cell Therapy-Promise and Challenges. *Cell Stem Cell* **2020**, *27*, 523–531. [CrossRef]
11. Kim, J.Y.; Nam, Y.; Rim, Y.A.; Ju, J.H. Review of the Current Trends in Clinical Trials Involving Induced Pluripotent Stem Cells. *Stem Cell Rev. Rep.* **2022**, *18*, 142–154. [CrossRef] [PubMed]
12. Mazzini, L.; De Marchi, F. iPSC-based research in ALS precision medicine. *Cell Stem Cell* **2023**, *30*, 748–749. [CrossRef] [PubMed]
13. Turan, S.; Farruggio, A.P.; Srifa, W.; Day, J.W.; Calos, M.P. Precise Correction of Disease Mutations in Induced Pluripotent Stem Cells Derived from Patients with Limb Girdle Muscular Dystrophy. *Mol. Ther.* **2016**, *24*, 685–696. [CrossRef]
14. Sumer, S.A.; Hoffmann, S.; Laue, S.; Campbell, B.; Raedecke, K.; Frajs, V.; Clauss, S.; Kaab, S.; Janssen, J.W.G.; Jauch, A.; et al. Precise Correction of Heterozygous SHOX2 Mutations in hiPSCs Derived from Patients with Atrial Fibrillation via Genome Editing and Sib Selection. *Stem Cell Rep.* **2020**, *15*, 999–1013. [CrossRef]
15. Li, Y.; Hermanson, D.L.; Moriarity, B.S.; Kaufman, D.S. Human iPSC-Derived Natural Killer Cells Engineered with Chimeric Antigen Receptors Enhance Anti-tumor Activity. *Cell Stem Cell* **2018**, *23*, 181–192.e5. [CrossRef]
16. Mattapally, S.; Pawlik, K.M.; Fast, V.G.; Zumaquero, E.; Lund, F.E.; Randall, T.D.; Townes, T.M.; Zhang, J. Human Leukocyte Antigen Class I and II Knockout Human Induced Pluripotent Stem Cell-Derived Cells: Universal Donor for Cell Therapy. *J. Am. Heart Assoc.* **2018**, *7*, e010239. [CrossRef] [PubMed]
17. Shi, Y.; Inoue, H.; Wu, J.C.; Yamanaka, S. Induced pluripotent stem cell technology: A decade of progress. *Nat. Rev. Drug Discov.* **2017**, *16*, 115–130. [CrossRef] [PubMed]
18. Aurora, M.; Spence, J.R. hPSC-derived lung and intestinal organoids as models of human fetal tissue. *Dev. Biol.* **2016**, *420*, 230–238. [CrossRef]
19. Frum, T.; Spence, J.R. hPSC-derived organoids: Models of human development and disease. *J. Mol. Med.* **2021**, *99*, 463–473. [CrossRef]
20. Huch, M.; Dorrell, C.; Boj, S.F.; van Es, J.H.; Li, V.S.; van de Wetering, M.; Sato, T.; Hamer, K.; Sasaki, N.; Finegold, M.J.; et al. In vitro expansion of single Lgr5+ liver stem cells induced by Wnt-driven regeneration. *Nature* **2013**, *494*, 247–250. [CrossRef]
21. Lancaster, M.A.; Renner, M.; Martin, C.A.; Wenzel, D.; Bicknell, L.S.; Hurles, M.E.; Homfray, T.; Penninger, J.M.; Jackson, A.P.; Knoblich, J.A. Cerebral organoids model human brain development and microcephaly. *Nature* **2013**, *501*, 373–379. [CrossRef] [PubMed]
22. Driehuis, E.; Kretzschmar, K.; Clevers, H. Establishment of patient-derived cancer organoids for drug-screening applications. *Nat. Protoc.* **2020**, *15*, 3380–3409. [CrossRef] [PubMed]
23. Bar-Ephraim, Y.E.; Kretzschmar, K.; Clevers, H. Organoids in immunological research. *Nat. Rev. Immunol.* **2020**, *20*, 279–293. [CrossRef] [PubMed]
24. Li, C.; Huang, J.; Yu, Y.; Wan, Z.; Chiu, M.C.; Liu, X.; Zhang, S.; Cai, J.P.; Chu, H.; Li, G.; et al. Human airway and nasal organoids reveal escalating replicative fitness of SARS-CoV-2 emerging variants. *Proc. Natl. Acad. Sci. USA* **2023**, *120*, e2300376120. [CrossRef]

25. Achberger, K.; Probst, C.; Haderspeck, J.; Bolz, S.; Rogal, J.; Chuchuy, J.; Nikolova, M.; Cora, V.; Antkowiak, L.; Haq, W.; et al. Merging organoid and organ-on-a-chip technology to generate complex multi-layer tissue models in a human retina-on-a-chip platform. *eLife* **2019**, *8*, e46188. [CrossRef]
26. Chang, C.Y.; Ting, H.C.; Liu, C.A.; Su, H.L.; Chiou, T.W.; Lin, S.Z.; Harn, H.J.; Ho, T.J. Induced Pluripotent Stem Cell (iPSC)-Based Neurodegenerative Disease Models for Phenotype Recapitulation and Drug Screening. *Molecules* **2020**, *25*, 2000. [CrossRef]
27. He, Z.; Maynard, A.; Jain, A.; Gerber, T.; Petri, R.; Lin, H.C.; Santel, M.; Ly, K.; Dupre, J.S.; Sidow, L.; et al. Lineage recording in human cerebral organoids. *Nat. Methods* **2022**, *19*, 90–99. [CrossRef]
28. Daoud, A.; Munera, J.O. Insights into Human Development and Disease from Human Pluripotent Stem Cell Derived Intestinal Organoids. *Front. Med.* **2019**, *6*, 297. [CrossRef]
29. Zhou, H.; Wang, Y.; Liu, L.P.; Li, Y.M.; Zheng, Y.W. Gene Editing in Pluripotent Stem Cells and Their Derived Organoids. *Stem Cells Int.* **2021**, *2021*, 8130828. [CrossRef]
30. Hendriks, D.; Clevers, H.; Artegiani, B. CRISPR-Cas Tools and Their Application in Genetic Engineering of Human Stem Cells and Organoids. *Cell Stem Cell* **2020**, *27*, 705–731. [CrossRef] [PubMed]
31. De Masi, C.; Spitalieri, P.; Murdocca, M.; Novelli, G.; Sangiuolo, F. Application of CRISPR/Cas9 to human-induced pluripotent stem cells: From gene editing to drug discovery. *Hum. Genom.* **2020**, *14*, 25. [CrossRef] [PubMed]
32. Haapaniemi, E.; Botla, S.; Persson, J.; Schmierer, B.; Taipale, J. CRISPR-Cas9 genome editing induces a p53-mediated DNA damage response. *Nat. Med.* **2018**, *24*, 927–930. [CrossRef] [PubMed]
33. Ihry, R.J.; Worringer, K.A.; Salick, M.R.; Frias, E.; Ho, D.; Theriault, K.; Kommineni, S.; Chen, J.; Sondey, M.; Ye, C.; et al. p53 inhibits CRISPR-Cas9 engineering in human pluripotent stem cells. *Nat. Med.* **2018**, *24*, 939–946. [CrossRef] [PubMed]
34. Merkle, F.T.; Ghosh, S.; Kamitaki, N.; Mitchell, J.; Avior, Y.; Mello, C.; Kashin, S.; Mekhoubad, S.; Ilic, D.; Charlton, M.; et al. Human pluripotent stem cells recurrently acquire and expand dominant negative P53 mutations. *Nature* **2017**, *545*, 229–233. [CrossRef]
35. Capecchi, M.R. Altering the genome by homologous recombination. *Science* **1989**, *244*, 1288–1292. [CrossRef]
36. Koller, B.H.; Smithies, O. Inactivating the beta 2-microglobulin locus in mouse embryonic stem cells by homologous recombination. *Proc. Natl. Acad. Sci. USA* **1989**, *86*, 8932–8935. [CrossRef]
37. Rudin, N.; Sugarman, E.; Haber, J.E. Genetic and physical analysis of double-strand break repair and recombination in Saccharomyces cerevisiae. *Genetics* **1989**, *122*, 519–534. [CrossRef]
38. Rouet, P.; Smih, F.; Jasin, M. Introduction of double-strand breaks into the genome of mouse cells by expression of a rare-cutting endonuclease. *Mol. Cell. Biol.* **1994**, *14*, 8096–8106. [CrossRef]
39. Saretzki, G.; Armstrong, L.; Leake, A.; Lako, M.; von Zglinicki, T. Stress defense in murine embryonic stem cells is superior to that of various differentiated murine cells. *Stem Cells* **2004**, *22*, 962–971. [CrossRef]
40. Maynard, S.; Swistowska, A.M.; Lee, J.W.; Liu, Y.; Liu, S.T.; Da Cruz, A.B.; Rao, M.; de Souza-Pinto, N.C.; Zeng, X.; Bohr, V.A. Human embryonic stem cells have enhanced repair of multiple forms of DNA damage. *Stem Cells* **2008**, *26*, 2266–2274. [CrossRef]
41. Fu, X.; Cui, K.; Yi, Q.; Yu, L.; Xu, Y. DNA repair mechanisms in embryonic stem cells. *Cell. Mol. Life Sci.* **2017**, *74*, 487–493. [CrossRef] [PubMed]
42. Tichy, E.D.; Pillai, R.; Deng, L.; Liang, L.; Tischfield, J.; Schwemberger, S.J.; Babcock, G.F.; Stambrook, P.J. Mouse embryonic stem cells, but not somatic cells, predominantly use homologous recombination to repair double-strand DNA breaks. *Stem Cells Dev.* **2010**, *19*, 1699–1711. [CrossRef] [PubMed]
43. Novo, N.; Romero-Tamayo, S.; Marcuello, C.; Boneta, S.; Blasco-Machin, I.; Velazquez-Campoy, A.; Villanueva, R.; Moreno-Loshuertos, R.; Lostao, A.; Medina, M.; et al. Beyond a platform protein for the degradosome assembly: The Apoptosis-Inducing Factor as an efficient nuclease involved in chromatinolysis. *PNAS Nexus* **2023**, *2*, pgac312. [CrossRef] [PubMed]
44. Artus, C.; Boujrad, H.; Bouharrour, A.; Brunelle, M.N.; Hoos, S.; Yuste, V.J.; Lenormand, P.; Rousselle, J.C.; Namane, A.; England, P.; et al. AIF promotes chromatinolysis and caspase-independent programmed necrosis by interacting with histone H2AX. *EMBO J.* **2010**, *29*, 1585–1599. [CrossRef]
45. Shivram, H.; Cress, B.F.; Knott, G.J.; Doudna, J.A. Controlling and enhancing CRISPR systems. *Nat. Chem. Biol.* **2021**, *17*, 10–19. [CrossRef] [PubMed]
46. Liu, G.; Lin, Q.; Jin, S.; Gao, C. The CRISPR-Cas toolbox and gene editing technologies. *Mol. Cell* **2022**, *82*, 333–347. [CrossRef]
47. Doudna, J.A. The promise and challenge of therapeutic genome editing. *Nature* **2020**, *578*, 229–236. [CrossRef]
48. Wang, J.Y.; Doudna, J.A. CRISPR technology: A decade of genome editing is only the beginning. *Science* **2023**, *379*, eadd8643. [CrossRef]
49. Katti, A.; Diaz, B.J.; Caragine, C.M.; Sanjana, N.E.; Dow, L.E. CRISPR in cancer biology and therapy. *Nat. Rev. Cancer* **2022**, *22*, 259–279. [CrossRef]
50. Durai, S.; Mani, M.; Kandavelou, K.; Wu, J.; Porteus, M.H.; Chandrasegaran, S. Zinc finger nucleases: Custom-designed molecular scissors for genome engineering of plant and mammalian cells. *Nucleic Acids Res.* **2005**, *33*, 5978–5990. [CrossRef]
51. Miller, J.; McLachlan, A.D.; Klug, A. Repetitive zinc-binding domains in the protein transcription factor IIIA from Xenopus oocytes. *EMBO J.* **1985**, *4*, 1609–1614. [CrossRef] [PubMed]
52. Kim, Y.G.; Cha, J.; Chandrasegaran, S. Hybrid restriction enzymes: Zinc finger fusions to Fok I cleavage domain. *Proc. Natl. Acad. Sci. USA* **1996**, *93*, 1156–1160. [CrossRef] [PubMed]

53. Paschon, D.E.; Lussier, S.; Wangzor, T.; Xia, D.F.; Li, P.W.; Hinkley, S.J.; Scarlott, N.A.; Lam, S.C.; Waite, A.J.; Truong, L.N.; et al. Diversifying the structure of zinc finger nucleases for high-precision genome editing. *Nat. Commun.* **2019**, *10*, 1133. [CrossRef] [PubMed]
54. Lombardo, A.; Genovese, P.; Beausejour, C.M.; Colleoni, S.; Lee, Y.L.; Kim, K.A.; Ando, D.; Urnov, F.D.; Galli, C.; Gregory, P.D.; et al. Gene editing in human stem cells using zinc finger nucleases and integrase-defective lentiviral vector delivery. *Nat. Biotechnol.* **2007**, *25*, 1298–1306. [CrossRef]
55. Zou, J.; Maeder, M.L.; Mali, P.; Pruett-Miller, S.M.; Thibodeau-Beganny, S.; Chou, B.K.; Chen, G.; Ye, Z.; Park, I.H.; Daley, G.Q.; et al. Gene targeting of a disease-related gene in human induced pluripotent stem and embryonic stem cells. *Cell Stem Cell* **2009**, *5*, 97–110. [CrossRef]
56. Hockemeyer, D.; Soldner, F.; Beard, C.; Gao, Q.; Mitalipova, M.; DeKelver, R.C.; Katibah, G.E.; Amora, R.; Boydston, E.A.; Zeitler, B.; et al. Efficient targeting of expressed and silent genes in human ESCs and iPSCs using zinc-finger nucleases. *Nat. Biotechnol.* **2009**, *27*, 851–857. [CrossRef]
57. Miller, J.C.; Holmes, M.C.; Wang, J.; Guschin, D.Y.; Lee, Y.L.; Rupniewski, I.; Beausejour, C.M.; Waite, A.J.; Wang, N.S.; Kim, K.A.; et al. An improved zinc-finger nuclease architecture for highly specific genome editing. *Nat. Biotechnol.* **2007**, *25*, 778–785. [CrossRef]
58. Cong, L.; Ran, F.A.; Cox, D.; Lin, S.; Barretto, R.; Habib, N.; Hsu, P.D.; Wu, X.; Jiang, W.; Marraffini, L.A.; et al. Multiplex genome engineering using CRISPR/Cas systems. *Science* **2013**, *339*, 819–823. [CrossRef]
59. Wang, Z.; Gerstein, M.; Snyder, M. RNA-Seq: A revolutionary tool for transcriptomics. *Nat. Rev. Genet.* **2009**, *10*, 57–63. [CrossRef]
60. Yusa, K.; Rashid, S.T.; Strick-Marchand, H.; Varela, I.; Liu, P.Q.; Paschon, D.E.; Miranda, E.; Ordonez, A.; Hannan, N.R.; Rouhani, F.J.; et al. Targeted gene correction of alpha1-antitrypsin deficiency in induced pluripotent stem cells. *Nature* **2011**, *478*, 391–394. [CrossRef]
61. Pattanayak, V.; Ramirez, C.L.; Joung, J.K.; Liu, D.R. Revealing off-target cleavage specificities of zinc-finger nucleases by in vitro selection. *Nat. Methods* **2011**, *8*, 765–770. [CrossRef] [PubMed]
62. Gabriel, R.; Lombardo, A.; Arens, A.; Miller, J.C.; Genovese, P.; Kaeppel, C.; Nowrouzi, A.; Bartholomae, C.C.; Wang, J.; Friedman, G.; et al. An unbiased genome-wide analysis of zinc-finger nuclease specificity. *Nat. Biotechnol.* **2011**, *29*, 816–823. [CrossRef] [PubMed]
63. Lee, H.J.; Kim, E.; Kim, J.S. Targeted chromosomal deletions in human cells using zinc finger nucleases. *Genome Res.* **2010**, *20*, 81–89. [CrossRef] [PubMed]
64. Lee, H.J.; Kweon, J.; Kim, E.; Kim, S.; Kim, J.S. Targeted chromosomal duplications and inversions in the human genome using zinc finger nucleases. *Genome Res.* **2012**, *22*, 539–548. [CrossRef] [PubMed]
65. Boch, J.; Bonas, U. Xanthomonas AvrBs3 family-type III effectors: Discovery and function. *Annu. Rev. Phytopathol.* **2010**, *48*, 419–436. [CrossRef]
66. Miller, J.C.; Tan, S.; Qiao, G.; Barlow, K.A.; Wang, J.; Xia, D.F.; Meng, X.; Paschon, D.E.; Leung, E.; Hinkley, S.J.; et al. A TALE nuclease architecture for efficient genome editing. *Nat. Biotechnol.* **2011**, *29*, 143–148. [CrossRef]
67. Boch, J. TALEs of genome targeting. *Nat. Biotechnol.* **2011**, *29*, 135–136. [CrossRef]
68. Qasim, W.; Zhan, H.; Samarasinghe, S.; Adams, S.; Amrolia, P.; Stafford, S.; Butler, K.; Rivat, C.; Wright, G.; Somana, K.; et al. Molecular remission of infant B-ALL after infusion of universal TALEN gene-edited CAR T cells. *Sci. Transl. Med.* **2017**, *9*, eaaj2013. [CrossRef]
69. Shahryari, A.; Burtscher, I.; Nazari, Z.; Lickert, H. Engineering Gene Therapy: Advances and Barriers. *Adv. Ther.-Ger.* **2021**, *4*, 2100040. [CrossRef]
70. Yahata, N.; Matsumoto, Y.; Omi, M.; Yamamoto, N.; Hata, R. TALEN-mediated shift of mitochondrial DNA heteroplasmy in MELAS-iPSCs with m.13513G>A mutation. *Sci. Rep.* **2017**, *7*, 15557. [CrossRef]
71. Karakikes, I.; Termglinchan, V.; Cepeda, D.A.; Lee, J.; Diecke, S.; Hendel, A.; Itzhaki, I.; Ameen, M.; Shrestha, R.; Wu, H.; et al. A Comprehensive TALEN-Based Knockout Library for Generating Human-Induced Pluripotent Stem Cell-Based Models for Cardiovascular Diseases. *Circ. Res.* **2017**, *120*, 1561–1571. [CrossRef] [PubMed]
72. Dreyer, A.K.; Hoffmann, D.; Lachmann, N.; Ackermann, M.; Steinemann, D.; Timm, B.; Siler, U.; Reichenbach, J.; Grez, M.; Moritz, T.; et al. TALEN-mediated functional correction of X-linked chronic granulomatous disease in patient-derived induced pluripotent stem cells. *Biomaterials* **2015**, *69*, 191–200. [CrossRef] [PubMed]
73. Ramalingam, S.; Annaluru, N.; Kandavelou, K.; Chandrasegaran, S. TALEN-mediated generation and genetic correction of disease-specific human induced pluripotent stem cells. *Curr. Gene Ther.* **2014**, *14*, 461–472. [CrossRef]
74. Mussolino, C.; Morbitzer, R.; Lutge, F.; Dannemann, N.; Lahaye, T.; Cathomen, T. A novel TALE nuclease scaffold enables high genome editing activity in combination with low toxicity. *Nucleic Acids Res.* **2011**, *39*, 9283–9293. [CrossRef] [PubMed]
75. Kim, Y.; Kweon, J.; Kim, J.S. TALENs and ZFNs are associated with different mutation signatures. *Nat. Methods* **2013**, *10*, 185. [CrossRef]
76. Kim, Y.; Kweon, J.; Kim, A.; Chon, J.K.; Yoo, J.Y.; Kim, H.J.; Kim, S.; Lee, C.; Jeong, E.; Chung, E.; et al. A library of TAL effector nucleases spanning the human genome. *Nat. Biotechnol.* **2013**, *31*, 251–258. [CrossRef]
77. Veres, A.; Gosis, B.S.; Ding, Q.; Collins, R.; Ragavendran, A.; Brand, H.; Erdin, S.; Cowan, C.A.; Talkowski, M.E.; Musunuru, K. Low incidence of off-target mutations in individual CRISPR-Cas9 and TALEN targeted human stem cell clones detected by whole-genome sequencing. *Cell Stem Cell* **2014**, *15*, 27–30. [CrossRef]

78. Smith, C.; Gore, A.; Yan, W.; Abalde-Atristain, L.; Li, Z.; He, C.; Wang, Y.; Brodsky, R.A.; Zhang, K.; Cheng, L.; et al. Whole-genome sequencing analysis reveals high specificity of CRISPR/Cas9 and TALEN-based genome editing in human iPSCs. *Cell Stem Cell* **2014**, *15*, 12–13. [CrossRef] [PubMed]
79. Barrangou, R.; Fremaux, C.; Deveau, H.; Richards, M.; Boyaval, P.; Moineau, S.; Romero, D.A.; Horvath, P. CRISPR provides acquired resistance against viruses in prokaryotes. *Science* **2007**, *315*, 1709–1712. [CrossRef]
80. Bolotin, A.; Quinquis, B.; Sorokin, A.; Ehrlich, S.D. Clustered regularly interspaced short palindrome repeats (CRISPRs) have spacers of extrachromosomal origin. *Microbiology* **2005**, *151*, 2551–2561. [CrossRef] [PubMed]
81. Jinek, M.; Chylinski, K.; Fonfara, I.; Hauer, M.; Doudna, J.A.; Charpentier, E. A programmable dual-RNA-guided DNA endonuclease in adaptive bacterial immunity. *Science* **2012**, *337*, 816–821. [CrossRef] [PubMed]
82. Mali, P.; Yang, L.; Esvelt, K.M.; Aach, J.; Guell, M.; DiCarlo, J.E.; Norville, J.E.; Church, G.M. RNA-guided human genome engineering via Cas9. *Science* **2013**, *339*, 823–826. [CrossRef] [PubMed]
83. Gasiunas, G.; Barrangou, R.; Horvath, P.; Siksnys, V. Cas9-crRNA ribonucleoprotein complex mediates specific DNA cleavage for adaptive immunity in bacteria. *Proc. Natl. Acad. Sci. USA* **2012**, *109*, E2579–E2586. [CrossRef] [PubMed]
84. Anders, C.; Niewoehner, O.; Duerst, A.; Jinek, M. Structural basis of PAM-dependent target DNA recognition by the Cas9 endonuclease. *Nature* **2014**, *513*, 569–573. [CrossRef] [PubMed]
85. Nakamura, M.; Gao, Y.; Dominguez, A.A.; Qi, L.S. CRISPR technologies for precise epigenome editing. *Nat. Cell. Biol.* **2021**, *23*, 11–22. [CrossRef] [PubMed]
86. Wang, H.; La Russa, M.; Qi, L.S. CRISPR/Cas9 in Genome Editing and Beyond. *Annu. Rev. Biochem.* **2016**, *85*, 227–264. [CrossRef] [PubMed]
87. Yano, N.; Fedulov, A.V. Targeted DNA Demethylation: Vectors, Effectors and Perspectives. *Biomedicines* **2023**, *11*, 1334. [CrossRef]
88. Brouns, S.J.; Jore, M.M.; Lundgren, M.; Westra, E.R.; Slijkhuis, R.J.; Snijders, A.P.; Dickman, M.J.; Makarova, K.S.; Koonin, E.V.; van der Oost, J. Small CRISPR RNAs guide antiviral defense in prokaryotes. *Science* **2008**, *321*, 960–964. [CrossRef]
89. Marraffini, L.A.; Sontheimer, E.J. CRISPR interference limits horizontal gene transfer in staphylococci by targeting DNA. *Science* **2008**, *322*, 1843–1845. [CrossRef]
90. Zetsche, B.; Gootenberg, J.S.; Abudayyeh, O.O.; Slaymaker, I.M.; Makarova, K.S.; Essletzbichler, P.; Volz, S.E.; Joung, J.; van der Oost, J.; Regev, A.; et al. Cpf1 is a single RNA-guided endonuclease of a class 2 CRISPR-Cas system. *Cell* **2015**, *163*, 759–771. [CrossRef] [PubMed]
91. Abudayyeh, O.O.; Gootenberg, J.S.; Essletzbichler, P.; Han, S.; Joung, J.; Belanto, J.J.; Verdine, V.; Cox, D.B.T.; Kellner, M.J.; Regev, A.; et al. RNA targeting with CRISPR-Cas13. *Nature* **2017**, *550*, 280–284. [CrossRef] [PubMed]
92. Pickar-Oliver, A.; Gersbach, C.A. The next generation of CRISPR-Cas technologies and applications. *Nat. Rev. Mol. Cell Biol.* **2019**, *20*, 490–507. [CrossRef]
93. Shalem, O.; Sanjana, N.E.; Zhang, F. High-throughput functional genomics using CRISPR-Cas9. *Nat. Rev. Genet.* **2015**, *16*, 299–311. [CrossRef] [PubMed]
94. Zhou, Y.; Zhu, S.; Cai, C.; Yuan, P.; Li, C.; Huang, Y.; Wei, W. High-throughput screening of a CRISPR/Cas9 library for functional genomics in human cells. *Nature* **2014**, *509*, 487–491. [CrossRef] [PubMed]
95. Michels, B.E.; Mosa, M.H.; Streibl, B.I.; Zhan, T.; Menche, C.; Abou-El-Ardat, K.; Darvishi, T.; Czlonka, E.; Wagner, S.; Winter, J.; et al. Pooled In Vitro and In Vivo CRISPR-Cas9 Screening Identifies Tumor Suppressors in Human Colon Organoids. *Cell Stem Cell* **2020**, *26*, 782–792.e7. [CrossRef] [PubMed]
96. Briganti, F.; Sun, H.; Wei, W.; Wu, J.; Zhu, C.; Liss, M.; Karakikes, I.; Rego, S.; Cipriano, A.; Snyder, M.; et al. iPSC Modeling of RBM20-Deficient DCM Identifies Upregulation of RBM20 as a Therapeutic Strategy. *Cell Rep.* **2020**, *32*, 108117. [CrossRef]
97. Jeong, J.; Jager, A.; Domizi, P.; Pavel-Dinu, M.; Gojenola, L.; Iwasaki, M.; Wei, M.C.; Pan, F.; Zehnder, J.L.; Porteus, M.H.; et al. High-efficiency CRISPR induction of t(9;11) chromosomal translocations and acute leukemias in human blood stem cells. *Blood Adv.* **2019**, *3*, 2825–2835. [CrossRef]
98. Maxwell, K.G.; Augsornworawat, P.; Velazco-Cruz, L.; Kim, M.H.; Asada, R.; Hogrebe, N.J.; Morikawa, S.; Urano, F.; Millman, J.R. Gene-edited human stem cell-derived beta cells from a patient with monogenic diabetes reverse preexisting diabetes in mice. *Sci. Transl. Med.* **2020**, *12*, eaax9106. [CrossRef]
99. Takasato, M.; Er, P.X.; Chiu, H.S.; Little, M.H. Generation of kidney organoids from human pluripotent stem cells. *Nat. Protoc.* **2016**, *11*, 1681–1692. [CrossRef]
100. Miller, A.J.; Dye, B.R.; Ferrer-Torres, D.; Hill, D.R.; Overeem, A.W.; Shea, L.D.; Spence, J.R. Generation of lung organoids from human pluripotent stem cells in vitro. *Nat. Protoc.* **2019**, *14*, 518–540. [CrossRef]
101. Drakhlis, L.; Devadas, S.B.; Zweigerdt, R. Generation of heart-forming organoids from human pluripotent stem cells. *Nat. Protoc.* **2021**, *16*, 5652–5672. [CrossRef] [PubMed]
102. Ouchi, R.; Togo, S.; Kimura, M.; Shinozawa, T.; Koido, M.; Koike, H.; Thompson, W.; Karns, R.A.; Mayhew, C.N.; McGrath, P.S.; et al. Modeling Steatohepatitis in Humans with Pluripotent Stem Cell-Derived Organoids. *Cell Metab.* **2019**, *30*, 374–384.e6. [CrossRef]
103. Xiang, Y.; Tanaka, Y.; Patterson, B.; Kang, Y.J.; Govindaiah, G.; Roselaar, N.; Cakir, B.; Kim, K.Y.; Lombroso, A.P.; Hwang, S.M.; et al. Fusion of Regionally Specified hPSC-Derived Organoids Models Human Brain Development and Interneuron Migration. *Cell Stem Cell* **2017**, *21*, 383–398.e7. [CrossRef] [PubMed]

104. Wimmer, R.A.; Leopoldi, A.; Aichinger, M.; Kerjaschki, D.; Penninger, J.M. Generation of blood vessel organoids from human pluripotent stem cells. *Nat. Protoc.* **2019**, *14*, 3082–3100. [CrossRef] [PubMed]
105. Freedman, B.S.; Brooks, C.R.; Lam, A.Q.; Fu, H.; Morizane, R.; Agrawal, V.; Saad, A.F.; Li, M.K.; Hughes, M.R.; Werff, R.V.; et al. Modelling kidney disease with CRISPR-mutant kidney organoids derived from human pluripotent epiblast spheroids. *Nat. Commun.* **2015**, *6*, 8715. [CrossRef] [PubMed]
106. Bian, S.; Repic, M.; Guo, Z.; Kavirayani, A.; Burkard, T.; Bagley, J.A.; Krauditsch, C.; Knoblich, J.A. Genetically engineered cerebral organoids model brain tumor formation. *Nat. Methods* **2018**, *15*, 631–639. [CrossRef] [PubMed]
107. VanderWall, K.B.; Huang, K.C.; Pan, Y.; Lavekar, S.S.; Fligor, C.M.; Allsop, A.R.; Lentsch, K.A.; Dang, P.; Zhang, C.; Tseng, H.C.; et al. Retinal Ganglion Cells with a Glaucoma OPTN(E50K) Mutation Exhibit Neurodegenerative Phenotypes when Derived from Three-Dimensional Retinal Organoids. *Stem Cell Rep.* **2020**, *15*, 52–66. [CrossRef]
108. Koehler, K.R.; Nie, J.; Longworth-Mills, E.; Liu, X.P.; Lee, J.; Holt, J.R.; Hashino, E. Generation of inner ear organoids containing functional hair cells from human pluripotent stem cells. *Nat. Biotechnol.* **2017**, *35*, 583–589. [CrossRef]
109. Zhu, H.; Blum, R.H.; Bernareggi, D.; Ask, E.H.; Wu, Z.; Hoel, H.J.; Meng, Z.; Wu, C.; Guan, K.L.; Malmberg, K.J.; et al. Metabolic Reprograming via Deletion of CISH in Human iPSC-Derived NK Cells Promotes In Vivo Persistence and Enhances Anti-tumor Activity. *Cell Stem Cell* **2020**, *27*, 224–237.e6. [CrossRef]
110. Woan, K.V.; Kim, H.; Bjordahl, R.; Davis, Z.B.; Gaidarova, S.; Goulding, J.; Hancock, B.; Mahmood, S.; Abujarour, R.; Wang, H.; et al. Harnessing features of adaptive NK cells to generate iPSC-derived NK cells for enhanced immunotherapy. *Cell Stem Cell* **2021**, *28*, 2062–2075.e5. [CrossRef]
111. Koo, T.; Lee, J.; Kim, J.S. Measuring and Reducing Off-Target Activities of Programmable Nucleases Including CRISPR-Cas9. *Mol. Cells* **2015**, *38*, 475–481. [CrossRef] [PubMed]
112. Cui, Z.; Liu, H.; Zhang, H.; Huang, Z.; Tian, R.; Li, L.; Fan, W.; Chen, Y.; Chen, L.; Zhang, S.; et al. The comparison of ZFNs, TALENs, and SpCas9 by GUIDE-seq in HPV-targeted gene therapy. *Mol. Ther. Nucleic Acids* **2021**, *26*, 1466–1478. [CrossRef] [PubMed]
113. Kim, D.; Bae, S.; Park, J.; Kim, E.; Kim, S.; Yu, H.R.; Hwang, J.; Kim, J.I.; Kim, J.S. Digenome-seq: Genome-wide profiling of CRISPR-Cas9 off-target effects in human cells. *Nat. Methods* **2015**, *12*, 237–243. [CrossRef]
114. Tsai, S.Q.; Nguyen, N.T.; Malagon-Lopez, J.; Topkar, V.V.; Aryee, M.J.; Joung, J.K. CIRCLE-seq: A highly sensitive in vitro screen for genome-wide CRISPR-Cas9 nuclease off-targets. *Nat. Methods* **2017**, *14*, 607–614. [CrossRef]
115. Tsai, S.Q.; Zheng, Z.; Nguyen, N.T.; Liebers, M.; Topkar, V.V.; Thapar, V.; Wyvekens, N.; Khayter, C.; Iafrate, A.J.; Le, L.P.; et al. GUIDE-seq enables genome-wide profiling of off-target cleavage by CRISPR-Cas nucleases. *Nat. Biotechnol.* **2015**, *33*, 187–197. [CrossRef] [PubMed]
116. Ran, F.A.; Hsu, P.D.; Lin, C.Y.; Gootenberg, J.S.; Konermann, S.; Trevino, A.E.; Scott, D.A.; Inoue, A.; Matoba, S.; Zhang, Y.; et al. Double nicking by RNA-guided CRISPR Cas9 for enhanced genome editing specificity. *Cell* **2013**, *154*, 1380–1389. [CrossRef] [PubMed]
117. Chen, J.S.; Dagdas, Y.S.; Kleinstiver, B.P.; Welch, M.M.; Sousa, A.A.; Harrington, L.B.; Sternberg, S.H.; Joung, J.K.; Yildiz, A.; Doudna, J.A. Enhanced proofreading governs CRISPR-Cas9 targeting accuracy. *Nature* **2017**, *550*, 407–410. [CrossRef]
118. Kleinstiver, B.P.; Pattanayak, V.; Prew, M.S.; Tsai, S.Q.; Nguyen, N.T.; Zheng, Z.; Joung, J.K. High-fidelity CRISPR-Cas9 nucleases with no detectable genome-wide off-target effects. *Nature* **2016**, *529*, 490–495. [CrossRef]
119. Lee, J.K.; Jeong, E.; Lee, J.; Jung, M.; Shin, E.; Kim, Y.H.; Lee, K.; Jung, I.; Kim, D.; Kim, S.; et al. Directed evolution of CRISPR-Cas9 to increase its specificity. *Nat. Commun.* **2018**, *9*, 3048. [CrossRef]
120. Fu, Y.; Sander, J.D.; Reyon, D.; Cascio, V.M.; Joung, J.K. Improving CRISPR-Cas nuclease specificity using truncated guide RNAs. *Nat. Biotechnol.* **2014**, *32*, 279–284. [CrossRef]
121. Kocak, D.D.; Josephs, E.A.; Bhandarkar, V.; Adkar, S.S.; Kwon, J.B.; Gersbach, C.A. Increasing the specificity of CRISPR systems with engineered RNA secondary structures. *Nat. Biotechnol.* **2019**, *37*, 657–666. [CrossRef] [PubMed]
122. Gaudelli, N.M.; Komor, A.C.; Rees, H.A.; Packer, M.S.; Badran, A.H.; Bryson, D.I.; Liu, D.R. Programmable base editing of A*T to G*C in genomic DNA without DNA cleavage. *Nature* **2017**, *551*, 464–471. [CrossRef]
123. Kurt, I.C.; Zhou, R.; Iyer, S.; Garcia, S.P.; Miller, B.R.; Langner, L.M.; Grunewald, J.; Joung, J.K. CRISPR C-to-G base editors for inducing targeted DNA transversions in human cells. *Nat. Biotechnol.* **2021**, *39*, 41–46. [CrossRef]
124. Zhao, D.; Li, J.; Li, S.; Xin, X.; Hu, M.; Price, M.A.; Rosser, S.J.; Bi, C.; Zhang, X. Glycosylase base editors enable C-to-A and C-to-G base changes. *Nat. Biotechnol.* **2021**, *39*, 35–40. [CrossRef] [PubMed]
125. Chen, L.; Hong, M.; Luan, C.; Gao, H.; Ru, G.; Guo, X.; Zhang, D.; Zhang, S.; Li, C.; Wu, J.; et al. Adenine transversion editors enable precise, efficient A*T-to-C*G base editing in mammalian cells and embryos. *Nat. Biotechnol.* **2023**, 1–13. [CrossRef] [PubMed]
126. Tong, H.; Wang, X.; Liu, Y.; Liu, N.; Li, Y.; Luo, J.; Ma, Q.; Wu, D.; Li, J.; Xu, C.; et al. Programmable A-to-Y base editing by fusing an adenine base editor with an N-methylpurine DNA glycosylase. *Nat. Biotechnol.* **2023**, 1–5. [CrossRef] [PubMed]
127. Grunewald, J.; Zhou, R.; Lareau, C.A.; Garcia, S.P.; Iyer, S.; Miller, B.R.; Langner, L.M.; Hsu, J.Y.; Aryee, M.J.; Joung, J.K. A dual-deaminase CRISPR base editor enables concurrent adenine and cytosine editing. *Nat. Biotechnol.* **2020**, *38*, 861–864. [CrossRef]
128. Sakata, R.C.; Ishiguro, S.; Mori, H.; Tanaka, M.; Tatsuno, K.; Ueda, H.; Yamamoto, S.; Seki, M.; Masuyama, N.; Nishida, K.; et al. Base editors for simultaneous introduction of C-to-T and A-to-G mutations. *Nat. Biotechnol.* **2020**, *38*, 865–869. [CrossRef]

129. Xie, J.; Huang, X.; Wang, X.; Gou, S.; Liang, Y.; Chen, F.; Li, N.; Ouyang, Z.; Zhang, Q.; Ge, W.; et al. ACBE, a new base editor for simultaneous C-to-T and A-to-G substitutions in mammalian systems. *BMC Biol.* **2020**, *18*, 131. [CrossRef]
130. Zhang, X.; Zhu, B.; Chen, L.; Xie, L.; Yu, W.; Wang, Y.; Li, L.; Yin, S.; Yang, L.; Hu, H.; et al. Dual base editor catalyzes both cytosine and adenine base conversions in human cells. *Nat. Biotechnol.* **2020**, *38*, 856–860. [CrossRef]
131. Komor, A.C.; Kim, Y.B.; Packer, M.S.; Zuris, J.A.; Liu, D.R. Programmable editing of a target base in genomic DNA without double-stranded DNA cleavage. *Nature* **2016**, *533*, 420–424. [CrossRef] [PubMed]
132. Nishida, K.; Arazoe, T.; Yachie, N.; Banno, S.; Kakimoto, M.; Tabata, M.; Mochizuki, M.; Miyabe, A.; Araki, M.; Hara, K.Y.; et al. Targeted nucleotide editing using hybrid prokaryotic and vertebrate adaptive immune systems. *Science* **2016**, *353*, aaf8729. [CrossRef]
133. Komor, A.C.; Zhao, K.T.; Packer, M.S.; Gaudelli, N.M.; Waterbury, A.L.; Koblan, L.W.; Kim, Y.B.; Badran, A.H.; Liu, D.R. Improved base excision repair inhibition and bacteriophage Mu Gam protein yields C:G-to-T:A base editors with higher efficiency and product purity. *Sci. Adv.* **2017**, *3*, eaao4774. [CrossRef]
134. Anzalone, A.V.; Koblan, L.W.; Liu, D.R. Genome editing with CRISPR-Cas nucleases, base editors, transposases and prime editors. *Nat. Biotechnol.* **2020**, *38*, 824–844. [CrossRef] [PubMed]
135. Chen, L.; Park, J.E.; Paa, P.; Rajakumar, P.D.; Prekop, H.T.; Chew, Y.T.; Manivannan, S.N.; Chew, W.L. Programmable C:G to G:C genome editing with CRISPR-Cas9-directed base excision repair proteins. *Nat. Commun.* **2021**, *12*, 1384. [CrossRef]
136. Zafra, M.P.; Schatoff, E.M.; Katti, A.; Foronda, M.; Breinig, M.; Schweitzer, A.Y.; Simon, A.; Han, T.; Goswami, S.; Montgomery, E.; et al. Optimized base editors enable efficient editing in cells, organoids and mice. *Nat. Biotechnol.* **2018**, *36*, 888–893. [CrossRef]
137. Koblan, L.W.; Doman, J.L.; Wilson, C.; Levy, J.M.; Tay, T.; Newby, G.A.; Maianti, J.P.; Raguram, A.; Liu, D.R. Improving cytidine and adenine base editors by expression optimization and ancestral reconstruction. *Nat. Biotechnol.* **2018**, *36*, 843–846. [CrossRef] [PubMed]
138. Gaudelli, N.M.; Lam, D.K.; Rees, H.A.; Sola-Esteves, N.M.; Barrera, L.A.; Born, D.A.; Edwards, A.; Gehrke, J.M.; Lee, S.J.; Liquori, A.J.; et al. Directed evolution of adenine base editors with increased activity and therapeutic application. *Nat. Biotechnol.* **2020**, *38*, 892–900. [CrossRef]
139. Liu, Y.; Zhou, C.; Huang, S.; Dang, L.; Wei, Y.; He, J.; Zhou, Y.; Mao, S.; Tao, W.; Zhang, Y.; et al. A Cas-embedding strategy for minimizing off-target effects of DNA base editors. *Nat. Commun.* **2020**, *11*, 6073. [CrossRef]
140. Rees, H.A.; Wilson, C.; Doman, J.L.; Liu, D.R. Analysis and minimization of cellular RNA editing by DNA adenine base editors. *Sci. Adv.* **2019**, *5*, eaax5717. [CrossRef]
141. Grunewald, J.; Zhou, R.; Iyer, S.; Lareau, C.A.; Garcia, S.P.; Aryee, M.J.; Joung, J.K. CRISPR DNA base editors with reduced RNA off-target and self-editing activities. *Nat. Biotechnol.* **2019**, *37*, 1041–1048. [CrossRef] [PubMed]
142. Jeong, Y.K.; Yu, J.; Bae, S. Construction of non-canonical PAM-targeting adenosine base editors by restriction enzyme-free DNA cloning using CRISPR-Cas9. *Sci. Rep.* **2019**, *9*, 4939. [CrossRef] [PubMed]
143. Zhang, Z.; Tao, W.; Huang, S.; Sun, W.; Wang, Y.; Jiang, W.; Huang, X.; Lin, C.P. Engineering an adenine base editor in human embryonic stem cells with minimal DNA and RNA off-target activities. *Mol. Ther. Nucleic Acids* **2022**, *29*, 502–510. [CrossRef] [PubMed]
144. Koblan, L.W.; Arbab, M.; Shen, M.W.; Hussmann, J.A.; Anzalone, A.V.; Doman, J.L.; Newby, G.A.; Yang, D.; Mok, B.; Replogle, J.M.; et al. Efficient C*G-to-G*C base editors developed using CRISPRi screens, target-library analysis, and machine learning. *Nat. Biotechnol.* **2021**, *39*, 1414–1425. [CrossRef]
145. Chen, S.; Liu, Z.; Lai, L.; Li, Z. Efficient C-to-G Base Editing with Improved Target Compatibility Using Engineered Deaminase-nCas9 Fusions. *CRISPR J.* **2022**, *5*, 389–396. [CrossRef]
146. Chen, L.; Zhu, B.; Ru, G.; Meng, H.; Yan, Y.; Hong, M.; Zhang, D.; Luan, C.; Zhang, S.; Wu, H.; et al. Re-engineering the adenine deaminase TadA-8e for efficient and specific CRISPR-based cytosine base editing. *Nat. Biotechnol.* **2023**, *41*, 663–672. [CrossRef]
147. Zuo, E.; Sun, Y.; Wei, W.; Yuan, T.; Ying, W.; Sun, H.; Yuan, L.; Steinmetz, L.M.; Li, Y.; Yang, H. Cytosine base editor generates substantial off-target single-nucleotide variants in mouse embryos. *Science* **2019**, *364*, 289–292. [CrossRef]
148. Yan, N.; Feng, H.; Sun, Y.; Xin, Y.; Zhang, H.; Lu, H.; Zheng, J.; He, C.; Zuo, Z.; Yuan, T.; et al. Cytosine base editors induce off-target mutations and adverse phenotypic effects in transgenic mice. *Nat. Commun.* **2023**, *14*, 1784. [CrossRef]
149. Jin, S.; Zong, Y.; Gao, Q.; Zhu, Z.; Wang, Y.; Qin, P.; Liang, C.; Wang, D.; Qiu, J.L.; Zhang, F.; et al. Cytosine, but not adenine, base editors induce genome-wide off-target mutations in rice. *Science* **2019**, *364*, 292–295. [CrossRef]
150. Li, A.; Mitsunobu, H.; Yoshioka, S.; Suzuki, T.; Kondo, A.; Nishida, K. Cytosine base editing systems with minimized off-target effect and molecular size. *Nat. Commun.* **2022**, *13*, 4531. [CrossRef]
151. McGrath, E.; Shin, H.; Zhang, L.; Phue, J.N.; Wu, W.W.; Shen, R.F.; Jang, Y.Y.; Revollo, J.; Ye, Z. Targeting specificity of APOBEC-based cytosine base editor in human iPSCs determined by whole genome sequencing. *Nat. Commun.* **2019**, *10*, 5353. [CrossRef] [PubMed]
152. Grunewald, J.; Zhou, R.; Garcia, S.P.; Iyer, S.; Lareau, C.A.; Aryee, M.J.; Joung, J.K. Transcriptome-wide off-target RNA editing induced by CRISPR-guided DNA base editors. *Nature* **2019**, *569*, 433–437. [CrossRef] [PubMed]
153. Kumar, R.; DiMenna, L.J.; Chaudhuri, J.; Evans, T. Biological function of activation-induced cytidine deaminase (AID). *Biomed. J.* **2014**, *37*, 269–283. [CrossRef]
154. Gehrke, J.M.; Cervantes, O.; Clement, M.K.; Wu, Y.; Zeng, J.; Bauer, D.E.; Pinello, L.; Joung, J.K. An APOBEC3A-Cas9 base editor with minimized bystander and off-target activities. *Nat. Biotechnol.* **2018**, *36*, 977–982. [CrossRef] [PubMed]

155. Zuo, E.; Sun, Y.; Yuan, T.; He, B.; Zhou, C.; Ying, W.; Liu, J.; Wei, W.; Zeng, R.; Li, Y.; et al. A rationally engineered cytosine base editor retains high on-target activity while reducing both DNA and RNA off-target effects. *Nat. Methods* **2020**, *17*, 600–604. [CrossRef] [PubMed]
156. Doman, J.L.; Raguram, A.; Newby, G.A.; Liu, D.R. Evaluation and minimization of Cas9-independent off-target DNA editing by cytosine base editors. *Nat. Biotechnol.* **2020**, *38*, 620–628. [CrossRef] [PubMed]
157. Kim, Y.B.; Komor, A.C.; Levy, J.M.; Packer, M.S.; Zhao, K.T.; Liu, D.R. Increasing the genome-targeting scope and precision of base editing with engineered Cas9-cytidine deaminase fusions. *Nat. Biotechnol.* **2017**, *35*, 371–376. [CrossRef]
158. Wang, L.; Xue, W.; Zhang, H.; Gao, R.; Qiu, H.; Wei, J.; Zhou, L.; Lei, Y.N.; Wu, X.; Li, X.; et al. Eliminating base-editor-induced genome-wide and transcriptome-wide off-target mutations. *Nat. Cell. Biol.* **2021**, *23*, 552–563. [CrossRef] [PubMed]
159. Neugebauer, M.E.; Hsu, A.; Arbab, M.; Krasnow, N.A.; McElroy, A.N.; Pandey, S.; Doman, J.L.; Huang, T.P.; Raguram, A.; Banskota, S.; et al. Evolution of an adenine base editor into a small, efficient cytosine base editor with low off-target activity. *Nat. Biotechnol.* **2023**, *41*, 673–685. [CrossRef] [PubMed]
160. Lam, D.K.; Feliciano, P.R.; Arif, A.; Bohnuud, T.; Fernandez, T.P.; Gehrke, J.M.; Grayson, P.; Lee, K.D.; Ortega, M.A.; Sawyer, C.; et al. Improved cytosine base editors generated from TadA variants. *Nat. Biotechnol.* **2023**, *41*, 686–697. [CrossRef]
161. Richter, M.F.; Zhao, K.T.; Eton, E.; Lapinaite, A.; Newby, G.A.; Thuronyi, B.W.; Wilson, C.; Koblan, L.W.; Zeng, J.; Bauer, D.E.; et al. Phage-assisted evolution of an adenine base editor with improved Cas domain compatibility and activity. *Nat. Biotechnol.* **2020**, *38*, 901. [CrossRef] [PubMed]
162. Li, J.A.; Yu, W.X.; Huang, S.S.; Wu, S.S.; Li, L.P.; Zhou, J.K.; Cao, Y.; Huang, X.X.; Qiao, Y.B. Structure-guided engineering of adenine base editor with minimized RNA off-targeting activity. *Nat. Commun.* **2021**, *12*, 2287. [CrossRef]
163. Chen, L.; Zhang, S.; Xue, N.; Hong, M.; Zhang, X.; Zhang, D.; Yang, J.; Bai, S.; Huang, Y.; Meng, H.; et al. Engineering a precise adenine base editor with minimal bystander editing. *Nat. Chem. Biol.* **2023**, *19*, 101–110. [CrossRef]
164. Tu, T.X.; Song, Z.M.; Liu, X.Y.; Wang, S.X.; He, X.X.; Xi, H.T.; Wang, J.H.; Yan, T.; Chen, H.R.; Zhang, Z.W.; et al. A precise and efficient adenine base editor. *Mol. Ther.* **2022**, *30*, 2933–2941. [CrossRef] [PubMed]
165. Park, J.C.; Jang, H.K.; Kim, J.; Han, J.H.; Jung, Y.; Kim, K.; Bae, S.; Cha, H.J. High expression of uracil DNA glycosylase determines C to T substitution in human pluripotent stem cells. *Mol. Ther. Nucleic Acids* **2022**, *27*, 175–183. [CrossRef]
166. Anzalone, A.V.; Randolph, P.B.; Davis, J.R.; Sousa, A.A.; Koblan, L.W.; Levy, J.M.; Chen, P.J.; Wilson, C.; Newby, G.A.; Raguram, A.; et al. Search-and-replace genome editing without double-strand breaks or donor DNA. *Nature* **2019**, *576*, 149–157. [CrossRef]
167. Chen, P.J.; Liu, D.R. Prime editing for precise and highly versatile genome manipulation. *Nat. Rev. Genet.* **2023**, *24*, 161–177. [CrossRef] [PubMed]
168. Chen, P.J.; Hussmann, J.A.; Yan, J.; Knipping, F.; Ravisankar, P.; Chen, P.F.; Chen, C.; Nelson, J.W.; Newby, G.A.; Sahin, M.; et al. Enhanced prime editing systems by manipulating cellular determinants of editing outcomes. *Cell* **2021**, *184*, 5635–5652.e29. [CrossRef] [PubMed]
169. Adikusuma, F.; Lushington, C.; Arudkumar, J.; Godahewa, G.I.; Chey, Y.C.J.; Gierus, L.; Piltz, S.; Geiger, A.; Jain, Y.; Reti, D.; et al. Optimized nickase- and nuclease-based prime editing in human and mouse cells. *Nucleic Acids Res.* **2021**, *49*, 10785–10795. [CrossRef] [PubMed]
170. Jiang, T.T.; Zhang, X.O.; Weng, Z.P.; Xue, W. Deletion and replacement of long genomic sequences using prime editing. *Nat. Biotechnol.* **2022**, *40*, 227–234. [CrossRef]
171. Tao, R.; Wang, Y.H.; Hu, Y.; Jiao, Y.G.; Zhou, L.F.; Jiang, L.R.; Li, L.; He, X.Y.; Li, M.; Yu, Y.M.; et al. WT-PE: Prime editing with nuclease wild-type Cas9 enables versatile large-scale genome editing. *Signal Transduct. Tar.* **2022**, *7*, 108. [CrossRef] [PubMed]
172. Li, X.; Zhang, G.; Huang, S.; Liu, Y.; Tang, J.; Zhong, M.; Wang, X.; Sun, W.; Yao, Y.; Ji, Q.; et al. Development of a versatile nuclease prime editor with upgraded precision. *Nat. Commun.* **2023**, *14*, 305. [CrossRef] [PubMed]
173. Song, M.; Lim, J.M.; Min, S.; Oh, J.S.; Kim, D.Y.; Woo, J.S.; Nishimasu, H.; Cho, S.R.; Yoon, S.; Kim, H.H. Generation of a more efficient prime editor 2 by addition of the Rad51 DNA-binding domain. *Nat. Commun.* **2021**, *12*, 5617. [CrossRef] [PubMed]
174. Park, S.J.; Jeong, T.Y.; Shin, S.K.; Yoon, D.E.; Lim, S.Y.; Kim, S.P.; Choi, J.; Lee, H.; Hong, J.I.; Ahn, J.; et al. Targeted mutagenesis in mouse cells and embryos using an enhanced prime editor. *Genome Biol.* **2021**, *22*, 170. [CrossRef] [PubMed]
175. Velimirovic, M.; Zanetti, L.C.; Shen, M.W.; Fife, J.D.; Lin, L.; Cha, M.; Akinci, E.; Barnum, D.; Yu, T.; Sherwood, R.I. Peptide fusion improves prime editing efficiency. *Nat. Commun.* **2022**, *13*, 3512. [CrossRef]
176. Nelson, J.W.; Randolph, P.B.; Shen, S.P.; Everette, K.A.; Chen, P.J.; Anzalone, A.V.; An, M.; Newby, G.A.; Chen, J.C.; Hsu, A.; et al. Engineered pegRNAs improve prime editing efficiency. *Nat. Biotechnol.* **2022**, *40*, 402–410. [CrossRef]
177. Chow, R.D.; Chen, J.S.; Shen, J.; Chen, S.D. A web tool for the design of prime-editing guide RNAs. *Nat. Biomed. Eng.* **2021**, *5*, 190–194. [CrossRef]
178. Hsu, J.Y.; Grunewald, J.; Szalay, R.; Shih, J.; Anzalone, A.V.; Lam, K.C.; Shen, M.W.; Petri, K.; Liu, D.R.; Joung, J.K.; et al. PrimeDesign software for rapid and simplified design of prime editing guide RNAs. *Nat. Commun.* **2021**, *12*, 1034. [CrossRef]
179. Hwang, G.H.; Jeong, Y.K.; Habib, O.; Hong, S.A.; Lim, K.; Kim, J.S.; Bae, S. PE-Designer and PE-Analyzer: Web-based design and analysis tools for CRISPR prime editing. *Nucleic Acids Res.* **2021**, *49*, W499–W504. [CrossRef]
180. Siegner, S.M.; Karasu, M.E.; Schroder, M.S.; Kontarakis, Z.; Corn, J.E. PnB Designer: A web application to design prime and base editor guide RNAs for animals and plants. *BMC Bioinform.* **2021**, *22*, 101. [CrossRef]
181. Anderson, M.V.; Haldrup, J.; Thomsen, E.A.; Wolff, J.H.; Mikkelsen, J.G. pegIT-a web-based design tool for prime editing. *Nucleic Acids Res.* **2021**, *49*, W505–W509. [CrossRef]

182. Yu, G.; Kim, H.K.; Park, J.; Kwak, H.; Cheong, Y.; Kim, D.; Kim, J.; Kim, J.; Kim, H.H. Prediction of efficiencies for diverse prime editing systems in multiple cell types. *Cell* **2023**, *186*, 2256–2272.e23. [CrossRef] [PubMed]
183. Li, X.; Zhou, L.; Gao, B.Q.; Li, G.; Wang, X.; Wang, Y.; Wei, J.; Han, W.; Wang, Z.; Li, J.; et al. Highly efficient prime editing by introducing same-sense mutations in pegRNA or stabilizing its structure. *Nat. Commun.* **2022**, *13*, 1669. [CrossRef] [PubMed]
184. Feng, Y.; Liu, S.; Mo, Q.; Liu, P.; Xiao, X.; Ma, H. Enhancing prime editing efficiency and flexibility with tethered and split pegRNAs. *Protein Cell* **2023**, *14*, 304–308. [CrossRef]
185. Liu, Y.; Yang, G.; Huang, S.; Li, X.; Wang, X.; Li, G.; Chi, T.; Chen, Y.; Huang, X.; Wang, X. Enhancing prime editing by Csy4-mediated processing of pegRNA. *Cell Res.* **2021**, *31*, 1134–1136. [CrossRef] [PubMed]
186. Zhang, G.; Liu, Y.; Huang, S.; Qu, S.; Cheng, D.; Yao, Y.; Ji, Q.; Wang, X.; Huang, X.; Liu, J. Enhancement of prime editing via xrRNA motif-joined pegRNA. *Nat. Commun.* **2022**, *13*, 1856. [CrossRef]
187. Huang, S.; Zhang, Z.; Tao, W.; Liu, Y.; Li, X.; Wang, X.; Harati, J.; Wang, P.Y.; Huang, X.; Lin, C.P. Broadening prime editing toolkits using RNA-Pol-II-driven engineered pegRNA. *Mol. Ther.* **2022**, *30*, 2923–2932. [CrossRef] [PubMed]
188. Habib, O.; Habib, G.; Hwang, G.H.; Bae, S. Comprehensive analysis of prime editing outcomes in human embryonic stem cells. *Nucleic Acids Res.* **2022**, *50*, 1187–1197. [CrossRef]
189. Zhou, M.; Tang, S.; Duan, N.; Xie, M.; Li, Z.; Feng, M.; Wu, L.; Hu, Z.; Liang, D. Targeted-Deletion of a Tiny Sequence via Prime Editing to Restore SMN Expression. *Int. J. Mol. Sci.* **2022**, *23*, 7941. [CrossRef] [PubMed]
190. Li, H.; Busquets, O.; Verma, Y.; Syed, K.M.; Kutnowski, N.; Pangilinan, G.R.; Gilbert, L.A.; Bateup, H.S.; Rio, D.C.; Hockemeyer, D.; et al. Highly efficient generation of isogenic pluripotent stem cell models using prime editing. *Elife* **2022**, *11*, e79208. [CrossRef] [PubMed]
191. Peters, J.E.; Makarova, K.S.; Shmakov, S.; Koonin, E.V. Recruitment of CRISPR-Cas systems by Tn7-like transposons. *Proc. Natl. Acad. Sci. USA* **2017**, *114*, E7358–E7366. [CrossRef] [PubMed]
192. Chavez, M.; Qi, L.S. Site-Programmable Transposition: Shifting the Paradigm for CRISPR-Cas Systems. *Mol. Cell* **2019**, *75*, 206–208. [CrossRef]
193. Strecker, J.; Ladha, A.; Gardner, Z.; Schmid-Burgk, J.L.; Makarova, K.S.; Koonin, E.V.; Zhang, F. RNA-guided DNA insertion with CRISPR-associated transposases. *Science* **2019**, *365*, 48–53. [CrossRef]
194. Tou, C.J.; Orr, B.; Kleinstiver, B.P. Precise cut-and-paste DNA insertion using engineered type V-K CRISPR-associated transposases. *Nat. Biotechnol.* **2023**, *41*, 968–979. [CrossRef] [PubMed]
195. Lampe, G.D.; King, R.T.; Halpin-Healy, T.S.; Klompe, S.E.; Hogan, M.I.; Vo, P.L.H.; Tang, S.; Chavez, A.; Sternberg, S.H. Targeted DNA integration in human cells without double-strand breaks using CRISPR-associated transposases. *Nat. Biotechnol.* **2023**, 1–12. [CrossRef]
196. Durrant, M.G.; Fanton, A.; Tycko, J.; Hinks, M.; Chandrasekaran, S.S.; Perry, N.T.; Schaepe, J.; Du, P.P.; Lotfy, P.; Bassik, M.C.; et al. Systematic discovery of recombinases for efficient integration of large DNA sequences into the human genome. *Nat. Biotechnol.* **2023**, *41*, 488–499. [CrossRef] [PubMed]
197. Anzalone, A.V.; Gao, X.D.; Podracky, C.J.; Nelson, A.T.; Koblan, L.W.; Raguram, A.; Levy, J.M.; Mercer, J.A.M.; Liu, D.R. Programmable deletion, replacement, integration and inversion of large DNA sequences with twin prime editing. *Nat. Biotechnol.* **2022**, *40*, 731–740. [CrossRef] [PubMed]
198. Yarnall, M.T.N.; Ioannidi, E.I.; Schmitt-Ulms, C.; Krajeski, R.N.; Lim, J.; Villiger, L.; Zhou, W.; Jiang, K.; Garushyants, S.K.; Roberts, N.; et al. Drag-and-drop genome insertion of large sequences without double-strand DNA cleavage using CRISPR-directed integrases. *Nat. Biotechnol.* **2023**, *41*, 500–512. [CrossRef] [PubMed]
199. Lampson, B.C.; Sun, J.; Hsu, M.Y.; Vallejo-Ramirez, J.; Inouye, S.; Inouye, M. Reverse transcriptase in a clinical strain of Escherichia coli: Production of branched RNA-linked msDNA. *Science* **1989**, *243*, 1033–1038. [CrossRef]
200. Hsu, M.Y.; Inouye, M.; Inouye, S. Retron for the 67-base multicopy single-stranded DNA from Escherichia coli: A potential transposable element encoding both reverse transcriptase and Dam methylase functions. *Proc. Natl. Acad. Sci. USA* **1990**, *87*, 9454–9458. [CrossRef]
201. Hsu, M.Y.; Eagle, S.G.; Inouye, M.; Inouye, S. Cell-free synthesis of the branched RNA-linked msDNA from retron-Ec67 of Escherichia coli. *J. Biol. Chem.* **1992**, *267*, 13823–13829. [CrossRef] [PubMed]
202. Linquist, S.; Cottenie, K.; Elliott, T.A.; Saylor, B.; Kremer, S.C.; Gregory, T.R. Applying ecological models to communities of genetic elements: The case of neutral theory. *Mol. Ecol.* **2015**, *24*, 3232–3242. [CrossRef]
203. Sharon, E.; Chen, S.A.; Khosla, N.M.; Smith, J.D.; Pritchard, J.K.; Fraser, H.B. Functional Genetic Variants Revealed by Massively Parallel Precise Genome Editing. *Cell* **2018**, *175*, 544–557.e16. [CrossRef] [PubMed]
204. Lopez, S.C.; Crawford, K.D.; Lear, S.K.; Bhattarai-Kline, S.; Shipman, S.L. Precise genome editing across kingdoms of life using retron-derived DNA. *Nat. Chem. Biol.* **2022**, *18*, 199–206. [CrossRef] [PubMed]
205. Kong, X.; Wang, Z.; Zhang, R.; Wang, X.; Zhou, Y.; Shi, L.; Yang, H. Precise genome editing without exogenous donor DNA via retron editing system in human cells. *Protein Cell* **2021**, *12*, 899–902. [CrossRef] [PubMed]
206. Allen, A.G.; Khan, S.Q.; Margulies, C.M.; Viswanathan, R.; Lele, S.; Blaha, L.; Scott, S.N.; Izzo, K.M.; Gerew, A.; Pattali, R.; et al. A highly efficient transgene knock-in technology in clinically relevant cell types. *Nat. Biotechnol.* **2023**, 1–12. [CrossRef] [PubMed]
207. Lin, S.; Staahl, B.T.; Alla, R.K.; Doudna, J.A. Enhanced homology-directed human genome engineering by controlled timing of CRISPR/Cas9 delivery. *eLife* **2014**, *3*, e04766. [CrossRef]

208. Li, M.; Zhong, A.; Wu, Y.; Sidharta, M.; Beaury, M.; Zhao, X.; Studer, L.; Zhou, T. Transient inhibition of p53 enhances prime editing and cytosine base-editing efficiencies in human pluripotent stem cells. *Nat. Commun.* **2022**, *13*, 6354. [CrossRef]
209. Zhang, Z.; Baxter, A.E.; Ren, D.; Qin, K.; Chen, Z.; Collins, S.M.; Huang, H.; Komar, C.A.; Bailer, P.F.; Parker, J.B.; et al. Efficient engineering of human and mouse primary cells using peptide-assisted genome editing. *Nat. Biotechnol.* **2023**, 1–11. [CrossRef]
210. Foss, D.V.; Muldoon, J.J.; Nguyen, D.N.; Carr, D.; Sahu, S.U.; Hunsinger, J.M.; Wyman, S.K.; Krishnappa, N.; Mendonsa, R.; Schanzer, E.V.; et al. Peptide-mediated delivery of CRISPR enzymes for the efficient editing of primary human lymphocytes. *Nat. Biomed. Eng.* **2023**, *7*, 647–660. [CrossRef]
211. Yu, C.; Liu, Y.; Ma, T.; Liu, K.; Xu, S.; Zhang, Y.; Liu, H.; La Russa, M.; Xie, M.; Ding, S.; et al. Small molecules enhance CRISPR genome editing in pluripotent stem cells. *Cell Stem Cell* **2015**, *16*, 142–147. [CrossRef]
212. Chu, V.T.; Weber, T.; Wefers, B.; Wurst, W.; Sander, S.; Rajewsky, K.; Kuhn, R. Increasing the efficiency of homology-directed repair for CRISPR-Cas9-induced precise gene editing in mammalian cells. *Nat. Biotechnol.* **2015**, *33*, 543–548. [CrossRef]
213. Maruyama, T.; Dougan, S.K.; Truttmann, M.C.; Bilate, A.M.; Ingram, J.R.; Ploegh, H.L. Increasing the efficiency of precise genome editing with CRISPR-Cas9 by inhibition of nonhomologous end joining. *Nat. Biotechnol.* **2015**, *33*, 538–542. [CrossRef]
214. Robert, F.; Barbeau, M.; Ethier, S.; Dostie, J.; Pelletier, J. Pharmacological inhibition of DNA-PK stimulates Cas9-mediated genome editing. *Genome Med.* **2015**, *7*, 93. [CrossRef]
215. Shin, H.R.; See, J.E.; Kweon, J.; Kim, H.S.; Sung, G.J.; Park, S.; Jang, A.H.; Jang, G.; Choi, K.C.; Kim, I.; et al. Small-molecule inhibitors of histone deacetylase improve CRISPR-based adenine base editing. *Nucleic Acids Res.* **2021**, *49*, 2390–2399. [CrossRef]
216. Perli, S.D.; Cui, C.H.; Lu, T.K. Continuous genetic recording with self-targeting CRISPR-Cas in human cells. *Science* **2016**, *353*, aag0511. [CrossRef]
217. Tang, W.; Liu, D.R. Rewritable multi-event analog recording in bacterial and mammalian cells. *Science* **2018**, *360*, aap8992. [CrossRef]
218. McKenna, A.; Findlay, G.M.; Gagnon, J.A.; Horwitz, M.S.; Schier, A.F.; Shendure, J. Whole-organism lineage tracing by combinatorial and cumulative genome editing. *Science* **2016**, *353*, aaf7907. [CrossRef]
219. Choi, J.; Chen, W.; Minkina, A.; Chardon, F.M.; Suiter, C.C.; Regalado, S.G.; Domcke, S.; Hamazaki, N.; Lee, C.; Martin, B.; et al. A time-resolved, multi-symbol molecular recorder via sequential genome editing. *Nature* **2022**, *608*, 98–107. [CrossRef]
220. Pausch, P.; Al-Shayeb, B.; Bisom-Rapp, E.; Tsuchida, C.A.; Li, Z.; Cress, B.F.; Knott, G.J.; Jacobsen, S.E.; Banfield, J.F.; Doudna, J.A. CRISPR-CasPhi from huge phages is a hypercompact genome editor. *Science* **2020**, *369*, 333–337. [CrossRef]
221. Li, Z.; Zhong, Z.; Wu, Z.; Pausch, P.; Al-Shayeb, B.; Amerasekera, J.; Doudna, J.A.; Jacobsen, S.E. Genome editing in plants using the compact editor CasPhi. *Proc. Natl. Acad. Sci. USA* **2023**, *120*, e2216822120. [CrossRef] [PubMed]
222. Al-Shayeb, B.; Skopintsev, P.; Soczek, K.M.; Stahl, E.C.; Li, Z.; Groover, E.; Smock, D.; Eggers, A.R.; Pausch, P.; Cress, B.F.; et al. Diverse virus-encoded CRISPR-Cas systems include streamlined genome editors. *Cell* **2022**, *185*, 4574–4586.e16. [CrossRef] [PubMed]
223. Karvelis, T.; Druteika, G.; Bigelyte, G.; Budre, K.; Zedaveinyte, R.; Silanskas, A.; Kazlauskas, D.; Venclovas, C.; Siksnys, V. Transposon-associated TnpB is a programmable RNA-guided DNA endonuclease. *Nature* **2021**, *599*, 692–696. [CrossRef]
224. Altae-Tran, H.; Kannan, S.; Demircioglu, F.E.; Oshiro, R.; Nety, S.P.; McKay, L.J.; Dlakic, M.; Inskeep, W.P.; Makarova, K.S.; Macrae, R.K.; et al. The widespread IS200/IS605 transposon family encodes diverse programmable RNA-guided endonucleases. *Science* **2021**, *374*, 57–65. [CrossRef] [PubMed]
225. Sasnauskas, G.; Tamulaitiene, G.; Druteika, G.; Carabias, A.; Silanskas, A.; Kazlauskas, D.; Venclovas, C.; Montoya, G.; Karvelis, T.; Siksnys, V. TnpB structure reveals minimal functional core of Cas12 nuclease family. *Nature* **2023**, *616*, 384–389. [CrossRef] [PubMed]
226. Han, D.; Xiao, Q.; Wang, Y.; Zhang, H.; Dong, X.; Li, G.; Kong, X.; Wang, S.; Song, J.; Zhang, W.; et al. Development of miniature base editors using engineered IscB nickase. *Nat. Methods* **2023**, *20*, 1029–1036. [CrossRef]
227. Saito, M.; Xu, P.; Faure, G.; Maguire, S.; Kannan, S.; Altae-Tran, H.; Vo, S.; Desimone, A.; Macrae, R.K.; Zhang, F. Fanzor is a eukaryotic programmable RNA-guided endonuclease. *Nature* **2023**, 1–3. [CrossRef] [PubMed]
228. Jiang, K.; Lim, J.; Sgrizzi, S.; Trinh, M.; Kayabolen, A.; Yutin, N.; Koonin, E.V.; Abudayyeh, O.O.; Gootenberg, J.S. Programmable RNA-guided endonucleases are widespread in eukaryotes and their viruses. *bioRxiv* **2023**. [CrossRef]
229. Wilkinson, M.E.; Frangieh, C.J.; Macrae, R.K.; Zhang, F. Structure of the R2 non-LTR retrotransposon initiating target-primed reverse transcription. *Science* **2023**, *380*, 301–308. [CrossRef]

Disclaimer/Publisher's Note: The statements, opinions and data contained in all publications are solely those of the individual author(s) and contributor(s) and not of MDPI and/or the editor(s). MDPI and/or the editor(s) disclaim responsibility for any injury to people or property resulting from any ideas, methods, instructions or products referred to in the content.

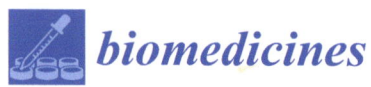
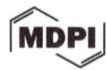

Article

Detection of ER Stress in iPSC-Derived Neurons Carrying the p.N370S Mutation in the *GBA1* Gene

Elena S. Yarkova [1,2,†], Elena V. Grigor'eva [1,*,†], Sergey P. Medvedev [1], Denis A. Tarasevich [1,2], Sophia V. Pavlova [1], Kamila R. Valetdinova [1], Julia M. Minina [1], Suren M. Zakian [1] and Anastasia A. Malakhova [1]

[1] Institute of Cytology and Genetics, Siberian Branch of Russian Academy of Sciences, Novosibirsk 630090, Russia; e.drozdova2@g.nsu.ru (E.S.Y.); medvedev@bionet.nsc.ru (S.P.M.); d.tarasevich1@g.nsu.ru (D.A.T.); spav@bionet.nsc.ru (S.V.P.); kamila23@list.ru (K.R.V.); minina_jul@bionet.nsc.ru (J.M.M.); zakian@bionet.nsc.ru (S.M.Z.); amal@bionet.nsc.ru (A.A.M.)

[2] Department of Natural Sciences, Novosibirsk State University, Novosibirsk 630090, Russia

* Correspondence: evlena@bionet.nsc.ru

† These authors contributed equally to this work.

Abstract: Endoplasmic reticulum (ER) stress is involved in the pathogenesis of many human diseases, such as cancer, type 2 diabetes, kidney disease, atherosclerosis and neurodegenerative diseases, in particular Parkinson's disease (PD). Since there is currently no treatment for PD, a better understanding of the molecular mechanisms underlying its pathogenesis, including the mechanisms of the switch from adaptation in the form of unfolded protein response (UPR) to apoptosis under ER stress conditions, may help in the search for treatment methods. Genetically encoded biosensors based on fluorescent proteins are suitable tools that facilitate the study of living cells and visualization of molecular events in real time. The combination of technologies to generate patient-specific iPSC lines and genetically encoded biosensors allows the creation of cell models with new properties. Using CRISPR-Cas9-mediated homologous recombination at the *AAVS1* locus of iPSC with the genetic variant p.N370S (rs76763715) in the *GBA1* gene, we created a cell model designed to study the activation conditions of the IRE1-XBP1 cascade of the UPR system. The cell lines obtained have a doxycycline-dependent expression of the genetically encoded biosensor XBP1-TagRFP, possess all the properties of human pluripotent cells, and can be used to test physical conditions and chemical compounds that affect the development of ER stress, the functioning of the UPR system, and in particular, the IRE1-XBP1 cascade.

Keywords: induced pluripotent stem cells; Parkinson's disease; *GBA1*; endoplasmic reticulum; ER stress; biosensors; CRISPR/Cas9

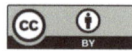

1. Introduction

The maintenance of protein homeostasis, or proteostasis, is one of the foundations of the normal functioning of a living cell. Dysregulation of proteostasis, in particular improper folding and pathological aggregation of protein molecules, leads to the development of many pathologies, including a variety of neurodegenerative diseases such as Alzheimer's, Huntington's or Parkinson's [1]. The accumulation of misfolded proteins in the lumen of the endoplasmic reticulum (ER) leads to the development of ER stress, which is directly linked to the signaling cascades that implement the programmed cell death, apoptosis. In response to ER stress, the unfolded protein response (UPR) system is activated. The UPR can contribute to an increase in chaperone activity and a decrease in protein synthesis. This mechanism is represented by proteins anchored in the ER membranes—PERK, IRE1 and ATF6 [2]. The study of ER function under normal and stress conditions is an urgent task in the study of molecular genetic mechanisms of various diseases pathogenesis. Currently, the main methods used to study ER stress and the UPR are methods that require the use of fixed cells or their lysates—immunocytochemical studies of marker protein expression, Western blot analysis or quantitative PCR [3,4]. Meanwhile, the tool set for in vivo studies of cellular physiology and biochemistry is very limited. Genetically encoded biosensors have been demonstrated to be a reliable alternative or additional method for analyzing various cellular processes and determining the concentration of different analytes. There are biosensors available for detecting oxidative stress [5–9], mitochondrial stress [10], apoptosis [11–14], and intracellular Ca^{2+} levels [15–17], among others. Experimental data also confirm the use of fluorescent biosensors for visualizing UPR in vitro and in vivo. These sensors detect mRNA splicing of the *XBP1* gene by the IRE1a protein or the relocation of the ATF6a protein from the ER to the cell nucleus [18,19].

Genetically encoded biosensors can be applied to various living systems, including cell cultures or animal models. One of the most promising systems for the application of protein biosensors are cellular disease models based on human-induced pluripotent stem cells (iPSCs) and their differentiated derivatives. Models of neurodegenerative diseases, such as Parkinson's disease, are particularly amenable to this approach. In cell models of Parkinson's disease, specifically those caused by the p.N370S variant in the *GBA1* gene, ER stress has been shown to actively manifest and cause dysfunction of patient-specific neurons [20]. In certain cases, such as with increased alpha-synuclein expression caused by triplications of the *SNCA* gene, UPR activity may be suppressed [21]. In both scenarios, UPR is a promising therapeutic target. This work presents the creation of a test model based on iPSC with the genetic variant p.N370S (rs76763715) in the *GBA1* gene (iPSC-GBA). The model was developed to study ER stress, which is the accumulation of denatured forms of proteins. To visualize the activation of the IRE1-XBP1 cascade and stress-dependent splicing of *XBP1* mRNA, a genetically encoded biosensor, XBP1-TagRFP, was used [18,22]. iPSCs carrying the XBP1-TagRFP biosensor transgene can be used to study the lifetime of UPR functioning in iPSC-derived dopaminergic (DA) neurons. They can also be used for screening small-molecule compounds aimed at modulating UPR activity.

2. Materials and Methods

2.1. Materials

The study utilized iPSCs derived from patients with the pathogenic mutation N370S in the *GBA1* gene, as well as iPSCs from healthy donors and iPSCs with an ER stress biosensor. Table 1 presents the data on the iPSC lines.

Table 1. Data on the iPSC lines used in the work.

iPSC Line Name (hPSCreg)	Alternative Name for iPSC Line	hPSCreg URL (All Accessed on 5 February 2024)	Genotype	Genetic Modifications	References
ICGi034-D	PD30-1	https://hpscreg.eu/cell-line/ICGi034-D	*GBA1* (c.1226A>G, p.N370S, rs76763715)	No	This study
ICGi034-E	PD30-3	https://hpscreg.eu/cell-line/ICGi034-E	*GBA1* (c.1226A>G, p.N370S, rs76763715)	No	This study
ICGi034-A	PD30-4-7	https://hpscreg.eu/cell-line/ICGi034-A	*GBA1* (c.1226A>G, p.N370S, rs76763715)	No	[23]
ICGi039-A	PD31-6	https://hpscreg.eu/cell-line/ICGi039-A	*GBA1* (c.1226A>G, p.N370S, rs76763715)	No	[24]
ICGi039-B	PD31-7	https://hpscreg.eu/cell-line/ICGi039-B	*GBA1* (c.1226A>G, p.N370S, rs76763715)	No	[24]
ICGi039-C	PD31-15	https://hpscreg.eu/cell-line/ICGi039-C	*GBA1* (c.1226A>G, p.N370S, rs76763715)	No	[24]
ICGi022-B	K7-2Lf	https://hpscreg.eu/cell-line/ICGi022-B	Healthy	No	This study
ICGi022-A	K7-4Lf	https://hpscreg.eu/cell-line/ICGi022-A	Healthy	No	[25]
ICGi021-A	K6-4f	https://hpscreg.eu/cell-line/ICGi021-A	Healthy	No	[25]
ICGi034-A-1	PD30-XBP-RFP-6	https://hpscreg.eu/cell-line/ICGi034-A-1	*GBA1* (c.1226A>G, p.N370S, rs76763715)	AAVS1 locus: pXBP1-TagRFP-ERSS, AAVS1-Neo-M2rtTA	This study
ICGi034-A-2	PD30-XBP-RFP-51	https://hpscreg.eu/cell-line/ICGi034-A-2	*GBA1* (c.1226A>G, p.N370S, rs76763715)	AAVS1 locus: pXBP1-TagRFP-ERSS, AAVS1-Neo-M2rtTA	This study
ICGi034-A-3	PD30-XBP-RFP-52	https://hpscreg.eu/cell-line/ICGi034-A-3	*GBA1* (c.1226A>G, p.N370S, rs76763715)	AAVS1 locus: pXBP1-TagRFP-ERSS, AAVS1-Neo-M2rtTA	This study

Table 1. *Cont.*

iPSC Line Name (hPSCreg)	Alternative Name for iPSC Line	hPSCreg URL (All Accessed on 5 February 2024)	Genotype	Genetic Modifications	References
ICGi034-A-4	PD30-XBP-RFP-86	https://hpscreg.eu/cell-line/ICGi034-A-4	GBA1 (c.1226A>G, p.N370S, rs76763715)	AAVS1 locus: pXBP1-TagRFP-ERSS, AAVS1-Neo-M2rtTA	This study
ICGi021-A-6	K6-XBP-RFP-62	https://hpscreg.eu/user/cellline/edit/ICGi021-A-6	Healthy	AAVS1 locus: pXBP1-TagRFP-ERSS, AAVS1-Neo-M2rtTA	This study
ICGi021-A-7	K6-XBP-RFP-68	https://hpscreg.eu/user/cellline/edit/ICGi021-A-7	Healthy	AAVS1 locus: pXBP1-TagRFP-ERSS, AAVS1-Neo-M2rtTA	This study

2.2. Isolation of Human Peripheral Blood Mononuclear Cells (PBMCs)

The research was approved by the Ethical Committee of the Federal Neurosurgical Center (Novosibirsk, Russia), protocol No. 1, dated 14 March 2017. Blood samples from patients and healthy donors were provided by the Federal Neurosurgical Center. All subjects signed the informed consent and information sheet.

Isolation and cultivation of mononuclear cells (PBMCs) was carried out according to the previously described technique [24]. Briefly, the blood was layered on a ficoll (Sigma-Aldrich, Darmstadt, Germany), centrifuged for 30 min at $400\times g$, interphase containing PBMCs was collected. PBMCs were washed twice with 10 mL of PBS.

Cultivation of 5×10^6 PBMCs 5 days before reprogramming was carried out in D35 mm Petri dishes on StemPro-34+ medium with the following composition: StemPro-34 Medium, Supplement StemPro-34, 1% penicillin-streptomycin (all Thermo Fisher Scientific, Waltham, MA, USA), 100 ng/mL SCF, 50 ng/mL IL-3, 40 ng/mL IGFI, 25 ng/mL GM-CSF (all SCI Store, Moscow, Russia), erythropoietin 3.6 µL/mL (PeproTech, Cranbury, NJ, USA), Dexamethasone 1 µm (Sigma-Aldrich, Darmstadt, Germany).

2.3. Obtaining and Cultivation of Induced Pluripotent Stem Cells (iPSCs)

IPSC was obtained using previously published methods [24]. PBMCs transfection was performed by electroporation using a Neon Transfection System device (Thermo Fisher Scientific, Waltham, MA, USA) with the following program: 1650 V, 10 ms, 3 pulses. Episomal vectors encoding *OCT4*, *KLF4*, *L-MYC*, *SOX2*, *LIN28*, and *mp53DD* (0.5 µg each; Addgene IDs #41813-14, #41855-57) were used [26]. Transfected cells were plated onto feeder layer of mitotically inactivated mouse embryonic fibroblasts (MEF) in StemPro-34+ medium with gradual addition of N2B27 from day 1 to day 8. On day 9, the medium was changed to iPSCs-medium containing KnockOut DMEM, 15% KnockOut SR, 2 mM GlutaMAX-I, 0.1 mM NEAA, 100 U/mL penicillin-streptomycin (all Thermo Fisher Scientific, Waltham, MA, USA), 0.1 mM 2-mce (Sigma-Aldrich, Darmstadt, Germany), and 10 ng/mL bFGF (SCI Store, Moscow, Russia).

The iPSC lines were cultured on a feeder monolayer of mitotically inactivated MEF using iPSCs-medium. Feeder cells were obtained by treating 3rd passage MEF with 10 µg/mL mitomycin C (Sigma-Aldrich, Darmstadt, Germany) for 2 h. The cells were cultured at 37 °C in a CO_2 incubator in a humid atmosphere containing 5% carbon dioxide, and the iPSCs-medium was changed daily.

The iPSC cells were passaged every 3–6 days using TrypLE Express (Thermo Fisher Scientific, Waltham, MA, USA) at a ratio of 1:10. Two µM thiazovivin was added to the transplanted cells for 24 h (ROCK inhibitor, Sigma-Aldrich, Darmstadt, Germany).

2.4. Karyotyping and G-Banding

Cells were expanded to a monolayer and seeded into 4 wells of a 12-well plate coated with Matrigel-GFR extracellular matrix (Corning, New York, NY, USA). Cells were cultured for 48–72 h, depending on the rate of cell proliferation. Two and a half h before fixation, the medium was changed to fresh medium, 3 µg/mL EtBr and 50 ng/mL colcemid were added, and the cells were left in a CO_2 incubator at 37 °C. Cells were then plated into tubes using TrypLE Express and centrifuged at 1300 rpm for 5 min. The cells were hypotonicized with 0.075 M KCl for 20 min at 37 °C, after which a few drops of Carnoy's solution (3 parts methanol, 1 part glacial acetic acid) were added, mixed, and the cells were centrifuged for 5 min at 1300 rpm. Cells were fixed by adding fresh Carnoy's solution to the supernatant for 15 min on ice. The cells were then centrifuged for 5 min at 1300 rpm, the Carnoy's solution was changed twice, and 70–80 µL of the cell suspension was dropped onto wet cooled slides from a height of 10–20 cm. The slides are dried at room temperature.

For chromosome G-banding, samples were stained with DAPI (4,6-diamino-2-phenylindole) solution (200 ng/mL, in 2xSSC) for 5 min. The slides were then rinsed in 2xSSC buffer and water. After air drying, 7–10 µL antifade (Vector, Burlingame, CA, USA) was applied under a coverslip.

Karyotype analysis was performed using an Axioplan 2 microscope (Zeiss, Oberkochen, Germany) equipped with a CV-M300 CCD camera (JAI Corp., Yokohama, Japan) at the Core Facility of Microscopic Analysis of Biological Objects at the Institute of Cytology and Genetics, SB RAS. ISIS 5 software (MetaSystems Group, Inc., Medford, MA, USA) was used for metaphase processing and chromosome folding.

2.5. Spontaneous Differentiation of iPSCs

Spontaneous differentiation of iPSCs was performed according to a previously published method [24]. Briefly, iPSCs were detached from the substrate using 0.15% collagenase IV (Thermo Fisher Scientific, Waltham, MA, USA) and seeded on 1% agarose in iPSCs medium without bFGF for 9–10 days. Embryoid cells were then seeded on Chambered Coverglass 8-well plates (Thermo Fisher Scientific, Waltham, MA, USA) pretreated with Matrigel-ESQ and cultured for another 7–9 days. Immunofluorescence analysis was then performed.

2.6. Immunofluorescence Analysis

Immunofluorescence staining was performed according to a previously published method [24]. Briefly, cells were fixed with 4% PFA (Sigma-Aldrich, Darmstadt, Germany), permeabilized with 0.5% Triton-X (Thermo Fisher Scientific, Waltham, MA, USA) for 30 min, and non-specific antibody binding was blocked with 1% BSA (Sigma-Aldrich, Darmstadt, Germany). Primary antibodies were incubated overnight at +4 °C, washed twice with PBS, and secondary antibodies were added for 1.5 h at room temperature. After two washes with PBS, the nuclei were stained with DAPI. All antibodies used in this work are summarized in Table 2.

Table 2. Reagents details.

	Antibodies Used for Immunocytochemistry		
	Antibody	Dilution	Company Cat. # and RRID
Pluripotency Markers	Rabbit IgG2b anti-OCT4	1:200	Abcam Cat. # ab18976, RRID:AB_444714
	Mouse IgG3 anti-SSEA4	1:200	Abcam Cat. # ab16287, RRID:AB_778073
	Mouse IgM anti-TRA-1-60	1:200	Abcam Cat. # ab16288, RRID:AB_778563
	Rabbit IgG anti-SOX2	1:500	Cell Signaling Cat. # 3579, RRID:AB_2195767
Differentiation Markers	Mouse IgG2a anti-αSMA	1:100	Dako Cat. # M0851, RRID:AB_2223500
	Mouse IgG2a anti-AFP	1:250	Sigma Cat. # A8452, RRID:AB_258392
	Mouse IgG2a anti-Tubulin β 3 (TUBB3)/Clone: TUJ1	1:1000	BioLegend Cat. # 801,201, RRID:AB_2313773

Table 2. Cont.

	Antibodies Used for Immunocytochemistry		
	Antibody	Dilution	Company Cat. # and RRID
	Rabbit IgG anti-NF200	1:1000	Sigma Cat. # N4142, RRID:AB_477272
	Mouse IgG1 anti-HNF3b (FOXA2)	1:50	Santa Cruz Biotechnology Cat. # sc-374,376, RRID:AB_10989742
	Goat IgG polyclonal anti-OTX2	1:400	R&D systems Cat. # AF1979, RRID:AB_2157172
	Rabbit IgG anti-TH	1:400	Millipore Cat. # AB152, RRID:AB_390204
	Rabbit IgG anti-LMX1A	1:50	Abcam Cat. # ab139726, RRID:AB_2827684
	CD29 (Integrin beta 1) Monoclonal Antibody (TS2/16)	1:100	Thermo Fisher Scientific Cat. # 14-0299-82, RRID:AB_1210468
	Mouse IgG1 anti-CK18	1:200	Millipore Cat. # MAB3234, RRID:AB_94763
Secondary antibodies	Goat anti-Mouse IgG (H + L) Secondary Antibody, Alexa Fluor 488	1:400	Thermo Fisher Scientific Cat. # A11029, RRID:AB_2534088
	Goat anti-Mouse IgG (H + L) Secondary Antibody, Alexa Fluor 568	1:400	Thermo Fisher Scientific Cat. # A11031, RRID:AB_144696
	Goat anti-Rabbit IgG (H + L) Highly Cross-Adsorbed Secondary Antibody, Alexa Fluor 488	1:400	Thermo Fisher Scientific Cat. # A11008, RRID:AB_143165
	Goat anti-Rabbit IgG (H + L) Secondary Antibody, Alexa Fluor 568	1:400	Thermo Fisher Scientific Cat. # A11011, RRID:AB_143157
	Goat anti-Mouse IgG1 Secondary Antibody, Alexa Fluor 568	1:400	Thermo Fisher Scientific Cat. # A21124, RRID:AB_2535766
	Goat anti-Mouse IgG3 Cross-Adsorbed Secondary Antibody, Alexa Fluor 488	1:400	Thermo Fisher Scientific Cat. # A21151, RRID: AB_2535784
	Goat anti-Mouse IgG1 Adsorbed Secondary Antibody, Alexa Fluor 488	1:400	Thermo Fisher Scientific Cat. # A21121, RRID: AB_2535764
	Goat anti-Mouse IgG3 Cross-Adsorbed Secondary Antibody, Alexa Fluor 488	1:400	Thermo Fisher Scientific Cat. # A21151, RRID:AB_2535784
	Goat anti-Mouse IgG2a Cross-Adsorbed Secondary Antibody, Alexa Fluor 568	1:400	Thermo Fisher Scientific Cat. # A21134, RRID:AB_2535773
	Goat anti-Mouse IgG2b Cross-Adsorbed Secondary Antibody, Alexa Fluor 568	1:400	Thermo Fisher Scientific Cat. # A21144, RRID:AB_2535780
	Goat anti-Mouse IgG2a Secondary Antibody, Alexa Fluor 488	1:400	Thermo Fisher Scientific Cat. # A21131, RRID:AB_2535771
	Primers		
	Target	Size of band	Forward/Reverse primer (5'-3')
Mycoplasma detection	16S ribosomal RNA gene	280 bp	GGGAGCAAACAGGATTAGATACCCT/ TGCACCATCTGTCACTCTGTTAACCTC
Targeted mutation analysis	GBA1	600 bp	CTGTTGCTACCTAGTCACTTCC/ CCCTATCTTCCCTTTCCTTCAC
Housekeeping gene (RT-qPCR)	B2M	90 bp	TAGCTGTGCTCGCGCTACT/ TCTCTGCTGGATGACGTGAG
	GAPDH	202 bp	TGTTGCCATCAATGACCCCTT/ CTCCACGACGTACTCAGCG
	ACTB	93 bp	GCACAGAGCCTCGCCTT/ GTTGTCGACGACGAGCG
Pluripotency marker (RT-qPCR)	NANOG	116 bp	TTTGTGGGCCTGAAGAAAACT/ AGGGCTGTCCTGAATAAGCAG
	OCT4	94 bp	CTTCTGCTTCAGGAGCTTGG/ GAAGGAGAAGCTGGAGCAAA
	SOX2	100 bp	GCTTAGCCTCGTCGATGAAC/ AACCCCAAGATGCACAACTC

Table 2. Cont.

	Antibodies Used for Immunocytochemistry		
	Antibody	Dilution	Company Cat. # and RRID
Neural differentiation markers (RT-qPCR)	LMX1A	150 bp	CAGCCTCAGACTCAGGTAAAAGTG/ TGAATGCTCGCCTCTGTTGA
	OTX2	82 bp	GGGTATGGACTTGCTGCAC/ CCGAGTGAACGTCGTCCT
	SOX6	76 bp	GCTTCTGGACTCAGCCCTTTA/ GGCCCTTTAGCCTTTGGTTA
	TH	125 bp	TCATCACCTGGTCACCAAGTT/ GGTCGCCGTGCCTGTACT
Gene expression analysis (RT-qPCR)	GBA1 [27]	160 bp	TCCAGGTCGTTCTTCTGACT/ ATTGGGTGCGTAACTTTGTC
	XBP1s [28]	231 bp	TCTGCTGAGTCCGCAGCAG/ GAAAAGGGAGGCTGGTAAGGAAC
	CHOP [28]	90 bp	AGCGACAGAGCCAAAATCAG/ TCTGCTTTCAGGTGTGGTGA
Gene expression analysis (RT-PCR)	XBP1 [29]	283 bp/ 257 bp	TTACGAGAGAAAACTCATGGC/ GGGTCCAAGTTGTCCAGAATGC
Detection of the wild-type AAVS1 allele	AAVS1	555 bp	CTCTGGCTCCATCGTAAGCAA/ CCCAAAGTACCCCGTCTCCC
Integration of the M2rtTA transgene into the AAVS1 locus	AAVS1-M2rtTA	1024 bp	CCGGACCACTTTGAGCTCTAC/ GCCCAGTCATAGCCGAATAG
Integration of the XBP1-TagRFP transgene into the AAVS1 locus	AAVS1-XBP1-TagRFP	1022 bp	CCGGACCACTTTGAGCTCTAC/ AGGCGCACCGTGGGCTTGTAC
Off-target integration of the AAVS1-Neo-M2rtTA plasmid into the genome	AAVS1-Neo-M2rtTA	1063 bp	CAGGAAACAGCTATGAC/ GCCCAGTCATAGCCGAATAG
Off-target integration of the pXBP1-TagRFP-ERSS-donor plasmid into the genome	pXBP1-TagRFP-ERSS-donor	1007 bp	CAGGAAACAGCTATGAC/ GCCCAGTCATAGCCGAATAG

Cell fluorescence was captured using a Nikon Eclipse Ti-E inverted fluorescence microscope (Nikon, Tokyo, Japan) and NIS Elements software Advanced Research version 4.30.

2.7. Directed Differentiation into Midbrain Neural Derivatives

Midbrain neural derivatives of iPSCs were obtained according to a previously published protocol [30] with modifications described in [24]. Briefly, for differentiation, iPSCs were plated on Matrigel-GFR coated plates and grown to 80–90% density for 24 h in Essential 8 medium (Thermo Fisher Scientific, Waltham, MA, USA). After 24 h, the medium was replaced with neural differentiation medium containing F12/DMEM:Neurobasal (1:1), $0.5\times$ N-2 supplement, $0.5\times$ B-27 supplement without vitamin A, 0.2 mM GlutaMAX™, 100 U/mL penicillin-streptomycin (all from Thermo Fisher Scientific, Waltham, MA, USA), and 200 µM ascorbic acid (Sigma-Aldrich, Darmstadt, Germany). Factors were then added:

100 ng/mL LDN193189 hydrochloride (LDN, Sigma-Aldrich, Darmstadt, Germany) from day 0 to day 11 of differentiation; 8µM SB431542 (SB, Abcam, Cambridge, UK) from day 0 to day 5; 2 µM purmorphamin (Tocris, Ellisville, MO, USA), 100 ng/mL SHH (C25II, PeproTech, Cranbury, NJ, USA) and 100 ng/mL FGF8b (PeproTech, Cranbury, NJ, USA) from day 1 to day 7; 3 µM CHIR99021 (Sigma-Aldrich, Darmstadt, Germany) from day 3 to day 13; 20 ng/mL BDNF (PeproTech, Cranbury, NJ, USA), 20 ng/mL GDNF (PeproTech, Cranbury, NJ, USA), 1 ng/mL TGFb3 (PeproTech, Cranbury, NJ, USA), 0. 5 mM dbcAMP (PeproTech, Cranbury, NJ, USA) from day 13. Compound E (0.1 µM) (Millipore, Burlington, VT, USA) was added at terminal differentiation.

Cell passaging was performed at days 11, 18 and 25 of differentiation using StemPro™ Accutase™ (Thermo Fisher Scientific, Waltham, MA, USA). Cells were seeded at a 1:2 ratio on Matrigel-ESQ with ROCK inhibitor.

2.8. Qualitative and Quantitative Polymerase Chain Reactions

Genomic DNA was extracted from iPSC using QuickExtract™ DNA Extraction Solution (Lucigen, Madison, WI, USA). PCR was performed using BioMaster HS-Taq PCR-Color (2×) (Biolabmix, Novosibirsk, Russia) and primers (Table 2) in a T100 Thermal Cycler Amplifier (Bio-Rad Laboratories, Singapore).

Program used to verify XBP1-TagRFP biosensor incorporation: 95 °C, 5 min; 35 cycles: 95 °C, 30 s, 62 °C (for detection of wild-type *AAVS1* allele: 64 °C), 30 s, 72 °C, 30 s.

Mycoplasma detection program: 95 °C, 5 min; 35 cycles: 95 °C, 15 s, 60 °C, 15 s, 72 °C, 20 s.

For RNA isolation, midbrain neural derivatives growing on a 35 mm Petri dish were harvested at day 55–60 after the onset of differentiation. Cells were lysed in 1 mL TRIzol reagent (Ambion by Life Technologies, Carlsbad, CA, USA) and RNA was isolated as described in the manufacturer's protocol. Reverse transcription of 1 µg RNA was performed using SuperScript III Reverse Transcriptase (Thermo Fisher Scientific, Waltham, MA, USA) according to the manufacturer's protocol.

Quantitative PCR (qPCR) was run on a LightCycler 480 II system (Roche, Basel, Switzerland) using BioMaster HS-qPCR SYBR Blue 2× (Biolabmix, Novosibirsk, Russia) according to the following program: 95 °C 5 min; 40 cycles: 95 °C 10 s, 62 °C 45 s.

When analyzing the expression of pluripotency markers, CT values were normalized to beta-2-microglobulin (B2M) (Table 2), and the results were processed using the ∆CT method.

When analyzing the expression of specific markers of differentiation in the culture of neural derivatives, the CT value was normalized to the geometric mean of three reference genes—*GAPDH*, *B2M* and *ACTB* (Table 2)—selected using the geNorm mathematical algorithm [31], embedded in the qbase+ program interface. The program allows to rank genes according to the stability of their expression, from the least stable to the most stable. The program is in the public domain: (https://cellcarta.com/genomic-data-analysis, accessed on 5 February 2024).

2.9. Sanger Sequencing

Sanger sequencing (Table 2) was used to confirm the mutation in the *GBA1* gene in PBMCs and iPSC lines obtained from the patients and healthy donor. PCR reactions were run on a T100 Thermal Cycler (Bio-Rad Laboratories, Singapore) using BioMaster HS-Taq PCR-Color (2×) (Biolabmix, Novosibirsk, Russia) with the following program: 95 °C for 3 min; 35 cycles: 95 °C for 30 s; 60 °C for 30 s; 72 °C for 30 s; and 72 °C for 5 min. Sanger sequencing reactions were performed using BigDye Terminator V. 3.1. Cycle Sequencing Kit (Applied Biosystems, Austin, TX, USA) and analyzed on ABI 3130XL Genetic Analyzer at the SB RAS Genomics Core Facility (http://www.niboch.nsc.ru/doku.php/corefacility, accessed on 5 February 2024).

2.10. Generation of Transgenic iPSCs

The donor plasmid AAVS1-Neo-M2rtTA, which encodes a reverse transactivator for doxycycline-controlled expression and a neomycin resistance gene (Addgene plasmid #60843; http://n2t.net/addgene:60843, accessed on 21 March 2024; RRID: Addgene_60843) [32], pXBP1-TagRFP-ERSS-donor (Supplementary Figure S1) with puromycin resistance gene [33], and pX458-AAVS1 with Cas9 nuclease and AAVS1 sgRNA (based on pSpCas9(BB)-2A-GFP (Addgene plasmid #48138; http://n2t.net/addgene:48138, accessed on 21 March 2024; RRID: Addgene_48138) [34] was electroporated using the Neon Transfection System 100 µL kit according to the instructions with the program 1100 V, 30 ms, 1 pulse. A total of 4–5 × 10^5 cells and 1.6 µg of each plasmid were used per 100 µL transfection reaction: After electroporation, cells were transferred to a layer of mitotically inactivated MEF in antibiotic-free iPSC culture medium in the presence of 2 µM thiazovivin. Forty-eight hours after transfection, 50 µg/mL geneticin (G418) sulfate (Santa Cruz Biotechnology, Dallas, TX, USA) was added for 72 h in culture medium without penicillin-streptomycin. Twenty-four hours after G418 withdrawal, cells were selected for resistance to 200 ng/mL puromycin (Santa Cruz Biotechnology, Dallas, TX, USA) for 3–4 days. After selection, surviving colonies were mechanically transferred to 48-well plates. Transgene integration was analyzed by PCR using primers (Table 2) as previously described [35].

2.11. Verifying the Performance of the XBP1-TagRFP Biosensor under ER Stress

Activation of the XBP1-TagRFP biosensor was performed by adding 2 µg/mL doxycycline (Santa Cruz Biotechnology, Dallas, TX, USA) to the medium for two days. ER stress was induced by adding 5–10 µg/mL tunicamycin (Abcam, Cambridge, UK) to the medium for one day. Images were taken using a Nikon Eclipse Ti-E microscope (Nikon, Tokyo, Japan) and NIS Elements software Advanced Research version 4.30.

2.12. Statistical Processing

Statistical analysis and construction of scatter plots were performed using R statistics 4.0.3 program. Median values were compared using the Wilcoxon signed-rank test. The significance level was set at $p < 0.05$. Graphs showing the expression of pluripotency and differentiation markers were generated in the Microsoft Office Excel 2016 program. The quantity of TH-positive neurons was determined in relation to the primary neuronal marker TUBB3 using the ImageJ 1.53c software.

3. Results
3.1. Obtaining and Characterization of Patient-Specific iPSCs

In the first part of the work, using transfection with episomal vectors encoding *OCT4*, *KLF4*, *L-MYC*, *SOX2*, *LIN28* and *mp53DD*, three lines of iPSCs were obtained, characterized in detail and registered in the Human Pluripotent Stem Cell Registry (hPSCreg): two lines from a patient with Parkinson's disease associated with a pathological mutation in the *GBA1* gene (p.N370S) (iPSC-GBA) PD30-1/ICGi034-D (https://hpscreg.eu/cell-line/ICGi034-D, accessed 5 February 2024) and PD30-3/ICGi034-E (https://hpscreg.eu/cell-line/ICGi034-E, accessed 5 February 2024); and an iPSC line from a conditionally healthy donor (iPSC-ctrl) K7-2Lf/ICGi022-B (https://hpscreg.eu/cell-line/ICGi022-B, accessed 5 February 2024). The cells have a morphology characteristic of human IPSCs (Figure 1A), express endogenous alkaline phosphatase (Figure 1B), and show the presence of pluripotency markers both in immunofluorescence analysis for specific transcription factors (SOX2 and OCT4) and surface markers (TRA-1-60 and SSEA-4) (Figure 1C) and in qPCR analysis (*OCT4*, *SOX2* and *NANOG*) (Figure 1D). The previously published IPSC line K7-4Lf/ICGi022-A was used as a reference line [25] (Malakhova et al., 2020; https://hpscreg.eu/cell-line/ICGi022-A, accessed 5 February 2024). G-staining of metaphase plates of all lines revealed a normal 46,XX karyotype in more than 65% of cells (Figure 1E).

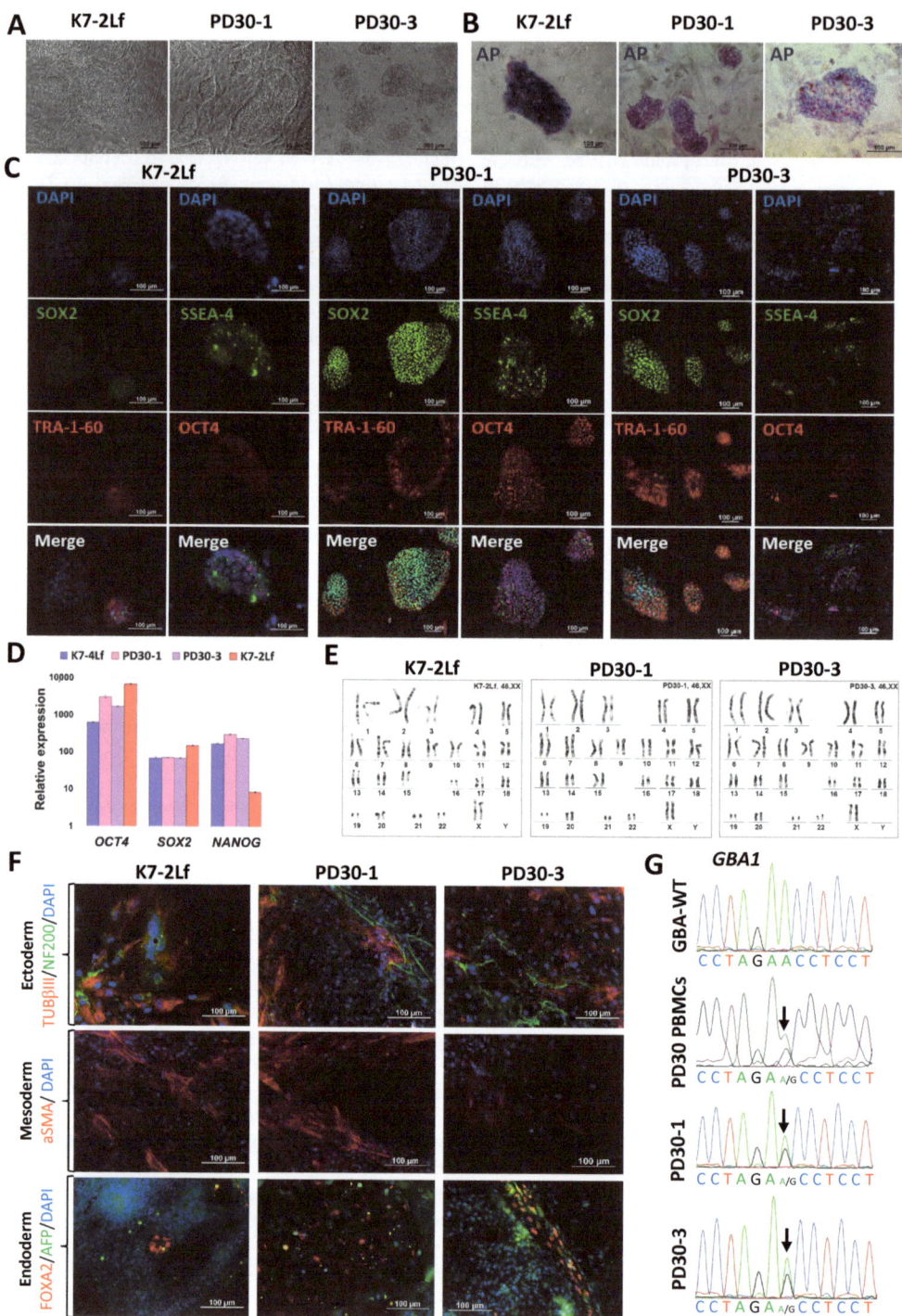

Figure 1. Characterization of the iPSC cell lines K7-2Lf, PD30-1 and PD30-3. (**A**) Cells exhibit typical iPSC morphology. (**B**) iPSC colonies are positively stained for alkaline phosphatase (AP). (**C**) Immunofluorescence analysis revealed expression of the pluripotency markers OCT4 (red signal),

SOX2 (green signal), SSEA-4 (green signal), TRA-1-60 (red signal). (**D**) Quantitative analysis of *NANOG*, *OCT4* and *SOX2* expression was performed by RT-qPCR. Error bars indicate the standard deviation. (**E**) Chromosome analysis demonstrated a normal karyotype (46,XX) for all three cell lines. (**F**) Immunofluorescence staining for differentiation markers in spontaneously differentiated cell cultures of K7-2Lf, PD30-1, and PD30-3 revealed derivatives of the three germ layers: mesoderm—αSMA (red signal); ectoderm—TUBB3 (red signal) and NF200 (green signal); and endoderm—FOXA2 (red signal) and AFP (green signal). Nuclei are stained with DAPI (blue signal). (**G**) Sequenograms of *GBA1* gene regions from PBMCs of a patient with Parkinson's disease, and a healthy donor (control, GBA-WT). The detected polymorphic position is indicated by arrows. All scale bars: 100 μm.

A test for spontaneous differentiation in embryoid bodies and immunofluorescence analysis of differentiated derivatives for specific markers revealed the ability of the lines to produce three germ layers: Ectoderm (microtubule protein βIII tubulin/TUBB3/TUJ1 and neurofilament 200 (NF200)), Mesoderm (α-smooth muscle actin (aSMA)) and Endoderm (alpha-fetoprotein (AFP) and hepatocyte nuclear factor 3 beta (HNF3β/FOXA2)) (Figure 1F). The presence of the pathogenic mutation N370S (c.1226 A>G) in the *GBA1* gene was confirmed by Sanger sequencing (Figure 1G). The PCR test for mycoplasma showed that all iPSC lines tested were negative for this contamination (Supplementary Figure S2A).

3.2. Differentiation of iPSCs into Neural Derivatives

Directed differentiation of the iPSC lines into DA neurons was performed to study the molecular genetic mechanisms of Parkinson's disease in relevant cell types. We performed directed differentiation of nine iPSC lines: three lines from a Parkinson's disease patient carrying the N370S *GBA1* mutation, 3 iPSC lines from an asymptomatic carrier of the mutation, and three iPSC lines from healthy donors. Three iPSC lines (K7-2Lf, PD30-1 and PD30-3) described in this study. We also used previously generated, characterized and registered in the Human Pluripotent Stem Cell Registry (hPSCreg; https://hpscreg.eu, accessed on 5 February 2024) iPSCs derived from: (1) healthy individuals (K6-4f/ICGi021-A and K7-4Lf/ICGi022-A) [25]; (2) a patient with Parkinson's disease associated with the pathogenic variant p.N370S in the *GBA1* gene (PD30-4-7/ICGi034-A) [23]; (3) an asymptomatic carrier of the N370S mutation in the *GBA1* gene (PD31-6/ICGi039-A, PD31-7/ICGi039-B, PD31-15/ICGi039-C) [24]. The efficacy of differentiation was confirmed by immunofluorescence analysis for specific neural markers. All lines showed the presence of the major neural marker TUBβIII, markers for midbrain precursors OTX2 and LMX1A, and a marker for mature DA neurons—tyrosine hydroxylase (TH)—at days 55–60 of differentiation (Figure 2A). The percentage of TH-positive neurons in culture ranges from 30 to 50%.

Quantitative PCR was used to evaluate the expression of specific neural markers (see Figure 2B). All lines express midbrain markers, including *OTX2*, *LMX1A*, and *SOX6*. It is worth noting that SOX6 is a marker of DA neurons in the substantia nigra, the brain region most severely affected by Parkinson's disease [36]. Additionally, the marker of mature DA neurons, TH, is present in all cultures.

A tendency towards an inverse relationship between the expression levels of the *TH* and *GBA1* genes can be observed (Figure 2C). The expression level of *GBA1* decreases as the percentage of mature DA neurons in the culture increases.

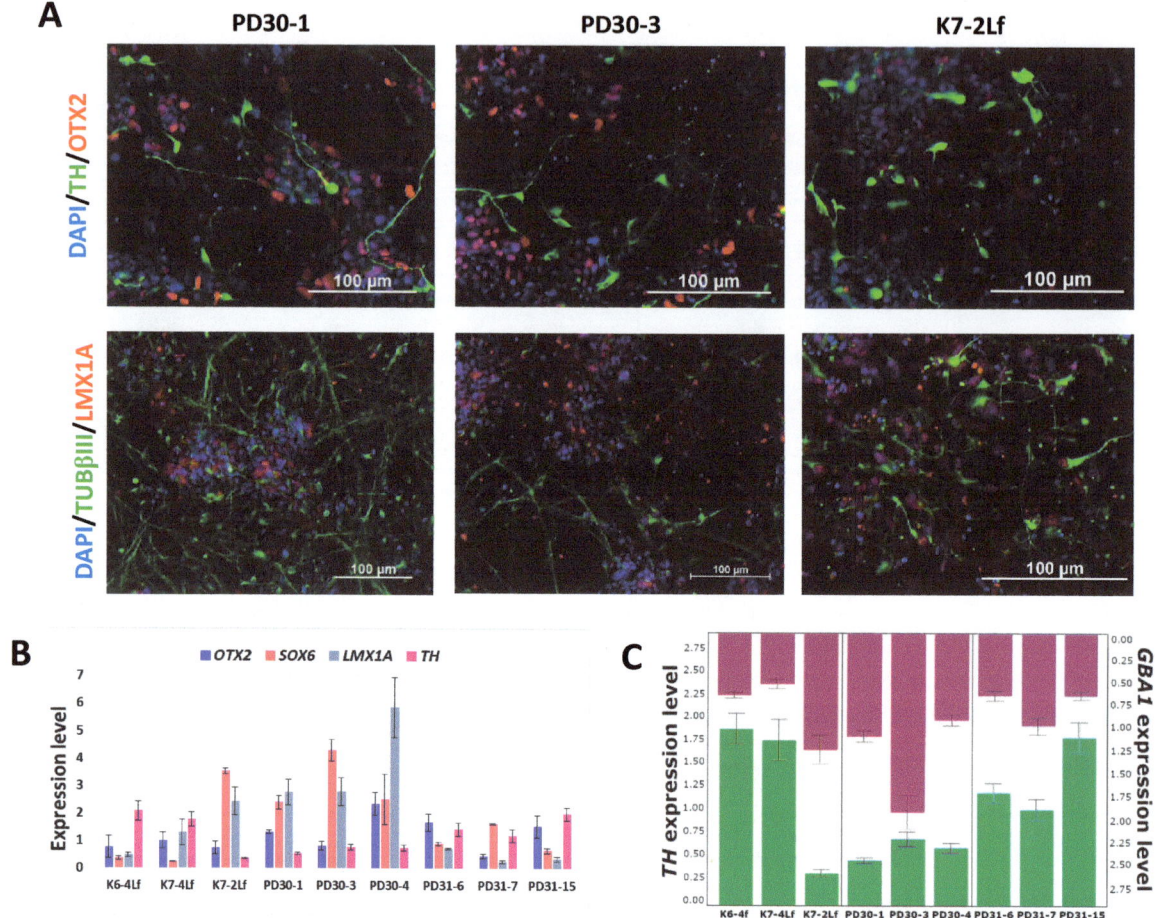

Figure 2. Characteristics of neural derivatives at days 55–60 of differentiation. (**A**) Immunofluorescence staining for markers of midbrain precursors OTX2 (red signal); a specific markers of DA neurons: tyrosine hydroxylase (TH, green signal) and LMX1A (red signal); and a common neural marker TUBβIII (green signal). Nuclei are stained with DAPI (blue signal). Scale bar: 100 µm. (**B**) Normalized expression level of dopaminergic neuron markers (*TH*, *LMX1A*, *OTX2* and *SOX6*) in neural derivatives (*n* = 4). (**C**) Correlation between *GBA1* (purple bars) and *TH* (green bars) expression level in neural derivatives.

3.3. Detection of ER Stress in Neural Derivatives Using qPCR

To investigate ER stress and UPR activation in neural derivatives and iPSCs, we conducted a qualitative and quantitative PCR analysis of the spliced mRNA variant of the *XBP1* gene that is specific for activated IRE1-XBP1 UPR cascade. Additionally, we examined the expression of the *CHOP* gene, which activates proapoptotic genes that induce cell death [37].

A PCR analysis was performed using primers for the spliced/unplaced form of the *XBP1* gene (*XBP1s* and *XBP1u*, respectively). The product was not detected in iPSC-GBA, DA neurons on day 60 of iPSC-GBA neural differentiation, or DA neurons from iPSC of healthy donors. This suggests the absence of activation of the IRE1-XBP1 cascade, as confirmed by the qPCR method using primers to identify the spliced variant *XBP1s* (Figure 3B). The IPSC samples treated with tunicamycin, an ER stress activator, were used as a positive control. Tunicamycin treatment induces the appearance of the spliced XBP1 variant, as indicated by the arrow in Figure 3A.

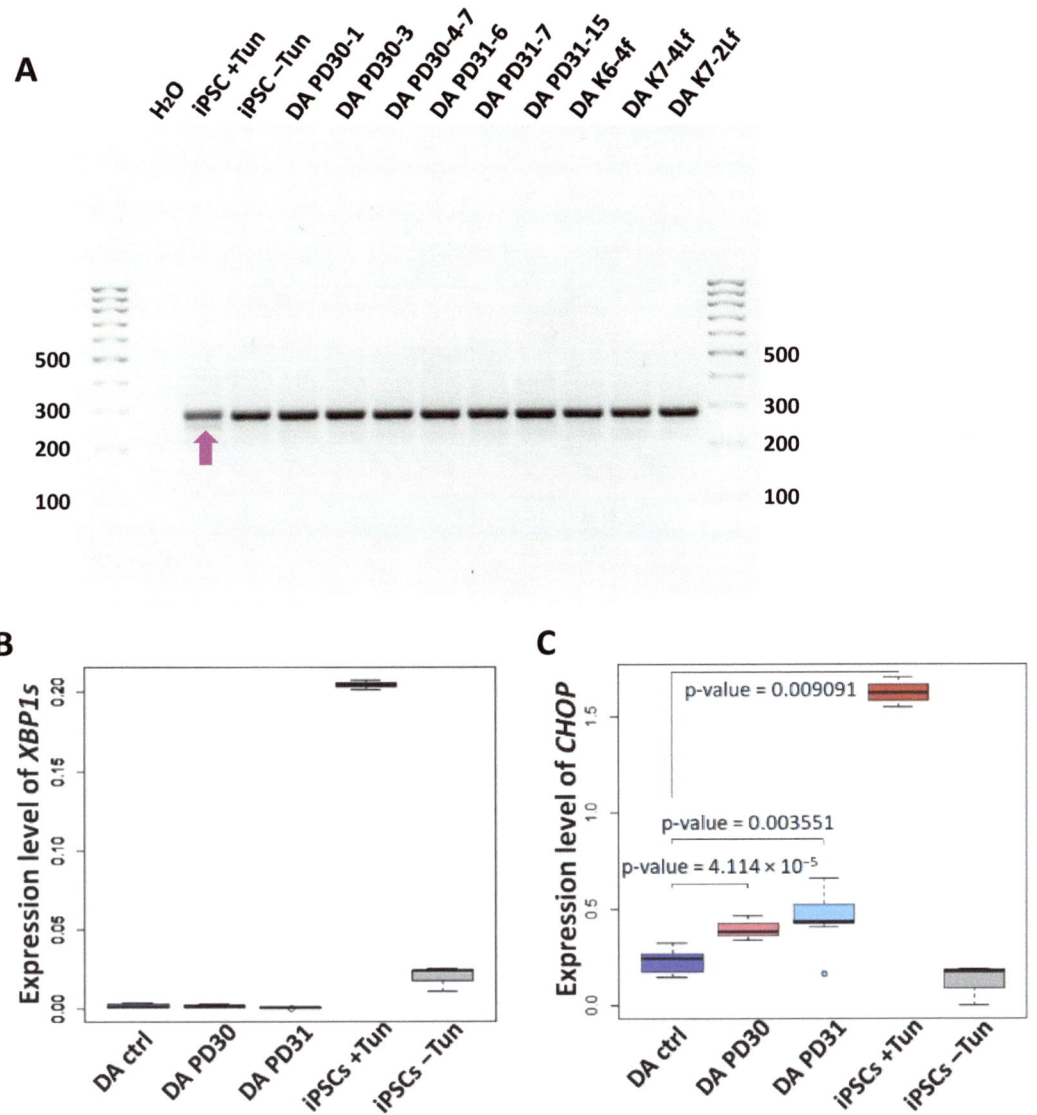

Figure 3. ER stress detection by evaluating the expression of *CHOP* and *XBP1* genes involved in UPR activation in iPSC-derived DA neurons and in iPSCs with and without tunicamycin treatment. (**A**) PCR analysis for the spliced form of *XBP1* (*XBP1s*, shown by arrow) in the iPSC-ctrl line after treatment with ER stress inducer tunicamycin (iPSCs +Tun). The spliced form of *XBP1* is absent in iPSC-ctrl without tunicamycin (iPSCs −Tun) and in neural derivatives derived from iPSC-GBA (DA PD30-1, DA PD30-3, DA PD30-4-7, DA PD31-6, DA PD31-7, DA PD31-15) and iPSC-ctrl (DA K6-4f, DA K7-4Lf, DA K7-2Lf) on days 55–60 of differentiation. (**B**) Detection of the *XBP1s* using qPCR. $n = 9$ for DA neurons. $n = 3$ for iPSC. (**C**) The expression level of the *CHOP* gene in DA-neurons and iPSCs +/−Tun estimated by qPCR. DA GBA—neurons obtained from iPSC-GBA, DA ctrl—DA -neurons obtained from iPSCs from healthy patients.

To determine if ER stress occurs in DA neurons with the N370S mutation in the *GBA1* gene, we conducted qPCR analysis of *CHOP* gene expression. The analysis revealed a significant increase in *CHOP* expression in DA neurons from iPSC-GBA compared to DA neurons from control 'healthy' iPSCs (Figure 3C). This suggests that neural derivatives carrying the N370S mutation in the *GBA1* gene respond to ER stress.

3.4. Preparation and Characterization of Transgenic iPSC Lines Carrying the XBP1-TagRFP ER Stress Biosensor at the AAVS1 Locus

To introduce transgenes of ER stress biosensor (XBP1-TagRFP) and doxycycline-dependent tetracycline reverse transactivator (M2rtTA) into the *AAVS1* locus using CRISPR-Cas9 technology, PD30-4-7 (ICGi034-A) iPSC lines [23] carrying a pathogenic heterozygous missense mutation c.1226A>G (p.N370S, rs76763715) in the *GBA1* gene were used. After selection of iPSCs for the antibiotics geneticin and puromycin, 99 individual surviving colonies were analyzed by PCR for the presence of transgenes at the *AAVS1* locus and the absence of non-specific integration of donor plasmids. After PCR screening, six transgenic subclones were selected (Figure 4).

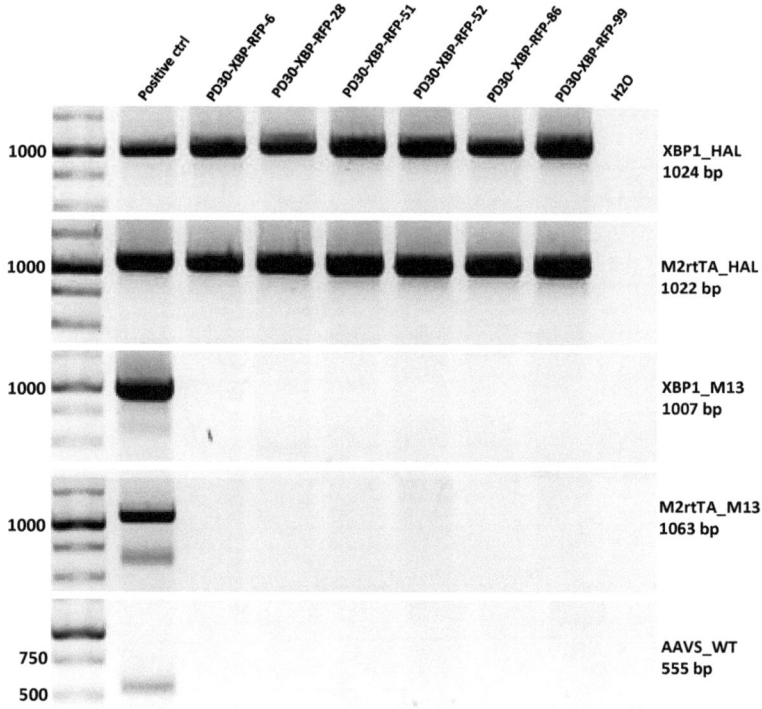

Figure 4. PCR assay for the integration of the XBP1-TagRFP biosensor and its doxycycline-dependent transactivator into the *AAVS1* locus. XBP1_HAL—screening for the integration of the XBP1-TagRFP biosensor into the *AAVS1* locus, M2rtTA_HAL—screening for the integration of the M2rtTA transgene with a transactivator into the *AAVS1* locus, XBP1_M13—screening for the presence of a non-target pXBP1-TagRFP-ERSS plasmid incorporating into the genome, M2rtTA_M13—screening for the presence of a non-target AAVS1-Neo-M2rtTA plasmid incorporating into the genome, AAVS_WT—screening against the wild type of the *AAVS1* locus.

Karyotyping was performed for subclones 6, 51, 52 and 86, which showed a normal 46,XX karyotype in more than 70% of the analyzed metaphases (Figure 5F). These subclones were characterized and registered in the Human Pluripotent Stem Cell Registry (hPSCreg).

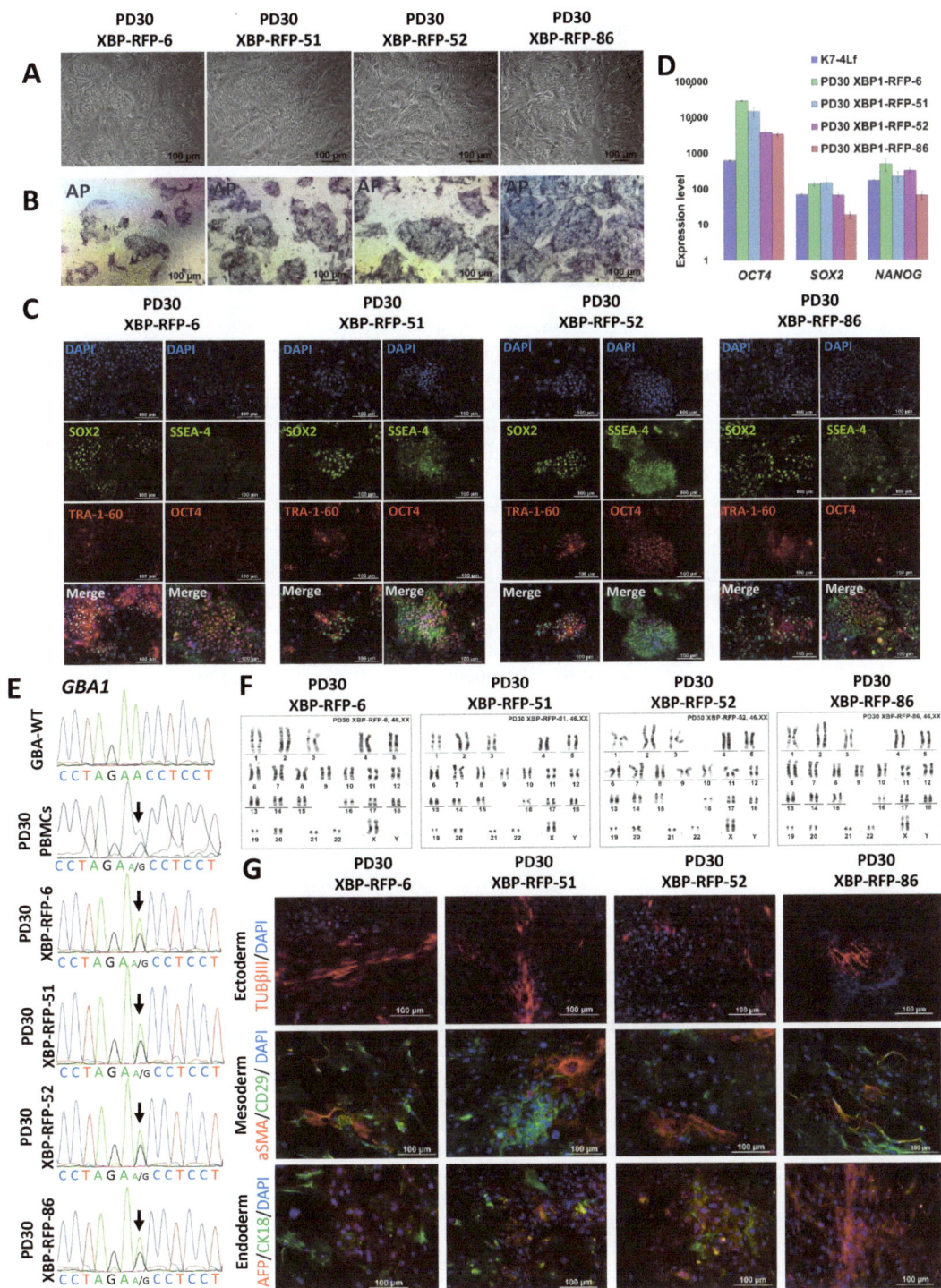

Figure 5. Characterization of the iPSC lines PD30-XBP-RFP-6, PD30-XBP-RFP-51, PD30-XBP-RFP-52 and PD30-XBP-RFP-86. (**A**) Typical morphology of iPSC colonies. (**B**) Cells demonstrate AP activity.

(**C**) Immunofluorescence staining reveals expression of the pluripotency markers OCT4 (red signal), SOX2 (green signal), SSEA-4 (green signal), TRA-1-60 (red signal). (**D**) Results of RT-qPCR analysis of the expression of pluripotency genes (*NANOG, OCT4, SOX2*) normalized to *B2M*. Error bars indicate standard deviation. (**E**) Sequenograms of *GBA1* gene regions from PBMCs of a patient with Parkinson's disease, transgenic iPSC lines, and a healthy donor (control, GBA-WT). The detected polymorphisms are marked with arrows. (**F**) Karyotype analysis shows a normal chromosome set (46,XX) in all four iPSC lines. (**G**) Immunofluorescence staining for differentiation markers in spontaneously differentiated cell cultures PD30-XBP-RFP-6, PD30-XBP-RFP-51, PD30-XBP-RFP-52 and PD30-XBP-RFP-86 revealed derivatives of the three germ layers: mesoderm—αSMA (red signal) and CD29 (green signal); ectoderm—TUBB3/TUJ1 (red signal); endoderm—cytokeratin 18 (CK18) (green signal) and AFP (red signal). Nuclei are stained with DAPI (blue signal). All scale bars: 100 μm.

A detailed characterization of the derived lines was carried out, after which they were registered in the Human Pluripotent Stem Cell Registry (https://hpscreg.eu/, accessed on 5 February 2024) with the assigned names ICGi034-A-1 (PD30-XBP-RFP-6, https://hpscreg.eu/cell-line/ICGi034-A-1); ICGi034-A-2 (PD30-XBP-RFP-51, https://hpscreg.eu/cell-line/ICGi034-A-2); ICGi034-A-3 (PD30-XBP-RFP-52, https://hpscreg.eu/cell-line/ICGi034-A-3); ICGi034-A-4 (PD30-XBP-RFP-86, https://hpscreg.eu/cell-line/ICGi034-A-4), all links accessed on 5 February 2024. It was shown that the morphology of the subclones is characteristic for iPSC (Figure 5A); the culture is positively stained for alkaline phosphatase (Figure 5B); the subclones express pluripotency markers, as shown by the results of immunofluorescence analysis (SOX2, TRA-1-60, OCT4, SSEA-4) (Figure 5C) and qPCR (Figure 5D). The previously characterized iPSC K7-4Lf line was used as a reference line for qPCR [25]. Sanger sequencing confirmed the presence of a pathogenic c.1226A>G substitution in the *GBA1* gene in transgenic subclones (Figure 5E). Spontaneous differentiation in embryoid bodies and subsequent immunofluorescence staining for markers of three germ layers revealed the presence of ectoderm (TUBB3/TUJ1), mesoderm (α-smooth muscle actin α-SMA and CD29), endoderm (alpha-fetoprotein (AFP) and cytokeratin 18 (CK18)) (Figure 5G). The PCR test for mycoplasma showed no contamination with this pathogen (Supplementary Figure S2B).

We also generated transgenic iPSC lines based on the previously obtained K6-4f control iPSC line [25] with the XBP1-TagRFP biosensor and doxycycline transactivator M2rtTA in the *AAVS1* locus. These lines meet all iPSC requirements, have iPSC-like cell colony morphology, and express markers of pluripotent cells OCT4, SOX2, SSEA-4 and TRA-1-60 (Supplement Figure S3).

3.5. Demonstration of XBP1-TagRFP Biosensor Operation in Transgenic iPSC Lines

The operating scheme of the UPR activation biosensor is shown in Figure 6. The XBP1-TagRFP sensor construct contains a 26 nucleotide intron that is cleaved by the endoribonuclease IRE1 upon ER stress [18]. Processing of the XBP1-TagRFP transcript results in a frameshift and the fluorescent protein TagRFP is translated. The red fluorescent signal indicates that the IRE1-XBP1 cascade of the UPR is activated.

To test the function of the biosensor, the obtained transgenic iPSC clones were cultured for 2 days in the presence of doxycycline to activate the expression of the XBP1-TagRFP biosensor transgene. However, since the cells are not stressed under normal culture conditions, we did not detect the fluorescent TagRFP signal in either iPSC-GBA or iPSC-ctrl (Figure 7A). To induce ER stress and activate the UPR in the cells, tunicamycin was added to the culture medium for 24 h (Figure 7B). We found that the stress inducer caused the appearance of red TagRFP fluorescence, indicating the correct functioning of the XBP1-TagRFP biosensor.

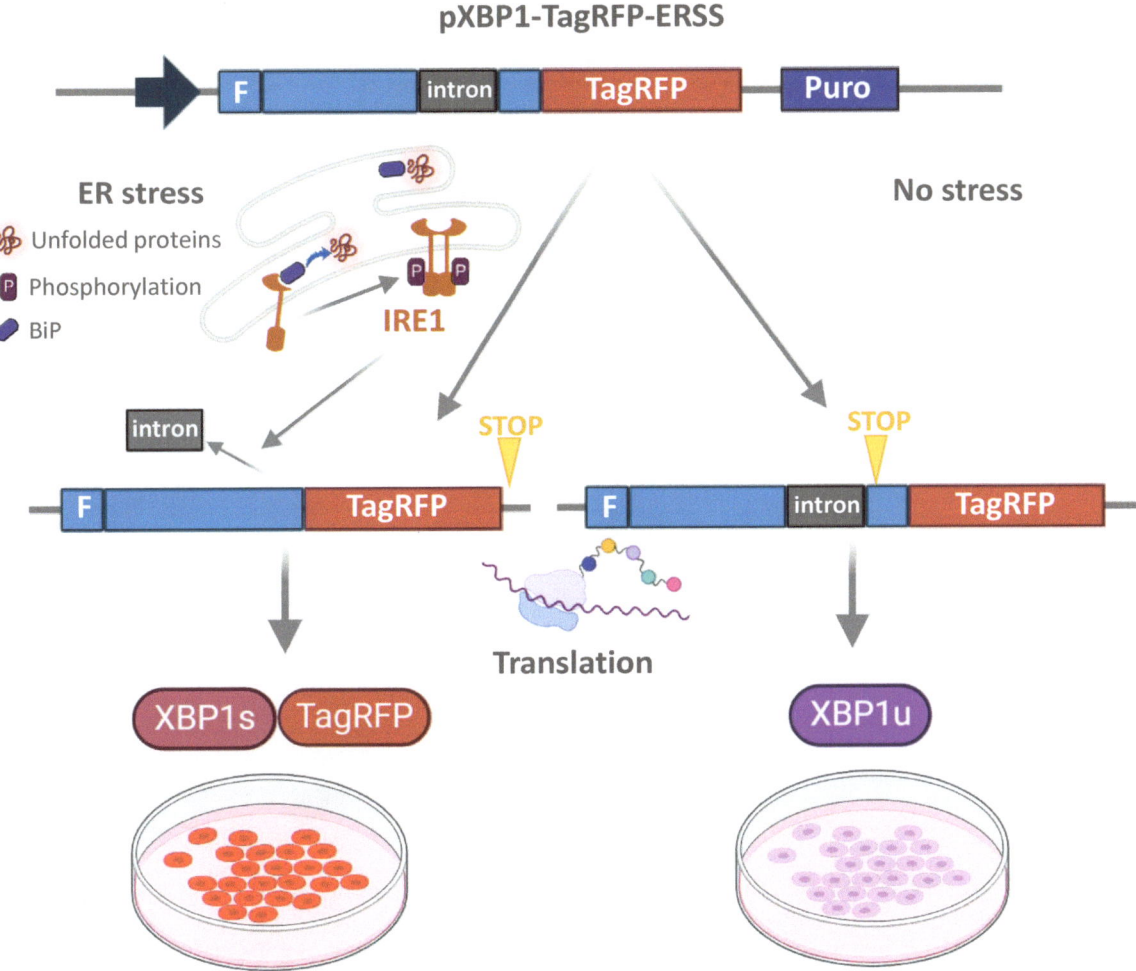

Figure 6. The scheme of operation of the ER stress biosensor XBP1-TagRFP. Under ER stress, the IRE1 protein is activated, forms a dimer, and begins to splice XBP1-TagRFP mRNA, i.e., to excise an intron of 26 base pairs (shown in gray), resulting in a frameshift and translation of the fluorescent TagRFP protein. A red fluorescent signal appears in transgenic cells, indicating activation of the UPR system. In the absence of ER stress, the chimeric mRNA XBP1-TagRFP is not spliced and translation of the sensory protein is terminated by the stop codon located after the intron. Thus, TagRFP synthesis is only provided from a spliced transcript.

It was also shown that the addition of doxycycline to transgenic K6-XBP iPSCs and further cultivation for one day in the presence of tunicamycin resulted in the appearance of intense fluorescence (Supplementary Figure S4).

The cells were further differentiated into neural derivatives (DA neurons and astrocytes) according to the protocols described in our previous work [24,38]. It was shown that the cultivation of transgenic neural derivatives in the presence of doxycycline and tunicamycin also leads to the appearance of the TagRFP fluorescence signal, i.e., activation of the UPR (Supplementary Figure S5).

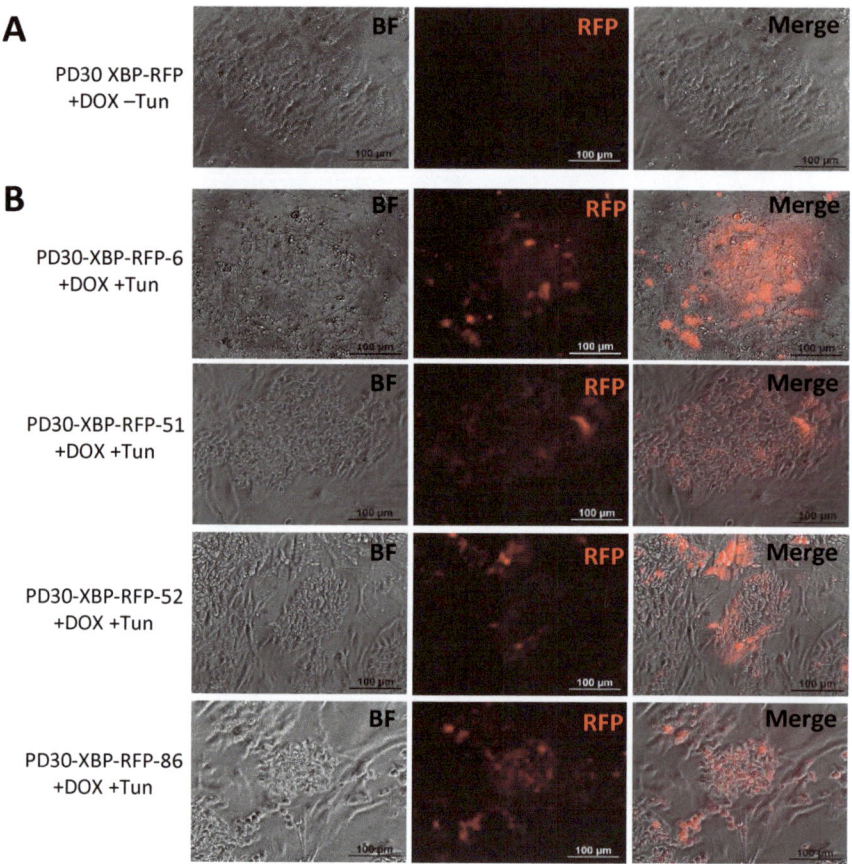

Figure 7. Operation of the ER stress biosensor in transgenic iPSC-GBA lines with integration of the XBP1-TagRFP biosensor. (**A**) Absence of TagRFP immunofluorescence signal in iPSCs without tunicamycin treatment. (**B**) Immunofluorescence lifetime glow of TagRFP in transgenic iPSCs after addition of tunicamycin. BF—bright field. All scale bars—100 μm.

4. Discussion

The study of pathological changes in cells caused by ER, mitochondrial or oxidative stress is an urgent task required to find targets to block these pathways that lead to dysfunction and death of various cell types.

The most important function of the granular ER is protein folding. The acquisition of the correct conformation of proteins is ensured by resident proteins and chaperones. However, the accumulation of misfolded proteins in the lumen of the ER can lead to a condition called "ER stress". To relieve ER stress and restore protein homeostasis, the UPR pathways are activated in the cell. The UPR is divided into three branches, each of which is activated by a specific transmembrane protein: protein kinase RNA (PKR)-like ER kinase (PERK), activating transcription factor-6 (ATF6), inositol-requiring enzyme 1 (IRE1) (Figure 8). All three UPR pathways contribute to the normalization of the ER in the early stages of the response by activating chaperone genes and expressing *XBP1*, which is processed at the RNA level by IRE1 to develop a functional protein [1,2,39–41].

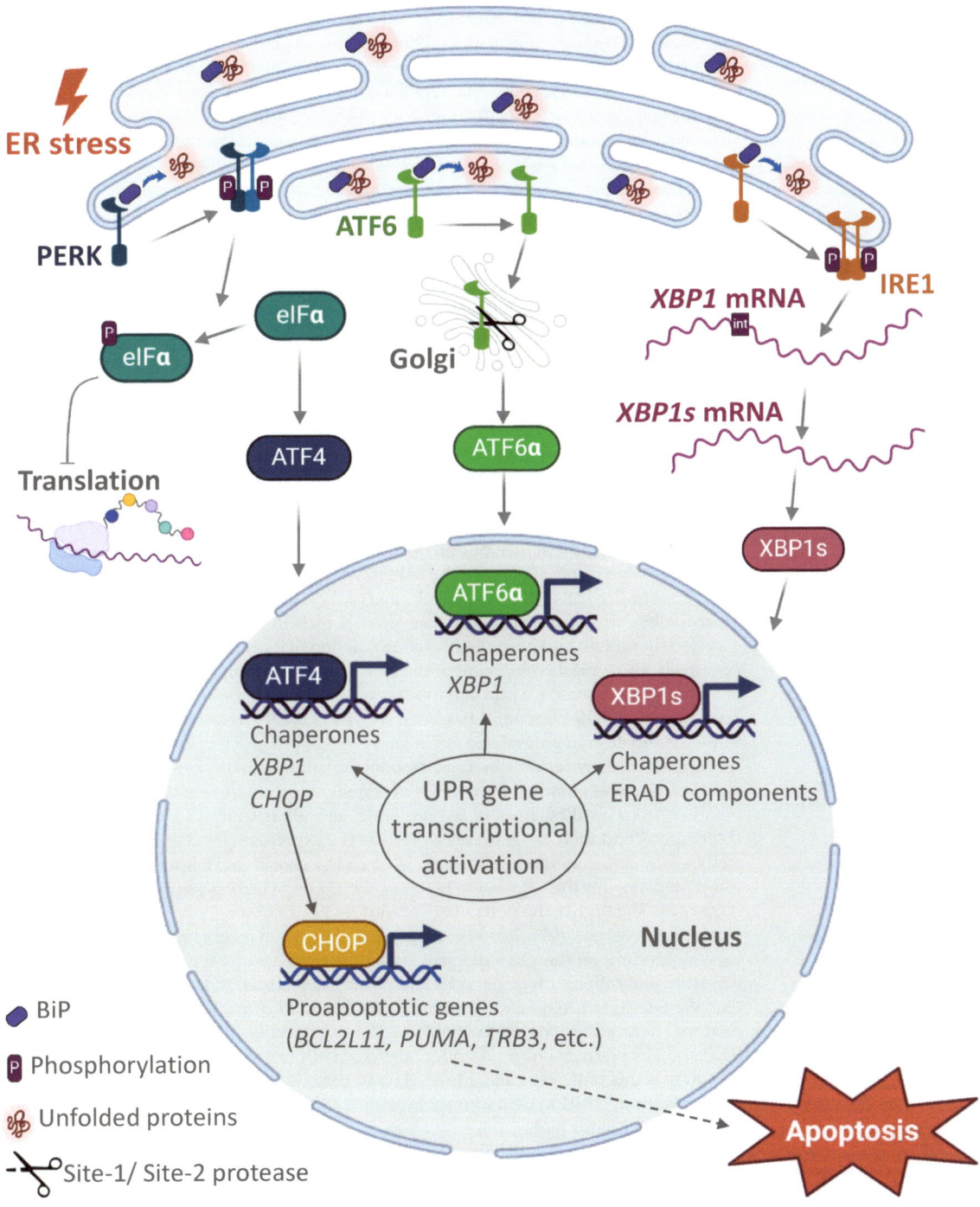

Figure 8. UPR systems activation under ER stress. The three major pathways of the UPR signaling cascade are determined by the key transmembrane proteins inositol-requiring protein 1α (IRE1α), activating transcription factor 6 (ATF6), and the protein kinase RNA-like ER kinase (PERK). In the

absence of stress, the transmembrane proteins IRE1a, ATF6 and PERK are associated with the chaperone-binding immunoglobulin (BiP), also known as the 78 kDa glucose regulatory protein (GRP78), in the lumen of the ER. In the presence of stress, BiP is released by binding to misfolded proteins, IRE1a and PERK proteins form homodimers, autophosphorylates and exit the ER. At the same time, phosphorylated IRE1a acquires ribonucleic acid endonuclease activity, cutting a 26-nucleotide intron from *XBP1* mRNA, resulting in the translation of the spliced form *XBP1* (XBP1s), a transcription factor that activates UPR chaperone response genes (including BiP) and ER components that contribute to peptide folding, ER lipid synthesis, and ER stress reduction. Under chronic ER stress, XBP1s induces an ER-related degradation (READ) pathway. Activated PERK phosphorylates the translation initiation factor eIF2α, inhibiting mRNA translation and protein synthesis, but activating transcription factor 4 (ATF4). ATF4 regulates the expression of chaperone genes and *XBP1*. Late in the development of the UPR response, ATF4 activates transcription of the master gene *CHOP*, which regulates the pro-apoptotic cascade of events. In the presence of ER stress, the ATP6 protein translocates to the Golgi apparatus, where the C-terminus of the protein is cleaved to form activated ATP6a, which enters the nucleus and activates the chaperone and *XBP1* genes [1,2,39–41].

As a model to study ER stress, we chose DA neurons derived from iPSC of a Parkinson's disease patient and an asymptomatic carrier of the N370S mutation in the *GBA1* gene. The most common heterozygous variants of the *GBA1* gene are c.1226A>G (N370S, rs76763715) and c.1448T>C (L444P, rs421016), which are associated with an increased risk of Parkinson's disease. These mutations disrupt the tertiary structure of GCase and lead to its dysfunction [42,43]. GCase with a perturbed tertiary structure can accumulate in the ER, leading to an imbalance of homeostasis and stress. A decrease in GCase activity in neurons obtained from iPSC with the heterozygous variant *GBA1* p.N370S has been shown in several studies [24,44,45]. As a result, due to the decrease in the amount of active GCase, glucocerebroside accumulates in lysosomes, which in turn disrupts the degradation of α-synuclein protein and promotes the accumulation of its neurotoxic aggregates [43], which negatively affect the development of the UPR in cells, possibly leading to the development of Parkinson's disease [21]. In cell models of Parkinson's disease caused by the p.N370S mutation in the *GBA1* gene, it has been shown that ER stress can actively manifest and cause dysfunction in patient-specific neurons [20,21].

In this work, we established a cell model of Parkinson's disease based on differentiated neural derivatives obtained from iPSCs. In a population of DA neurons with *GBA1* p.N370S obtained from six iPSC lines of two patients, as well as from iPCs-ctrl, genes specific to DA neurons and their progenitors, as well as the expression level of the *GBA1* gene, were analyzed by qPCR method. Although *GBA1* can be considered a housekeeping gene, there was a tendency for the expression levels of the *TH* and *GBA1* genes to be inversely related (Figure 2). The higher the percentage of mature DA neurons in the culture, the lower the expression level of *GBA1*. It is known that the expression level of housekeeping genes can vary depending on the physiological state of the cell and its type. It is also noted in the literature that different types of cells and tissues have different levels of *GBA1* mRNA [27].

We attempted to assess ER stress levels and UPR activation in IPSC-GBA and their neuronal derivatives. We were unable to identify the spliced form of *XBP1* in samples of iPSC and DA neurons cultured under normal conditions (Figure 3A), although it has been shown that this pathway can be turned on in patients with Parkinson's disease [21]. The spliced form of *XBP1* appeared only in samples treated with tunicamycin, a well-known ER stress modulator [46].

One explanation for the absence of the spliced form of *XBP1* may be that the culture of DA neurons obtained from iPSCs as a result of differentiation has a "young" phenotype and is more similar to embryonic cells than to adult cells, while Parkinson's disease is a disease that most often develops during the aging process [47].

However, we were able to detect the expression of the *CHOP* gene in neurons, which differed between samples derived from iPSC-GBA and iPSC-ctrl (Figure 3C). It is likely that the neurons obtained from iPSC-GBA underwent chronic ER stress during prolonged cultivation, in which the developmental stage of the CHOP cascade already prevailed.

For lifetime visualization of UPR events, it is convenient to use genetically encoded biosensors. The natural ability of the activated ER stress ribonuclease IRE1a to splice the 26-nucleotide intron in *XBP1* was exploited to create biologically encoded sensors based on the XBP1 protein without the DBD domain, fused to a fluorescent protein [18,33] (Figure 6). Using CRISPR-Cas9 technology, transgenic lines iPSC-GBA (based on the PD30-4-7 iPSC line) and iPSC-ctrl (based on the K6-4f iPSC line) with XBP1-RFP and doxycycline-dependent reverse transactivator transgenes introduced into the *AAVS1* locus were generated. It was shown that the biosensor function was observed in transgenic iPSCs after treatment with tunicamycin.

Thus, we have obtained a functional cellular test system for the in vitro study of ER stress-inducing factors that trigger a cell-saving UPR response by activating the IRE1-XBP1 pathway.

5. Conclusions

In this work, for the first time, iPSCs carrying the p.N370S genetic variant in the *GBA1* gene were used to create a test model for studying ER stress (accumulation of denatured forms of proteins) using the genetically encoded XBP1-TagRFP biosensor designed to visualize the activation of the IRE1-XBP1 cascade and the stress-dependent splicing of *XBP1* mRNA. iPSCs carrying the XBP1-TagRFP biosensor transgene can be used for lifetime studies of UPR function in different cell types, as well as for screening of small molecules aimed at modulating UPR function.

Supplementary Materials: The following supporting information can be downloaded at: https://www.mdpi.com/article/10.3390/biomedicines12040744/s1, Figure S1: Plasmid map pXBP1-TagRFP-ERSS-donor; Figure S2: PCR test for mycoplasma of the iPSC lines; Figure S3: Characteristics of transgenic iPSCs carrying an ER stress biosensor XBP1-TagRFP (K6-XBP-RFP-62, K6-XBP-RFP-68); Figure S4: Visualization of the XBP1-TagRFP biosensor in two transgenic iPSC lines (K6-XBP-RFP-62 and K6-XBP-RFP-68); Figure S5: Visualization of the XBP1-TagRFP biosensor in neural derivatives from K6-XBP-RFP iPSCs.

Author Contributions: Conceptualization, E.V.G., S.V.P., S.M.Z. and A.A.M.; methodology, E.V.G., S.P.M. and S.V.P.; validation, E.V.G. and A.A.M.; investigation, E.S.Y., E.V.G., J.M.M., D.A.T., K.R.V. and S.P.M.; writing—original draft preparation, E.S.Y., E.V.G. and D.A.T.; writing—review and editing, E.S.Y., E.V.G., D.A.T., S.V.P., S.P.M. and A.A.M.; visualization, E.S.Y., D.A.T., J.M.M. and E.V.G.; supervision, S.M.Z.; project administration, E.V.G.; funding acquisition, A.A.M. All authors have read and agreed to the published version of the manuscript.

Funding: This research was funded by Russian Science Foundation, grant number 23-15-00224 (https://rscf.ru/en/project/23-15-00224/, accessed on 21 March 2024).

Institutional Review Board Statement: The study was conducted in accordance with the Declaration of Helsinki and approved by the Ethics Committee of the FSBI Federal Neurosurgical Center (Protocol No. 1, 14 March 2017).

Informed Consent Statement: Informed consent was obtained from all subjects involved in the study.

Data Availability Statement: Characteristics of iPSCs is presented in the Human Pluripotent Stem Cell Registry (hPSCreg; https://hpscreg.eu/, accessed on 5 February 2024): for GBA-PD (PD30-1/ICGi034-D, https://hpscreg.eu/cell-line/ICGi034-D and PD30-3/ICGi034-E https://hpscreg.eu/cell-line/ICGi034-E; all accessed on 5 February 2024); for healthy donor K7-2Lf/ICGi022-B (https://hpscreg.eu/cell-line/ICGi022-B, accessed on 5 February 2024); for transgenic iPSC lines: ICGi034-A-1 (PD30-XBP-RFP-6, https://hpscreg.eu/cell-line/ICGi034-A-1); ICGi034-A-2 (PD30-XBP-RFP-51, https://hpscreg.eu/cell-line/ICGi034-A-2); ICGi034-A-3 (PD30-XBP-RFP-52, https://hpscreg.eu/cell-line/ICGi034-A-3); ICGi034-A-4 (PD30-XBP-RFP-86, https://hpscreg.eu/cell-line/ICGi034-A-4) all accessed on 5 February 2024.

Acknowledgments: The immunofluorescent imaging was performed using resources of the Common Facilities Center of Microscopic Analysis of Biological Objects, ICG SB RAS (https://ckp.icgen.ru/ckpmabo/, accessed on 31 January 2024), supported by the state project of the Institute of Cytology and Genetics (FWNR-2022-0015). Sanger sequencing was performed at the SB RAS Genomics Core Facility (http://www.niboch.nsc.ru/doku.php/corefacility, accessed on 5 February 2024).

Conflicts of Interest: The authors declare no conflicts of interests.

References

1. Hetz, C.; Zhang, K.; Kaufman, R.J. Mechanisms, regulation and functions of the unfolded protein response. *Nat. Rev. Mol. Cell Biol.* **2020**, *21*, 421–438. [CrossRef]
2. Frakes, A.E.; Dillin, A. The UPRER: Sensor and Coordinator of Organismal Homeostasis. *Mol. Cell* **2017**, *66*, 761–771. [CrossRef]
3. Oslowski, C.M.; Urano, F. Measuring ER stress and the unfolded protein response using mammalian tissue culture system. *Methods Enzymol.* **2011**, *490*, 71–92. [CrossRef]
4. Kennedy, D.; Samali, A.; Jäger, R. Methods for studying ER stress and UPR markers in human cells. *Methods Mol. Biol.* **2015**, *1292*, 3–18. [CrossRef]
5. Subach, O.M.; Kunitsyna, T.A.; Mineyeva, O.A.; Lazutkin, A.A.; Bezryadnov, D.V.; Barykina, N.V.; Piatkevich, K.D.; Ermakova, Y.G.; Bilan, D.S.; Belousov, V.V.; et al. Slowly reducible genetically encoded green fluorescent indicator for in vivo and ex vivo visualization of hydrogen peroxide. *Int. J. Mol. Sci.* **2019**, *20*, 3138. [CrossRef] [PubMed]
6. Schwarzländer, M.; Dick, T.P.; Meyer, A.J.; Morgan, B. Dissecting redox biology using fluorescent protein sensors. *Antioxid. Redox Signal.* **2016**, *24*, 680–712. [CrossRef] [PubMed]
7. Morgan, B.; Sobotta, M.C.; Dick, T.P. Measuring EGSH and H_2O_2 with roGFP2-based redox probes. *Free Radic. Biol. Med.* **2011**, *51*, 1943–1951. [CrossRef]
8. Gutscher, M.; Pauleau, A.L.; Marty, L.; Brach, T.; Wabnitz, G.H.; Samstag, Y.; Meyer, A.J.; Dick, T.P. Real-time imaging of the intracellular glutathione redox potential. *Nat. Methods* **2008**, *5*, 553–559. [CrossRef]
9. Pak, V.V.; Ezeriņa, D.; Lyublinskaya, O.G.; Pedre, B.; Tyurin-Kuzmin, P.A.; Mishina, N.M.; Thauvin, M.; Young, D.; Wahni, K.; Martínez Gache, S.A.; et al. Ultrasensitive Genetically Encoded Indicator for Hydrogen Peroxide Identifies Roles for the Oxidant in Cell Migration and Mitochondrial Function. *Cell Metab.* **2020**, *31*, 642–653.e6. [CrossRef] [PubMed]
10. Laker, R.C.; Xu, P.; Ryall, K.A.; Sujkowski, A.; Kenwood, B.M.; Chain, K.H.; Zhang, M.; Royal, M.A.; Hoehn, K.L.; Driscoll, M.; et al. A novel mitotimer reporter gene for mitochondrial content, structure, stress, and damage in vivo. *J. Biol. Chem.* **2014**, *289*, 12005–12015. [CrossRef]
11. Habif, M.; Corbat, A.A.; Silberberg, M.; Grecco, H.E. CASPAM: A Triple-Modality Biosensor for Multiplexed Imaging of Caspase Network Activity. *ACS Sens.* **2021**, *6*, 2642–2653. [CrossRef]
12. Zhang, Q.; Schepis, A.; Huang, H.; Yang, J.; Ma, W.; Torra, J.; Zhang, S.Q.; Yang, L.; Wu, H.; Nonell, S.; et al. Designing a Green Fluorogenic Protease Reporter by Flipping a Beta Strand of GFP for Imaging Apoptosis in Animals. *J. Am. Chem. Soc.* **2019**, *141*, 4526–4530. [CrossRef] [PubMed]
13. Zlobovskaya, O.A.; Sergeeva, T.F.; Shirmanova, M.V.; Dudenkova, V.V.; Sharonov, G.V.; Zagaynova, E.V.; Lukyanov, K.A. Genetically encoded far-red fluorescent sensors for caspase-3 activity. *Biotechniques* **2016**, *60*, 62–68. [CrossRef]
14. Takemoto, K.; Nagai, T.; Miyawaki, A.; Miura, M. Spatio-temporal activation of caspase revealed by indicator that is insensitive to environmental effects. *J. Cell Biol.* **2003**, *160*, 235–243. [CrossRef]
15. Chen, T.W.; Wardill, T.J.; Sun, Y.; Pulver, S.R.; Renninger, S.L.; Baohan, A.; Schreiter, E.R.; Kerr, R.A.; Orger, M.B.; Jayaraman, V.; et al. Ultrasensitive fluorescent proteins for imaging neuronal activity. *Nature* **2013**, *499*, 295–300. [CrossRef] [PubMed]
16. Zhang, Y.; Rózsa, M.; Liang, Y.; Bushey, D.; Wei, Z.; Zheng, J.; Reep, D.; Broussard, G.J.; Tsang, A.; Tsegaye, G.; et al. Fast and sensitive GCaMP calcium indicators for imaging neural populations. *Nature* **2023**, *615*, 884891. [CrossRef] [PubMed]
17. Dana, H.; Sun, Y.; Mohar, B.; Hulse, B.K.; Kerlin, A.M.; Hasseman, J.P.; Tsegaye, G.; Tsang, A.; Wong, A.; Patel, R.; et al. High-performance calcium sensors for imaging activity in neuronal populations and microcompartments. *Nat. Methods* **2019**, *16*, 649–657. [CrossRef]
18. Iwawaki, T.; Akai, R.; Kohno, K.; Miura, M. A transgenic mouse model for monitoring endoplasmic reticulum stress. *Nat. Med.* **2004**, *10*, 98–102. [CrossRef]
19. Helfand, B.T.; Mendez, M.G.; Pugh, J.; Delsert, C.; Goldman, R.D. Maintaining the Shape of Nerve Cells. *Mol. Biol. Cell* **2003**, *14*, 5069–5081. [CrossRef]
20. Fernandes, H.J.R.; Hartfield, E.M.; Christian, H.C.; Emmanoulidou, E.; Zheng, Y.; Booth, H.; Bogetofte, H.; Lang, C.; Ryan, B.J.; Sardi, S.P.; et al. ER Stress and Autophagic Perturbations Lead to Elevated Extracellular α-Synuclein in GBA-N370S Parkinson's iPSC-Derived Dopamine Neurons. *Stem Cell Rep.* **2016**, *6*, 342–356. [CrossRef]
21. Stojkovska, I.; Wani, W.Y.; Zunke, F.; Belur, N.R.; Pavlenko, E.A.; Mwenda, N.; Sharma, K.; Francelle, L.; Mazzulli, J.R. Rescue of α-synuclein aggregation in Parkinson's patient neurons by synergistic enhancement of ER proteostasis and protein trafficking. *Neuron* **2022**, *110*, 436–451.e11. [CrossRef]
22. Yoshida, H.; Matsui, T.; Yamamoto, A.; Okada, T.; Mori, K. XBP1 mRNA is induced by ATF6 and spliced by IRE1 in response to ER stress to produce a highly active transcription factor. *Cell* **2001**, *107*, 881–891. [CrossRef] [PubMed]

23. Grigor'eva, E.V.; Drozdova, E.S.; Sorogina, D.A.; Malakhova, A.A.; Pavlova, S.V.; Vyatkin, Y.V.; Khabarova, E.A.; Rzaev, J.A.; Medvedev, S.P.; Zakian, S.M. Generation of induced pluripotent stem cell line, ICGi034-A, by reprogramming peripheral blood mononuclear cells from a patient with Parkinson's disease associated with *GBA* mutation. *Stem Cell Res.* **2022**, *59*, 102651. [CrossRef] [PubMed]
24. Grigor'eva, E.V.; Kopytova, A.E.; Yarkova, E.S.; Pavlova, S.V.; Sorogina, D.A.; Malakhova, A.A.; Malankhanova, T.B.; Baydakova, G.V.; Zakharova, E.Y.; Medvedev, S.P.; et al. Biochemical Characteristics of iPSC-Derived Dopaminergic Neurons from N370S *GBA* Variant Carriers with and without Parkinson's Disease. *Int. J. Mol. Sci.* **2023**, *24*, 4437. [CrossRef] [PubMed]
25. Malakhova, A.A.; Grigor'eva, E.V.; Pavlova, S.V.; Malankhanova, T.B.; Valetdinova, K.R.; Vyatkin, Y.V.; Khabarova, E.A.; Rzaev, J.A.; Zakian, S.M.; Medvedev, S.P. Generation of induced pluripotent stem cell lines ICGi021-A and ICGi022-A from peripheral blood mononuclear cells of two healthy individuals from Siberian population. *Stem Cell Res.* **2020**, *48*, 101952. [CrossRef] [PubMed]
26. Okita, K.; Yamakawa, T.; Matsumura, Y.; Sato, Y.; Amano, N.; Watanabe, A.; Goshima, N.; Yamanaka, S. An efficient nonviral method to generate integration-free human-induced pluripotent stem cells from cord blood and peripheral blood cells. *Stem Cells* **2013**, *31*, 458–466. [CrossRef] [PubMed]
27. Straniero, L.; Rimoldi, V.; Samarani, M.; Goldwurm, S.; Di Fonzo, A.; Krüger, R.; Deleidi, M.; Aureli, M.; Soldà, G.; Duga, S.; et al. The *GBAP1* pseudogene acts as a ceRNA for the glucocerebrosidase gene *GBA* by sponging *miR-22-3p*. *Sci. Rep.* **2017**, *7*, 12702. [CrossRef] [PubMed]
28. Mu, T.W.; Ong, D.S.T.; Wang, Y.J.; Balch, W.E.; Yates, J.R.; Segatori, L.; Kelly, J.W. Chemical and Biological Approaches Synergize to Ameliorate Protein-Folding Diseases. *Cell* **2008**, *134*, 769–781. [CrossRef] [PubMed]
29. Maor, G.; Rencus-Lazar, S.; Filocamo, M.; Steller, H.; Segal, D.; Horowitz, M. Unfolded protein response in Gaucher disease: From human to *Drosophila*. *Orphanet J. Rare Dis.* **2013**, *8*, 140. [CrossRef]
30. de Rus Jacquet, A. Preparation and Co-Culture of iPSC-Derived Dopaminergic Neurons and Astrocytes. *Curr. Protoc. Cell Biol.* **2019**, *85*, e98. [CrossRef]
31. Vandesompele, J.; De Preter, K.; Pattyn, F.; Poppe, B.; Van Roy, N.; De Paepe, A.; Speleman, F. Accurate normalization of real-time quantitative RT-PCR data by geometric averaging of multiple internal control genes. *Genome Biol.* **2002**, *3*, research0034.1. [CrossRef]
32. DeKelver, R.C.; Choi, V.M.; Moehle, E.A.; Paschon, D.E.; Hockemeyer, D.; Meijsing, S.H.; Sancak, Y.; Cui, X.; Steine, E.J.; Miller, J.C.; et al. Functional genomics, proteomics, and regulatory DNA analysis in isogenic settings using zinc finger nuclease-driven transgenesis into a safe harbor locus in the human genome. *Genome Res.* **2010**, *20*, 1133–1142. [CrossRef]
33. Ustyantseva, E.I.; Medvedev, S.P.; Vetchinova, A.S.; Minina, J.M.; Illarioshkin, S.N.; Zakian, S.M.; Ustyantseva, E.I.; Medvedev, S.P.; Vetchinova, A.S.; Minina, J.M.; et al. A Platform for Studying Neurodegeneration Mechanisms Using Genetically Encoded Biosensors. *Biochemistry* **2019**, *84*, 299–309. [CrossRef]
34. Ran, F.A.; Hsu, P.D.; Wright, J.; Agarwala, V.; Scott, D.A.; Zhang, F. Genome engineering using the CRISPR-Cas9 system. *Nat. Protoc.* **2013**, *8*, 2281–2308. [CrossRef] [PubMed]
35. Ustyantseva, E.; Pavlova, S.V.; Malakhova, A.A.; Ustyantsev, K.; Zakian, S.M.; Medvedev, S.P. Oxidative stress monitoring in iPSC-derived motor neurons using genetically encoded biosensors of H_2O_2. *Sci. Rep.* **2022**, *12*, 8928. [CrossRef]
36. Oosterveen, T.; Garção, P.; Moles-Garcia, E.; Soleilhavoup, C.; Travaglio, M.; Sheraz, S.; Peltrini, R.; Patrick, K.; Labas, V.; Combes-Soia, L.; et al. Pluripotent stem cell derived dopaminergic subpopulations model the selective neuron degeneration in Parkinson's disease. *Stem Cell Rep.* **2021**, *16*, 2718–2735. [CrossRef] [PubMed]
37. McCullough, K.D.; Martindale, J.L.; Klotz, L.-O.; Aw, T.-Y.; Holbrook, N.J. Gadd153 Sensitizes Cells to Endoplasmic Reticulum Stress by Down-Regulating Bcl2 and Perturbing the Cellular Redox State. *Mol. Cell. Biol.* **2001**, *21*, 1249–1259. [CrossRef] [PubMed]
38. Yarkova, E.S.; Grigor'eva, E.V.; Medvedev, S.P.; Pavlova, S.V.; Zakian, S.M.; Malakhova, A.A. IPSC-Derived Astrocytes Contribute to In Vitro Modeling of Parkinson's Disease Caused by the *GBA1* N370S Mutation. *Int. J. Mol. Sci.* **2023**, *25*, 327. [CrossRef]
39. Tabas, I.; Ron, D. Integrating the mechanisms of apoptosis induced by endoplasmic reticulum stress. *Nat. Cell Biol.* **2011**, *13*, 184–190. [CrossRef]
40. Rozpedek, W.; Pytel, D.; Mucha, B.; Leszczynska, H.; Diehl, J.A.; Majsterek, I. The Role of the PERK/eIF2α/ATF4/CHOP Signaling Pathway in Tumor Progression During Endoplasmic Reticulum Stress. *Curr. Mol. Med.* **2016**, *16*, 533–544. [CrossRef]
41. Huang, W.; Gong, Y.; Yan, L. ER Stress, the Unfolded Protein Response and Osteoclastogenesis: A Review. *Biomolecules* **2023**, *13*, 1050. [CrossRef] [PubMed]
42. Senkevich, K.A.; Kopytova, A.E.; Usenko, T.S.; Emelyanov, A.K.; Pchelina, S.N. Parkinson's Disease Associated with *GBA* Gene Mutations: Molecular Aspects and Potential Treatment Approaches. *Acta Naturae* **2021**, *13*, 70–78. [CrossRef]
43. Chatterjee, D.; Krainc, D. Mechanisms of Glucocerebrosidase Dysfunction in Parkinson's Disease: Mechanisms of GBA1-PD. *J. Mol. Biol.* **2023**, *435*, 168023. [CrossRef] [PubMed]
44. Alcalay, R.N.; Levy, O.A.; Waters, C.C.; Fahn, S.; Ford, B.; Kuo, S.H.; Mazzoni, P.; Pauciulo, M.W.; Nichols, W.C.; Gan-Or, Z.; et al. Glucocerebrosidase activity in Parkinson's disease with and without *GBA* mutations. *Brain* **2015**, *138*, 2648–2658. [CrossRef] [PubMed]

45. Woodard, C.M.; Campos, B.A.; Kuo, S.-H.; Nirenberg, M.J.; Nestor, M.W.; Zimmer, M.; Mosharov, E.V.; Sulzer, D.; Zhou, H.; Paull, D.; et al. iPSC-Derived Dopamine Neurons Reveal Differences between Monozygotic Twins Discordant for Parkinson's Disease. *Cell Rep.* **2014**, *9*, 1173–1182. [CrossRef] [PubMed]
46. Guha, P.; Kaptan, E.; Gade, P.; Kalvakolanu, D.V.; Ahmed, H. Tunicamycin induced endoplasmic reticulum stress promotes apoptosis of prostate cancer cells by activating mTORC1. *Oncotarget* **2017**, *8*, 68191–68207. [CrossRef]
47. Studer, L.; Vera, E.; Cornacchia, D. Programming and reprogramming cellular age in the era of induced pluripotency. *Cell Stem Cell* **2015**, *16*, 591–600. [CrossRef]

Disclaimer/Publisher's Note: The statements, opinions and data contained in all publications are solely those of the individual author(s) and contributor(s) and not of MDPI and/or the editor(s). MDPI and/or the editor(s) disclaim responsibility for any injury to people or property resulting from any ideas, methods, instructions or products referred to in the content.

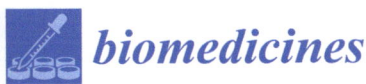

Review

Timing and Graded BMP Signalling Determines Fate of Neural Crest and Ectodermal Placode Derivatives from Pluripotent Stem Cells

Keshi Chung [1,*], Malvina Millet [1,2], Ludivine Rouillon [1] and Azel Zine [1,*]

1 LBN, Laboratory of Bioengineering and Nanoscience, University of Montpellier, 34193 Montpellier, France
2 Harvard Medical School, Massachusetts Eye and Ear Infirmary, Boston, MA 02114, USA
* Correspondence: keshi.chung@umontpellier.fr (K.C.); azel.zine@umontpellier.fr (A.Z.)

Abstract: Pluripotent stem cells (PSCs) offer many potential research and clinical benefits due to their ability to differentiate into nearly every cell type in the body. They are often used as model systems to study early stages of ontogenesis to better understand key developmental pathways, as well as for drug screening. However, in order to fully realise the potential of PSCs and their translational applications, a deeper understanding of developmental pathways, especially in humans, is required. Several signalling molecules play important roles during development and are required for proper differentiation of PSCs. The concentration and timing of signal activation are important, with perturbations resulting in improper development and/or pathology. Bone morphogenetic proteins (BMPs) are one such key group of signalling molecules involved in the specification and differentiation of various cell types and tissues in the human body, including those related to tooth and otic development. In this review, we describe the role of BMP signalling and its regulation, the consequences of BMP dysregulation in disease and differentiation, and how PSCs can be used to investigate the effects of BMP modulation during development, mainly focusing on otic development. Finally, we emphasise the unique role of BMP4 in otic specification and how refined understanding of controlling its regulation could lead to the generation of more robust and reproducible human PSC-derived otic organoids for research and translational applications.

Keywords: bone morphogenetic proteins; human pluripotent stem cells; human cell models; organoids; pre-placodal ectoderm; otic lineage

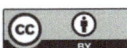

1. Introduction

Many features of early human development can be recapitulated in vitro using pluripotent stem cells (PSCs). The embryonic specification of various domains arising from the different germ layers is achieved by the activation of complex and pleiotropic signalling pathways and inhibitors which interact with one another at critical times during development. Similarly, the addition of numerous small molecules that can either activate or inhibit signalling pathways in cultures of PSCs can lead to their specification and subsequent differentiation into cell types from any of the three germ layers: endoderm, mesoderm, or ectoderm.

Several in vitro protocols have been developed and refined in recent years for the generation of diverse cell types from human PSCs into complex tissue-like structures and organoids, including brain [1,2], cardiac [3–6], blood vessel [7], retina [8–12], lens [13–16], inner ear [17–24], etc. However, variations either across labs or between cell lines exist, suggesting the need for further optimisation of differentiation protocols in order to better understand the complex dynamics of signalling molecules involved in specific developmental pathways.

Bone morphogenetic proteins (BMPs) are one such class of signalling molecules that act in a timed manner across concentration gradients during development. Most BMPs are members of the transforming growth factor β (TGFβ) superfamily of ligands that play critical roles in a multitude of processes during the specification and development of nearly all tissue and cell types. Originally named for their ability to induce bone and cartilage formation [25], they have since been found to be involved in many aspects of development, such as extraembryonic and mesodermal specification [26,27], dorsoventral axis formation (reviewed in [28]), ectodermal patterning, and subsequent specification of ectodermal fates including neuronal, epidermal, and pre-placodal lineages [26,29–32]. Several types of BMP ligands (BMP1, BMP2, BMP4, BMP6, BMP7) have additional roles during early development and interact with multiple receptors (BMPR1A, BMPR1B, BMPR2) and mediators (SMAD proteins) for further specification of various cell types.

For BMP signalling in particular, endogenous levels of expression and activity within cell lines have previously been shown to affect the concentration of BMPs that are required to be added to cultures of PSCs in order to direct differentiation into specific lineages, such as otic lineages [17,18,20,24]. Different levels of BMP and Activin/Nodal signalling are also required for cardiac differentiation of many mouse and human PSC lines [33,34]. A similar observation has been made in human retinal organoids derived from induced PSCs, whereby activation of BMP4 had different effects on different PSC lines, resulting in the generation of different retinal cell types in organoids from each cell line [10]. Differing levels of endogenous BMP4 and BMP4 signalling activity have also been shown to affect differentiation of PSC lines into corneal epithelial-like cells [12]. This suggests that the effects of BMP4 are dependent on the PSC line used, and that in vitro differentiation protocols that are both robust and efficient require optimisation for each cell line.

In addition, the interplay between BMP signalling and other signalling pathways is complex and likely critical in determining cell fate. Indeed, induction of ectodermal placodal fate by exogenous BMP4 in human ES cell lines can be abolished by the addition of WNT3a and rescued when the concentration of BMP4 is increased relative to that of WNT3a [26]. Similarly, Camacho-Aguilar et al. [27] demonstrated the requirement of upregulation of WNT signalling in addition to BMP for conversion of human PSCs from the pluripotent state to mesodermal and extraembryonic fates. Importantly, they observed that the timing of BMP exposure was critical for the specification of different fates, with long and medium culture period duration of exposure to BMP4 driving extraembryonic and mesodermal fates, respectively, due to activation of endogenous WNT, while short pulses of BMP4 caused cells to remain in the pluripotent state. Indeed, recent studies have indicated that it is not necessarily the concentration of BMPs that is important for determining cell fate per se, but rather the integrated signalling level (i.e., concentration and duration) that determines cell fate. Recently, elegant experiments performed by Teague et al. [35] demonstrated that lower levels of BMP signalling over long durations resulted in differentiation similar to that of hPSCs exposed to higher signalling levels over shorter durations, highlighting that the timing of BMP signalling also needs to be taken into account when designing hPSC in vitro differentiation protocols.

2. Role and Function of BMP Signalling during Development

2.1. Dorsoventral Patterning and Ectodermal Derivatives

A gradient of BMP signalling is required for the mechanisms of dorsoventral axis determination during gastrulation (reviewed in [28]). In zebrafish, overexpression of BMP can rescue dorsalised mutants [36], while inhibiting BMP by overexpression of either human *TAPT1* or zebrafish *tapt1a/tapt1b* results in dorsalised embryos [37]. Similarly, in *Xenopus*, inhibition of BMP signalling by injection of the BMP antagonist USAG1 into embryos causes them to become more dorsalised [38], supporting a conserved role of BMPs in dorsoventral axis patterning during embryonic development. R-spondin 2 (RSPO2) has also been shown to regulate dorsoventral axis formation in *Xenopus* by antagonising BMP signalling [39,40]; whether R-spondins are similarly involved in mammalian dorsoventral patterning is not known. Later in development, this BMP gradient appears to be inverted in the ectodermal layer: epidermal specification occurs in the most dorsal region, where BMP concentration is highest; non-neural ectoderm (NNE), which gives rise to pre-placodal ectoderm (PPE), and neural crest in the ventral underlying regions where BMP concentration is lower; and neuronal cell fate where BMP concentration is the lowest [41–43] (Figure 1).

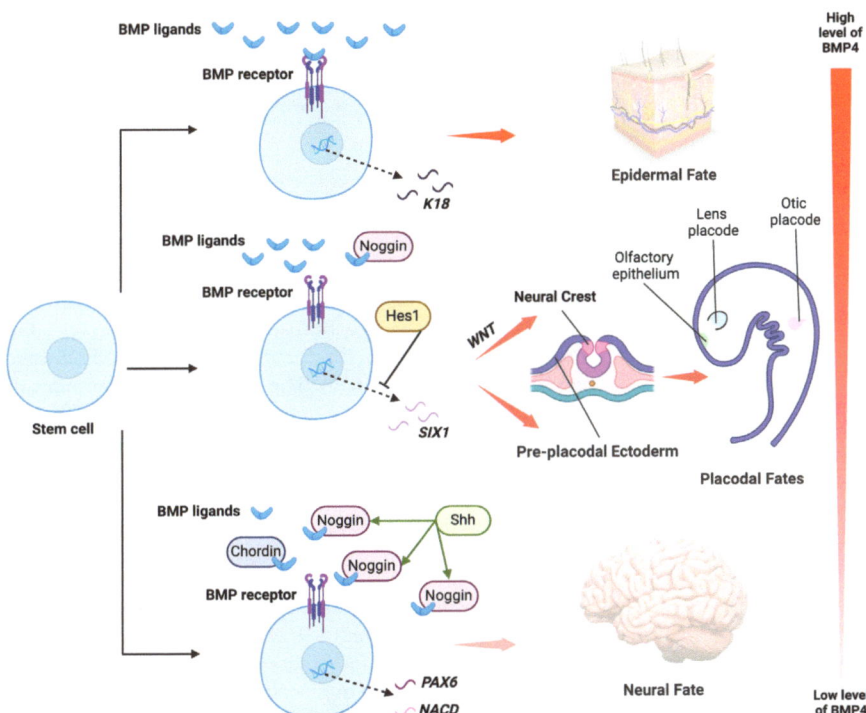

Figure 1. Effects of BMP concentration on fate of ectodermal cells to induce epidermal, placodal, neural crest, and neural derivatives. Exposure of pluripotent stem cells to different concentrations of BMP4 results in differentiation towards different cell fates via activation of various downstream genes. High concentration of BMP4 results in activation of genes such as *K18*, which causes cells to differentiate towards epidermal fate. Medium concentration of BMP4, which can be due to the presence of some inhibitors such as Noggin, causes activation of *SIX1* for differentiation towards pre-placodal ectoderm and subsequent placodal lineages including lens, olfactory, and otic placodes. However, in the presence of WNT, neural crest fate is induced. Activation of genes such as *Hes1* can have an inhibitory effect on this pathway. Low concentration of BMP4, which can be the result of high levels of Noggin due to Shh signalling or the presence of Chordin, results in activation of *PAX6*, *NCAD*, and other genes that result in neural fate. (Generated using Biorender.com, accessed 6 September 2024).

BMPs are required for the expression of NNE genes and PPE competence factors, and previous work with human stem cell lines has demonstrated that this expression requires transient BMP signalling at an optimal concentration for the generation of the desired cell types [26,30,44]. Blocking BMP signalling by the addition of Noggin abolished expression of PPE competence genes and induced expression of the neural precursor marker *HES5* [30], supporting the notion that a reduction of BMPs induces neuronal fate. Conversely, removal of Noggin in human PSCs undergoing neural induction using dual-SMAD inhibition resulted in induction of placodal fate at the expense of neuronal fate [14]. Neuroectodermal cells express several transcription factors that regulate their competency to respond to neural inducing signals and inhibit the effects of BMP and WNT signalling (reviewed in [45,46]). In contrast, high BMP levels have been found to induce epithelial differentiation of human ES cells, and addition of Noggin to these cells can increase the population of Nestin-positive neuroectodermal cells in culture at the expense of keratinocyte differentiation [47]. BMPs appear to block neural differentiation, possibly through induction of *DeltaNp63*, a transcriptional target of BMP signalling that can block neuronal development in zebrafish upon its forced expression in this model organism [48].

The PPE in turn gives rise to the sensory placodes of the head region, including the lens, inner ear, olfactory epithelium, etc. (reviewed in [49]). The development of the placodal structures and their subsequent tissues involves BMP signalling and will be discussed in detail below.

2.2. Placodal Lineages

Sensory placodes derived from the PPE reutilize many of the same signalling molecules and pathways that operate during earlier developmental stages to give rise to a diverse range of cell and tissue types, including the anterior pituitary gland, lens, olfactory epithelium, trigeminal ganglia, otic epithelium, and epibranchial neurons (reviewed in [49]). Studies in *Xenopus* and zebrafish have shown that, once the PPE has been specified, BMPs must then be inhibited by dorsally expressed BMP antagonists in order for placodal development to occur [29,50]. The expression of non-neural genes such as *DLX* and *GATA* inhibits the expression of neural genes such as *SOX2*, and vice versa, resulting in the establishment of distinct non-neural and neural boundaries [51]. PPE cells generated from human iPSCs and ES cells can be further differentiated in vitro to produce various placodally-derived cells, including trigeminal ganglia, lens fibres, and anterior pituitary hormone-producing cells [14,30].

2.2.1. Lens Development

The specification of the PPE into PAX6-expressing anterior placode is required for the development of the eye. BMP induces expression of MAF, a downstream target of PAX6 that is required for the elongation of lens fibre cells and the expression of crystalline [52,53]. Experiments with human ES cell lines have shown that BMP inhibition is required for the induction of the anterior placode from PPE, and that addition of BMP4 is subsequently required for the induction of lens placode from these cells [30]. The addition of recombinant BMP4 or the inhibition of FGF signalling were both also able to induce expression of the lens precursor marker *PITX3* in human PSC-derived pre-placodal cells, which could be further differentiated into crystalline-positive cells containing mature lens fibres [14]. Lentoid bodies can also be generated from hiPSCs and ES cells through continuous stimulation with BMP4 and BMP7, followed by WNT activation [13,15,16], and have recently been employed in drug screening for cataract treatments [16].

2.2.2. Olfactory Epithelium Development

The anterior placode appears to default to lens placode in the absence of additional signals such as FGF, which is required for the development of olfactory epithelium [54]. Loss of BMP signalling is also sufficient to cause prospective lens placodal cells to switch to an olfactory placodal fate [52]. Although BMPs play important roles in the development of the embryonic olfactory epithelium and bulb, where they are expressed along with their receptors [55–57], studies in mouse and chick embryos demonstrate that the expression of SOX2 is required to downregulate BMP4 in the developing olfactory epithelium for subsequent formation of the olfactory pit [56]. Downregulation of BMPs also appears to be required for the development of odorant-responsive olfactory sensory neurons derived from hiPSCs [58]. Nevertheless, BMPs continue to be expressed in the olfactory epithelium throughout adulthood, where they are thought to be important for adult neurogenesis in the olfactory system [57].

2.2.3. Inner Ear Development

The posterior placodal region gives rise to the otic-epibranchial progenitor domain (OEPD), from which both the otic and epibranchial placodes are generated. The otic placode invaginates into the underlying mesenchyme to form the otic vesicle. This involves inhibition of BMP signalling, which is recapitulated in human pluripotent stem cell-derived otic organoids using the BMP inhibitor LDN193189 [17,18,22–24]. Such inhibition of BMP signalling could be mediated by LMO4, which was recently found to negatively regulate BMP2 and BMP4 signalling in the zebrafish inner ear [59].

BMP signalling is also important at later stages of otic development. In chick otic vesicles dissected from E3.5-4 embryos, the addition of recombinant BMP4 reduced the number of hair cells due to decreased proliferation of otic progenitor cells and increased cell death, while the addition of the BMP inhibitor Noggin increased the number of sensory hair cells [60]. Similarly, treatment of chick organotypic cultures with BMP4 during hair cell destruction prevented regeneration of hair cells from supporting cells, while Noggin was able to increase the number of regenerated hair cells [61]. In contrast, another study using chick otocyst cultures reported that blocking BMP signalling reduced generation of hair cells and supporting cells, and that exogenous BMP4 treatment increased the number of hair cells by downregulation of PAX2 in proliferating sensory epithelial progenitor cells [62]. It has been proposed that differences in the concentrations of BMP4 might be responsible for these discrepancies between studies, as the concentration of BMP4 is also found to affect patterning of sensory and nonsensory tissue in the mouse cochlea, with intermediate levels of BMP signalling required to increase the number of sensory hair cells [63]. Similar experiments have not yet been performed in stem cell-derived otic organoids to investigate whether modulation of BMP signalling could alter the number of hair cells (or indeed other otic cell types) produced within these 3D-cell structures.

2.2.4. Epibranchial Placodes

The epibranchial placodes, derived from the posterior placode, give rise to sensory neurons in ganglia associated with the facial, glossopharyngeal, and vagal nerves. While the OEPD is routinely generated during production of otic organoids, and the generation of epibranchial-like neurons has been reported in these cultures [18,22], there are currently no known established models for specific and directed differentiation of epibranchial neurons from human pluripotent stem cells. Interestingly, development of epibranchial-like neurons (and other off-target neurons including neural crest) appears to occur earlier than otic neurons in these cell culture systems [22]. Treatment of stem cell aggregates with FGF, the TGFβ inhibitor SB431542, and the pan-BMP inhibitor LDN193189 was found to be sufficient for the generation of cells expressing posterior placodal markers including PAX8, SOX2, TFAP2A, ECAD, and NCAD, but not the otic marker PAX2 [18], suggesting it may be possible to generate epibranchial neurons separately from otic cells. Moreover, these cells could mature into BRN3A/POU4F1 and TUJ1-positive sensory-like neurons with a morphology more similar to epibranchial neurons than inner ear ganglia neurons. More directed differentiation and maturation of these neurons have not been investigated, although BMP signalling could be involved. Recent experiments in mice have found that blocking BMP signalling using LDN193189 strongly reduced the numbers of neuroblasts in epibranchial placode 1 and moderately in epibranchial placode 3 [64], suggesting a differential requirement for BMP signalling in neurogenesis in the epibranchial placodes.

2.2.5. Trigeminal Neurons

The trigeminal ganglia are derived from the intermediate placode and contain neurons responsible for transmitting sensory information such as pain and temperature from the face. BMP signalling is implicated in the development of trigeminal ganglion neurons, possibly via interaction with MEGF8 [65]. Trigeminal sensory neurons have been generated from hiPSCs by initial activation of BMP signalling. In one protocol, trigeminal fate was subsequently induced by maintaining cells in N2 medium supplemented with ascorbic acid and BDNF [14], while another protocol used CHIR to activate WNT signalling followed by maturation in neurobasal medium supplemented with NGF, BDNF, and GDNF [66]. Engraftment of hiPSC-derived trigeminal ganglia into chicks and mice have shown their survival and ability to establish axonal projections to their target regions [14].

2.3. Tooth Development

Teeth are another ectodermally derived tissue, and their development requires reciprocal interactions between the epithelium and mesenchyme [67]. BMPs, in particular, play a role and have been shown to interact with other signalling pathways such as SHH [68] and WNT [69] during tooth development. Experiments in mice at embryonic days E14 and E15 have confirmed the expression of BMP2 in the oral epithelium, and of BMP4, BMP6, and BMP7 in both the epithelium and mesenchyme [70,71]. Uterine sensitization associated gene-1 (USAG1) is an antagonist of BMP signalling which is also expressed in the epithelium and mesenchyme during tooth formation [70,72]. Mice lacking USAG1 have an increased number of teeth (supernumerary teeth) which is due to enhanced BMP signalling [71,72], suggesting that BMPs are involved in regulating tooth number. Indeed, topical administration of BMP7 can result in partial supernumerary incisor formation in mouse dental explant cultures [70]. Modulation of BMP signalling has also been used to recover tooth development in mice [73]. By using antibodies to block USAG1 in a mouse model of tooth agenesis, Murashima-Suginami and colleagues were able to induce tooth formation in these mice.

Human ES cells have been used to generate oral ectoderm and dental epithelium following a differentiation protocol with increasing concentration of BMP4 [74]. These cells could be mixed with cultures of mouse dental mesenchyme and, when transplanted into murine hosts, were capable of forming tooth-like structures in vivo. Recently developed in vitro protocols have enabled the rapid generation of dental epithelial cells from hiPSCs in just over one week, by simultaneously inhibiting BMP signalling and activating SHH signalling to generate oral ectoderm from NNE, followed by activation of BMP and SHH pathways and inhibition of WNT signalling [75]. It is not clear why the induction of Pitx1-expressing oral epithelium required a low concentration of BMPs in one protocol and BMP inhibition in the other, although differences in endogenous BMP signalling and activity between the cell lines used in these studies may account for this discrepancy.

2.4. Neural Crest

BMP signalling, in conjunction with WNT and FGF, is also important for development of the neural crest [76–79], and WNT signalling appears to be key in determining whether ectodermal cells become NNE/PPE or neural crest. Neural crest cells, localised at the dorsolateral position of the neural tube, give rise to the neurons and glia of the peripheral nervous system, the enteric nervous system, as well as non-neural derivatives. Low concentrations of BMP4 in combination with WNT activation have been shown to generate SOX10-expressing neural crest cells from human PSC cultures [44]. Similarly, treatment of neural crest stem cell-like cells isolated from human skin with BMP2 and an activator of WNT signalling improves their multipotency and differentiation potential to neural crest lineage cells [80]. Conversely, in cultures of human ES cells, BMP signalling in combination with the inhibition of WNT signalling resulted in increased expression of SIX1-positive PPE cells and a reduced number of cells expressing PAX3 and SOX9 neural crest markers [26]. The low levels of BMP required for neural crest induction may be mediated by Gremlin 1, which acts as a BMP antagonist during early neural crest development, and also interacts with heparan sulfate proteoglycans during later stages of neural crest development [81].

2.5. Cardiac Development

BMPs act with other signalling pathways, including WNT, Nodal, and FGF, to induce early mesoderm (reviewed in [82]). Specification of later mesodermal fates, such as cardiac, requires additional BMP signalling. BMP2 and BMP4 are involved in cardiomyogenesis, with exogeneous application of either BMP2 or BMP4 proving sufficient to induce ectopic cardiomyocyte differentiation in chick embryos [83]. Experiments performed in precardiac spheroids generated from PSCs found that the specification of two separate populations of cardiac progenitor cells (termed first and second heart fields) requires BMP signalling, but that cells of the first heart field are specified via the BMP/SMAD pathway, while cells of the second heart field are specified through the SMAD-independent BMP/WNT pathway [3]. Moreover, blocking BMP signalling abolished the specification of both populations of cardiac progenitor cells, highlighting the importance of BMPs for early cardiac development. Nevertheless, modulation of WNT signalling is sufficient to generate heart organoids from PSCs, although the addition of BMP4 and Activin A was found to improve the size and vascularisation of organoids [5].

Certain cardiac structures, such as the cardiac outflow tract and aortic arch, are derived from neural crest cells (reviewed in [84]). Cardiac neural crest cells have also been proposed to contribute to regeneration of the myocardium following injury in zebrafish and mice [85–87]. In mice, cKit-positive cardiac neural crest cells possess full cardiomyogenic capacity and give rise to several cardiac cell types, which is a process dependent on BMP antagonism [88]. The suppression of BMP activity is also involved in fate specification of cardiac neural crest cells, via Adam19-mediated cleavage of ACVR1 and suppression of the BMP-SOX9 cascade [89]. In contrast, BMP activity is required for delamination of neural crest cells from the dorsal neural tube [90,91], via cleavage of N-cadherin allowing these cells to migrate [92]. Stem cell therapies based on cardiac neural crest cells derived from hiPSCs could offer a promising therapy for heart repair following disease or injury, but further investigation is required to better understand the processes involved in the specification of cardiac neural crest cells as distinct from other types of neural crest cells, and to determine how to differentiate these cells into the various cardiac cell types.

2.6. Bone

The role of BMPs in bone development, homeostasis, and remodelling has been extensively reviewed elsewhere [93,94]. Exposure of mesenchymal stem cells (MSCs) to BMP2 is able to induce osteogenic differentiation of these cells both in vitro and in vivo and promote bone formation [95–98]. Hydrogels containing BMP2 mimetics were found to induce bone formation when injected into rats, which was enhanced when these hydrogels were injected in combination with MSCs [95,97]. In addition to BMP2, BMP9 may also be important for bone formation and regeneration. Overexpression of BMP9 in MSCs increased their osteogenic potential and resulted in increased bone formation and bone mineral density when injected into rats with calvarial bone defects [99]. This BMP9-induced differentiation of MSCs towards osteogenic fate seems to require Notch signalling, as the inhibition of Notch prevents BMP9-induced osteogenic differentiation [100]. A recent study revealed that conditioned media from MSCs overexpressing BMP9 also enhanced bone repair of mouse calvarial defects, compared with media from MSCs that did not overexpress BMP9 [101], suggesting the presence of additional trophic factors released by these cells. BMP9 was additionally able to induce osteogenic differentiation in spheroids derived from human gingival stem cells [102], indicating that osteogenesis can be induced in several types of stem cells.

More recently, attempts have been made to induce bone formation from iPSCs, due to their greater proliferative and differentiation capabilities over MSCs. Bone formation has successfully been induced in hiPSCs using retinoic acid, which results in activation of BMP and WNT signalling pathways and differentiation of hiPSCs into osteoblast-like and osteocyte-like cells [103]. These cells were able to form bone tissue when injected into mice with calvarial defects, and also recapitulated the phenotype of osteogenesis-imperfecta when cultured from patient-derived iPSCs. Undifferentiated muscle-derived hiPSCs loaded onto an osteoconductive scaffold and implanted into mice can induce ectopic bone formation [104]. Analysis of the scaffolds at 15 and 30 days post-implantation revealed the absence of mRNA of human origin, suggesting that the implanted cells were able to induce bone formation via a paracrine communication. Indeed, conditioned media from these cells was able to induce expression of osteogenesis-related genes, upregulation of BMP2, BMP4, and BMP6, increased phosphorylation of SMAD 1/5/8, and the appearance of calcium-containing deposits in the extracellular matrix of cultured human MSCs. Further analysis of these undifferentiated hiPSCs in culture revealed higher expression of BMPs relative to expression in fibroblasts, with BMP2 levels being particularly elevated. It is unclear whether this high expression of BMPs is due to the muscle-derived origin of these cells, or whether hiPSCs derived from other cell types would have similarly high BMP expression. It also cannot be ruled out that the high BMP levels are a feature of the cell line that was used in the study. Further experiments in additional hiPSC lines derived from cells of different origins would help to clarify this issue.

Unlike bone formation in the rest of the body, the bone and cartilage of craniofacial structures are derived from cranial neural crest cells, a process which relies heavily on BMP signalling (reviewed in [105]). Treatment of human PSCs with BMP4 from day 8 after neural crest specification induces the expression of cranial neural crest markers such as *TFAP2A*, *MSX1*, and *DLX1* [106]. Increased BMP signalling in cranial neural crest cells has been shown to cause premature fusion of cranial sutures and skull bass deformities in mice [107–109]. As a result of this difference in embryonic origin, the MSCs found in cranial structures have different characteristics from those in the long bones. For instance, orofacial MSCs and iliac crest MSCs from the same donor have been found to behave differently when cultured in vitro. Orofacial MSCs proliferated more rapidly and had delayed senescence compared with iliac crest MSCs. Moreover, iliac crest MSCs were more responsive to osteogenic and adipogenic inductions than orofacial MSCs [110]. Recently, ectodermal MSCs, derived from human ES cells via a neural crest intermediate, have been compared with adult bone marrow-derived MSCs. They were found to have comparable osteogenic and chondrogenic abilities in culture, although ectodermal MSCs had greater proliferation and formed more dense osseous constructs in a rat calvarial defect model [111].

3. Regulation of BMP Signalling during Development

3.1. BMP Signalling Pathways and Downstream Effects on Gene Expression

BMPs act on their receptors, which are typically heterotetrameric complexes composed of type I and type II serine/threonine kinase receptors. Upon ligand binding, type II receptors phosphorylate type I receptors, which then activate SMAD1, SMAD5, and SMAD8 (Figure 2). These receptor-regulated SMADs pair with SMAD4 and translocate to the nucleus to influence the transcription of target genes. This signalling affects gene expression linked to cell growth, differentiation, and apoptosis, which is crucial during embryonic development [112,113]. Certain subclasses of BMPs, such as BMP4, have specific effects on developmental pathways, including those of inner ear hair cells and spiral ganglion neurons, highlighting their importance for neurosensory differentiation [62,114].

3.2. Endogenous Activators and Inhibitors of BMP Signalling

BMP signalling is finely tuned by endogenous molecules and its role in the differentiation of many cell types, including neural differentiation, is complex. While BMPs are generally antagonistic to neural differentiation at early stages of development, they promote the formation of autonomic and sensory neurons from neural crest progenitors at later stages. Extracellular antagonists like Noggin, Chordin, Gremlin, and Follistatin bind BMP proteins (Figure 2), inhibiting receptor interaction and modulating processes such as neural and limb development. Conversely, modulators like Twisted Gastrulation (TWSG1) can either enhance or inhibit BMP signalling depending on the developmental context. For instance, TWSG1 can enhance BMP signalling in the context of early neural development, promoting neural crest cell formation, while it can inhibit BMP signalling during limb formation to prevent excessive growth. USAG1 directly binds to BMPs to antagonise BMP signalling and has been shown to be important for tooth and kidney development [38,71–73]. Transmembrane anterior posterior transformation 1 (TAPT1), involved in axial skeletal patterning, causes proteasomal degradation of SMAD1/5, thereby inhibiting BMP signalling [37]. R-spondin 2 and 3 (RSPO2 and RSPO3) act as BMP antagonists by binding to the BMP receptor BMPR1A, resulting in their internalisation and degradation [39,40]. Intracellular inhibitors such as SMAD6 and SMAD7 prevent R-SMAD phosphorylation or promote receptor degradation, ensuring balanced BMP4 activity for normal development [115,116]. BMP4 specifically promotes glial differentiation while inhibiting oligodendrocyte formation, but this can be overridden by Notch signalling, which favours Schwann cell differentiation [117–119].

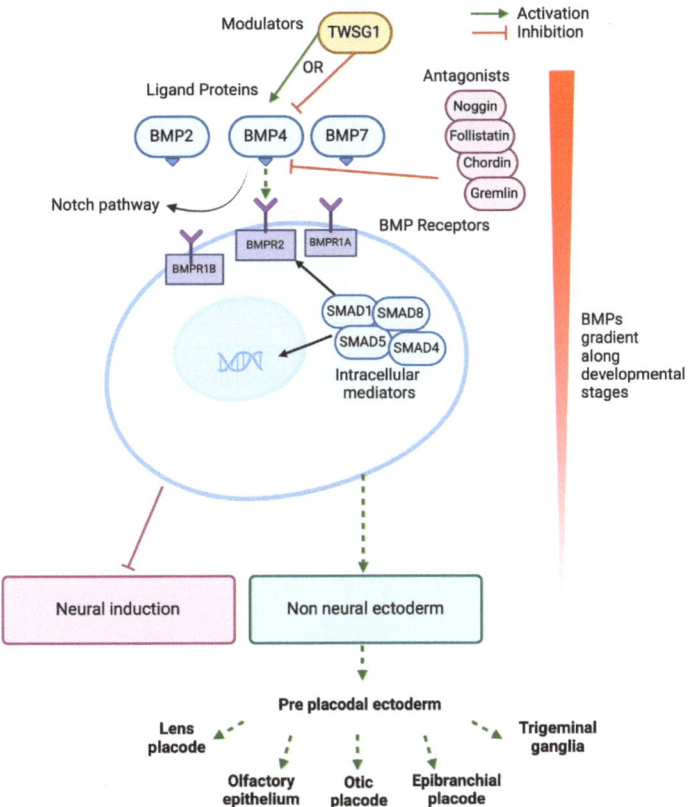

Figure 2. Overview of BMP signalling pathway and modulators during development of pre-placodal ectoderm. BMPs such as BMP4 bind to their receptors BMPR1A, BMPR1B, and BMPR2 on the cell surface, resulting in activation of SMADs which translocate to the nucleus to influence transcription of genes directing cell fate towards non-neural ectoderm/pre-placodal and subsequent placodal fates, and inhibiting differentiation towards neural fate. The presence of antagonists and modulators such as Noggin, Follistatin, Chordin, Gremlin, and TWSG1 alter the level of BMP activity on the cell and hence can also influence cell fate. (Generated using Biorender.com, accessed 6 September 2024).

4. Consequences of BMP Dysregulation

Because of their diverse roles in development and differentiation of many cell types, dysregulation of BMPs, their receptors, and their endogenous modulators can have a spectrum of effects on nearly every tissue type involving all three germ layers. Indeed, BMPs are essential for development, with embryonic lethality reported in mice lacking expression of either BMP2 or BMP4 [120,121], while mice deficient in BMP7 experience eye, kidney, and skeletal patterning defects and die shortly after birth [122,123]. Expression of BMP4 is found to be strong in mouse caudal tissues, and loss of BMP4 in this region resulted in hindlimb fusion and lethality [124].

The effects of dysregulation of BMP signalling and its links to various diseases have been extensively reviewed elsewhere [125–129], highlighting the need for improved understanding of the roles of BMPs, their receptors, and their modulators in development and disease. Considering the importance of BMP signalling for development and differentiation of tissues, studying the effects of BMPs in whole model organisms is challenging, due to the lack of viability and early arrest of growth and development of embryos following perturbation of BMP signalling. Moreover, many different tissues and organs may be affected, which further complicates interpretation of the effects of loss, mutation, or forced expression of BMP and/or its receptors and modulators in the whole organism. Some of these effects are likely to be secondary, arising from gross defects caused by dysregulation of BMP signalling, rather than as a direct consequence of BMP signalling itself. Conditional knockouts (and other similar targeting of specific tissues) might overcome some of these limitations. For instance, while loss of BMP4 results in embryonic lethality, Suzuki et al. [124] were able to use a conditional knockout *Isl1*-Cre mouse line in which BMP4 expression was reduced in the caudal body region only, allowing their mice to survive to a developmental stage late enough to investigate the caudalising effects of BMP4. Likewise, Chang et al. [130] conditionally deleted BMP4 expression in the mouse inner ear and were able to demonstrate the importance of BMP4 for the formation of the vestibular cristae and canals. They also succeeded in electroporating expression vectors to inhibit BMP signalling directly into the otocyst of the developing chick, and observed that downregulation of BMPs resulted in patterning defects in the crista, although they cautioned that some of the effects could also be due to electroporation rather than reduced BMP signalling.

Using pluripotent stem cells to investigate BMP signalling could also be used to overcome some of the limitations mentioned above, although care must be taken to ensure that perturbations of BMP signalling do not affect their overall survival, maintenance, and differentiation potential. Indeed, the ability of cells to differentiate towards the desired lineage is likely to be affected in conditions of abnormal BMP signalling or if cells are unable to respond to exogenous BMP. The maintenance of murine ES cell pluripotency has been shown to require BMP4, which induces the expression of *Klf2* [131], although direct BMP signalling is unlikely to be involved in the maintenance of human ES and iPS cell pluripotency, as these cells are primed, unlike mouse ES, and require Activin A for their maintenance [132–134].

Generation of pluripotent stem cells may also be affected by perturbation of BMP activity. For instance, fibroblasts from fibrodysplasia ossificans progressiva patients carrying a mutation in the *ACVR1* gene, which resulted in hyperactivation of BMP-SMAD signalling, were found to have increased iPSC reprogramming efficiency [135]. The addition of exogenous BMP4 to cultures during the early stages of reprogramming was found to have a similar effect. Recently, modulation of the stiffness of the hydrogels on which fibroblasts were cultured during reprogramming to iPSCs was found to upregulate BMP2 and several genes involved in BMP signalling, as well as improve reprogramming of the cells. Increased hydrogel stiffness upregulated *Phactr3*, which then resulted in increased BMP2 and improved reprogramming efficiency [136]. How *Phactr3* causes an increase in BMP2 is not known, although *Phactr3* is known to associate with nuclear nonchromatin structure [137], where it might influence expression of genes involved in reprogramming. Alternatively, *Phactr3* may exert its effects by inhibiting polymerisation of actin within the cell, resulting in increased cell spreading [138]. Recent studies have shown that changes in cell shape can affect the distribution of BMP receptors on the cell membrane [139].

5. Uses of Pluripotent Stem Cells to Investigate the Role of BMP in Development
5.1. Advantages and Limitations of Human PSCs

Stem cells, particularly human-derived stem cells, are invaluable tools for studying development and disease mechanisms without the need for fetal samples, which are difficult to acquire. They provide the opportunity to study aspects of development that are specific to humans. Indeed, previous studies have demonstrated differences in development and disease mechanisms between humans and animal models [140,141]. For instance, in the case of the inner ear, development and maturation are nearly complete by approximately 36 weeks of gestation in humans [142,143], whereas in mice, the cells of the cochlea of the inner ear continue to develop and mature after birth until about the third post-natal week [144,145]. This highlights the need for human-specific models to study development. Moreover, patient-derived stem cells can be used to study development in a patient-specific or disease context, without the need for generating mutant cell lines that might not behave in the same manner or may fail to recapitulate some aspects of the disease. Gene correction of such patient-derived stem cells can also be used to correct mutations to investigate whether proper functioning of the gene is regained, opening the way for gene therapy treatments. For instance, patient-derived hiPSCs have recently been used to model mutations in *TMC1*, which are associated with a type of progressive hearing loss termed DFNA36 [146]. While differentiation of pluripotent stem cells to sensory hair cells was not affected by the TMC1 mutation, the morphology and electrophysiological properties of the derived hair cells were altered. Additionally, using CRISPR/Cas9 genome editing technique to generate an isogenic cell line, in which the mutated gene was corrected, resulted in the recovery of hair cell morphology and electrophysiology. Similar works have been done using patient-derived lines carrying mutations for several genes associated with hearing loss, including *USH2A* [147,148], *TRMU* [149], *ELMOD3* [150], *MYO7A* [151], and *AIFM1* [152], highlighting the potential strength of this approach for therapeutic genome editing.

In spite of recent developments and advances in stem cell technologies, numerous barriers must still be overcome before stem cells can reach their optimal potential in research and clinical applications. Many stem cell differentiation protocols result in batch-to-batch variability and also variation between labs, necessitating further refinements to produce more uniform and homogenous populations of the desired cell and tissue types being investigated. Furthermore, unlike studying development in animal models, such in vitro differentiation often occurs in isolation from other cell types, which might provide trophic and supportive factors beneficial to generating the cells under investigation. For instance, differentiation and development of inner ear hair cells require the support of the surrounding connective tissue and mesenchymal cells [153–155]. Indeed, otic mesenchyme cells comprise a diverse array of cell types that make up several important cell types in the inner ear, including spiral limbus fibrocytes and modiolar osteoblasts [156]. Since hair cells rely on neurons to transmit auditory signals to the brain, co-culturing stem cell-derived hair cells with spiral ganglion neurons should be considered to establish functional circuits. Additionally, the generation of vascularised organoids would be beneficial to enable the growth of larger and healthier organoids. Incorporation of such tissues in the form of co-cultures and assembloids can lead to the development of more robust and mature models, which have already shown promising results [157,158]. However, this may also complicate the system, especially if looking for populations of pure and mature cells with the intention of being able to transplant the generated cells into patients. Finally, different biomaterials should also be tested to investigate their roles and potential benefits in constructing more physiologically relevant 3D culture systems that better recapitulate the tissue microenvironment (reviewed in [159]), as remodelling of the extracellular matrix plays an important role during maturation of the cochlea (reviewed in [160]).

5.2. Otic Neurosensory Specification as a Model to Study BMP4 Signalling

Because BMPs are involved in many steps of inner ear development and are required at specific concentrations over precise durations [161], otic lineages provide an interesting model system to investigate the effects of BMP signalling during development. Human PSCs can be differentiated under either 2D or 3D culture systems to give rise to otic progenitors that express several of the markers and components of activation pathways found during early otic development, and eventually hair cells, supporting cells, and neurons in inner ear otic organoids that have been allowed to mature in long-term culture [17,18,20,22,24,162]. Recent advances in 3D-otic organoids have additionally been able to generate both cochlear and vestibular type hair cells [20], demonstrating the ability to finely control the generation of inner ear hair cells in such 3D-cell culture systems.

Mutations in some genes involved in BMP signalling are associated with hearing loss (Table 1). Nager syndrome is associated with hearing loss as a result of mutations in the *SF3B4* gene, which codes for a spliceosome that affects expression of Noggin and BMPs and may be directly involved in neural crest and otic development [163]. Mutations in chondroitin synthase 1 (*CHSY1*), involved in the synthesis of chondroitin sulfate, are characterised by limb malformations, short stature, and hearing loss [164], and studies in the inner ears of zebrafish larvae have found that *Chsy1* expression is similar to that of the BMP inhibitor *dan* and complementary to *Bmp2b* expression, suggesting a role for this gene in BMP signalling and otic development [165]. In cultures of mouse chondrocytes, knockdown of *Chsy1* resulted in increased BMP signalling, while overexpression of *Chsy1* reduced BMP signalling [166]. Whether similar effects of *Sf3b4*, *Chsy1*, and other genes potentially involved in BMP signalling (Table 1) can be observed in cultures of PSC-derived otic progenitors remains to be investigated.

Table 1. Genes involved in BMP signalling that are associated with hearing loss in humans.

Gene	Role in BMP Signalling	Inner Ear Deficits	Additional Symptoms	References
ACVR1 (Activin A receptor type 1)	Type 1 BMP receptor	Sensorineural hearing loss; conductive hearing loss	Bone and skeletal disorders	[167–170]
BMP2	BMP ligand	Conductive hearing loss (otosclerosis)	Craniofacial, cardiac, and skeletal anomalies	[171–175]
BMP4	BMP ligand	Sensorineural hearing loss; conductive hearing loss (otosclerosis)	Eye, joint, and craniofacial disorders, renal dysplasia	[171,172,174,176]
BMP7	BMP ligand	Sensorineural hearing loss	Eye anomalies, developmental delay, scoliosis, cleft palate	[177]
CHD7	Promotes Col2a1 expression; regulation of BMPR1B expression	Sensorineural hearing loss; some conductive hearing loss due to enlargement of vestibular aqueduct	Vestibular dysfunctions, hypogonadotropic hypogonadism	[178–180]
CHSY1 (Chondroitin synthase 1)	BMP inhibition	Sensorineural hearing loss	Facial dysmorphism, dental anomalies, digital anomalies, delayed motor development, delayed mental development, growth retardation	[164]
COL2A1	Binds BMPs	Sensorineural hearing loss	Short stature, bone and joint dysplasias, ocular problems	[181–183]
GDF6 (Growth and differentiation factor 6)	Forms heterodimers with BMPs	Conductive hearing loss (otosclerosis); cochlear aplasia	Wrist and ankle deformities, tarsal–carpal fusion, vertebral fusion, speech impairment	[184–187]
NOG (Noggin)	BMP antagonist	Conductive hearing loss (stapes ankylosis and incus short process fixation)	Bone and joint disorders, digital and eye anomalies	[188–197]
SF3B4 (Splicing factor 3B subunit 4)	Spliceosome that affects Noggin and BMP expression	Conductive, sensorineural, and mixed hearing loss	Craniofacial defects, limb defects	[163]
SMAD4	Downstream effector of BMP signalling	Conductive, sensorineural, and mixed hearing loss	Short stature, facial dysmorphism, muscular hypertrophy, cognitive delay	[198–204]
TMEM53 (Transmembrane protein 53)	Inhibits BMP/SMAD signalling	Sensorineural hearing loss	Bone and eye disorders	[205,206]

One of the consequences of suboptimal BMP4 signalling during the early specification of otic progenitors under these pluripotent cell culture systems is the generation of off-target cell types, such as neurons and surface epidermis [8,20,24,171]. Current methods for detecting subtle differences in off-target differentiation are mostly restricted to immunolabelling and qPCR analyses for off-target genes, most of which are transcription factors. It has also been reported that the epithelial thickness of organoids after just 3 days in vitro can be used as a proxy to optimise BMP4 concentration in such cultures [24]. However, the link between BMP4 concentration and epidermal thickness is not clear, and this method requires the production and screening of many otic organoids. New methods that can allow for the rapid detection of off-target differentiation using fewer samples would enable researchers to detect such off-target effects more efficiently and gain a better understanding of the variations between different lineages, beyond the expression of transcription factors, for example, in the biochemical and metabolic properties of such in vitro differentiated cells.

Pluripotent stem cells also offer the opportunity to study the effects of BMP signalling at later stages of development. Several studies have reported conductive hearing loss in patients with mutations in the *NOG* gene, which encodes for the BMP antagonist Noggin, resulting from auditory-ossicle fusion [188–197]. As these patients exhibit additional symptoms, including bone and joint disorders and digital anomalies, patient-derived stem cells may facilitate the study of these mutations specifically in inner ear development. This approach could help determine at which stages in development these symptoms begin to appear, as well as follow disease progression and test the effects of potential therapeutics. PSC-derived otic organoids could also be used to investigate the role of different BMPs in cochlear and vestibular development in humans, as these organs have been shown to require differential BMP signalling in chick embryos [114].

6. Conclusions and Future Perspectives

Advances in stem cell research have greatly expanded our knowledge and understanding of development and the signalling pathways involved in developmental processes, while also prompting new questions and lines of investigation. Nevertheless, as the role of BMP signalling in the development of the inner ear and other tissues has demonstrated, further work is needed to better understand general human-specific developmental and disease pathways and mechanisms, rather than potentially batch or cell line-specific features. As signalling pathways other than BMP are likely to differ among cell types and perhaps among culture conditions, the starting state of stem cell cultures should be determined before initiating any cell differentiation protocol, in order to ensure that the optimal conditions for differentiation of the desired tissues are being met. New technologies could help to simplify the determination of endogenous levels of signalling molecules and signalling activity in cell lines, allowing for more robust and homogeneous cultures that better recapitulate in vivo conditions.

Author Contributions: Conceptualization, A.Z. and K.C.; writing—original draft preparation, K.C. and M.M.; writing—review and editing, K.C., A.Z., M.M. and L.R.; visualization, K.C., A.Z., M.M. and L.R.; supervision, A.Z.; project administration, A.Z.; funding acquisition, A.Z. All authors have read and agreed to the published version of the manuscript.

Funding: This research has been financially supported by la Fondation pour l'Audition (Paris) to A.Z., grant number FPA RD-2022-8.

Acknowledgments: We sincerely apologize for the articles that could not be referenced due to space limitations. We thank several collaborators, in particular, Frederic Cuisinier (LBN, University of Montpellier), Hanae Lahlou, and Albert Edge (Harvard Medical School).

Conflicts of Interest: The authors declare no conflicts of interest.

Abbreviations

ACVR1	Activin A receptor type 1
BMP	Bone morphogenetic protein
CHSY1	Chondroitin synthase 1
ES	Embryonic stem cell
FGF	Fibroblast growth factor
hiPSC	Human induced pluripotent stem cell
OEPD	Otic-epibranchial progenitor domain
MSC	Mesenchymal stem cell
NNE	Non-neural ectoderm
PPE	Pre-placodal ectoderm
PSC	Pluripotent stem cell
SHH	Sonic hedgehog
TAPT1	Transmembrane anterior posterior transformation 1
TGFβ	Transforming growth factor beta
TMEM53	Transmembrane protein 53
TWSG1	Twisted Gastrulation 1
USAG1	Uterine sensitization associated gene-1

References

1. Chiaradia, I.; Lancaster, M.A. Brain Organoids for the Study of Human Neurobiology at the Interface of In Vitro and In Vivo. *Nat. Neurosci.* **2020**, *23*, 1496–1508. [CrossRef] [PubMed]
2. Lancaster, M.A.; Renner, M.; Martin, C.-A.; Wenzel, D.; Bicknell, L.S.; Hurles, M.E.; Homfray, T.; Penninger, J.M.; Jackson, A.P.; Knoblich, J.A. Cerebral Organoids Model Human Brain Development and Microcephaly. *Nature* **2013**, *501*, 373–379. [CrossRef] [PubMed]
3. Andersen, P.; Tampakakis, E.; Jimenez, D.V.; Kannan, S.; Miyamoto, M.; Shin, H.K.; Saberi, A.; Murphy, S.; Sulistio, E.; Chelko, S.P.; et al. Precardiac Organoids Form Two Heart Fields via Bmp/Wnt Signaling. *Nat. Commun.* **2018**, *9*, 3140. [CrossRef] [PubMed]
4. Kostina, A.; Lewis-Israeli, Y.R.; Abdelhamid, M.; Gabalski, M.A.; Kiselev, A.; Volmert, B.D.; Lankerd, H.; Huang, A.R.; Wasserman, A.H.; Lydic, T.; et al. ER Stress and Lipid Imbalance Drive Diabetic Embryonic Cardiomyopathy in an Organoid Model of Human Heart Development. *Stem Cell Rep.* **2024**, *19*, 317–330. [CrossRef] [PubMed]
5. Lewis-Israeli, Y.R.; Wasserman, A.H.; Gabalski, M.A.; Volmert, B.D.; Ming, Y.; Ball, K.A.; Yang, W.; Zou, J.; Ni, G.; Pajares, N.; et al. Self-Assembling Human Heart Organoids for the Modeling of Cardiac Development and Congenital Heart Disease. *Nat. Commun.* **2021**, *12*, 5142. [CrossRef]
6. Lewis-Israeli, Y.R.; Abdelhamid, M.; Olomu, I.; Aguirre, A. Modeling the Effects of Maternal Diabetes on the Developing Human Heart Using Pluripotent Stem Cell–Derived Heart Organoids. *Curr. Protoc.* **2022**, *2*, e461. [CrossRef]
7. Wimmer, R.A.; Leopoldi, A.; Aichinger, M.; Wick, N.; Hantusch, B.; Novatchkova, M.; Taubenschmid, J.; Hämmerle, M.; Esk, C.; Bagley, J.A.; et al. Human Blood Vessel Organoids as a Model of Diabetic Vasculopathy. *Nature* **2019**, *565*, 505–510. [CrossRef]
8. Agarwal, D.; Dash, N.; Mazo, K.W.; Chopra, M.; Avila, M.P.; Patel, A.; Wong, R.M.; Jia, C.; Do, H.; Cheng, J.; et al. Human Retinal Ganglion Cell Neurons Generated by Synchronous BMP Inhibition and Transcription Factor Mediated Reprogramming. *NPJ Regen. Med.* **2023**, *8*, 55. [CrossRef]
9. Capowski, E.E.; Samimi, K.; Mayerl, S.J.; Phillips, M.J.; Pinilla, I.; Howden, S.E.; Saha, J.; Jansen, A.D.; Edwards, K.L.; Jager, L.D.; et al. Reproducibility and Staging of 3D Human Retinal Organoids across Multiple Pluripotent Stem Cell Lines. *Development* **2018**, *146*, dev171686. [CrossRef]
10. Chichagova, V.; Hilgen, G.; Ghareeb, A.; Georgiou, M.; Carter, M.; Sernagor, E.; Lako, M.; Armstrong, L. Human IPSC Differentiation to Retinal Organoids in Response to IGF1 and BMP4 Activation Is Line- and Method-Dependent. *Stem Cells* **2020**, *38*, 195–201. [CrossRef]
11. Hallam, D.; Hilgen, G.; Dorgau, B.; Zhu, L.; Yu, M.; Bojic, S.; Hewitt, P.; Schmitt, M.; Uteng, M.; Kustermann, S.; et al. Human-Induced Pluripotent Stem Cells Generate Light Responsive Retinal Organoids with Variable and Nutrient-Dependent Efficiency. *Stem Cells* **2018**, *36*, 1535–1551. [CrossRef] [PubMed]
12. Kamarudin, T.A.; Bojic, S.; Collin, J.; Yu, M.; Alharthi, S.; Buck, H.; Shortt, A.; Armstrong, L.; Figueiredo, F.C.; Lako, M. Differences in the Activity of Endogenous Bone Morphogenetic Protein Signaling Impact on the Ability of Induced Pluripotent Stem Cells to Differentiate to Corneal Epithelial-Like Cells. *Stem Cells* **2018**, *36*, 337–348. [CrossRef] [PubMed]
13. Ali, M.; Kabir, F.; Thomson, J.J.; Ma, Y.; Qiu, C.; Delannoy, M.; Khan, S.Y.; Riazuddin, S.A. Comparative Transcriptome Analysis of HESC- and IPSC-Derived Lentoid Bodies. *Sci. Rep.* **2019**, *9*, 18552. [CrossRef] [PubMed]
14. Dincer, Z.; Piao, J.; Niu, L.; Ganat, Y.; Kriks, S.; Zimmer, B.; Shi, S.-H.; Tabar, V.; Studer, L. Specification of Functional Cranial Placode Derivatives from Human Pluripotent Stem Cells. *Cell Rep.* **2013**, *5*, 1387–1402. [CrossRef]
15. Fu, Q.; Qin, Z.; Jin, X.; Zhang, L.; Chen, Z.; He, J.; Ji, J.; Yao, K. Generation of Functional Lentoid Bodies from Human Induced Pluripotent Stem Cells Derived from Urinary Cells. *Investig. Opthalmol. Vis. Sci.* **2017**, *58*, 517. [CrossRef]

16. Zhang, L.; Qin, Z.; Lyu, D.; Lu, B.; Chen, Z.; Fu, Q.; Yao, K. Postponement of the Opacification of Lentoid Bodies Derived from Human Induced Pluripotent Stem Cells after Lanosterol Treatment—The First Use of the Lens Aging Model in Vitro in Cataract Drug Screening. *Front. Pharmacol.* **2022**, *13*, 959978. [CrossRef]
17. Doda, D.; Alonso Jimenez, S.; Rehrauer, H.; Carreño, J.F.; Valsamides, V.; Di Santo, S.; Widmer, H.R.; Edge, A.; Locher, H.; van der Valk, W.H.; et al. Human Pluripotent Stem Cell-Derived Inner Ear Organoids Recapitulate Otic Development In Vitro. *Development* **2023**, *150*, dev201865. [CrossRef]
18. Koehler, K.R.; Nie, J.; Longworth-Mills, E.; Liu, X.-P.; Lee, J.; Holt, J.R.; Hashino, E. Generation of Inner Ear Organoids Containing Functional Hair Cells from Human Pluripotent Stem Cells. *Nat. Biotechnol.* **2017**, *35*, 583–589. [CrossRef]
19. Kurihara, S.; Fujioka, M.; Hirabayashi, M.; Yoshida, T.; Hosoya, M.; Nagase, M.; Kato, F.; Ogawa, K.; Okano, H.; Kojima, H.; et al. Otic Organoids Containing Spiral Ganglion Neuron-like Cells Derived from Human-Induced Pluripotent Stem Cells as a Model of Drug-Induced Neuropathy. *Stem Cells Transl. Med.* **2022**, *11*, 282–296. [CrossRef]
20. Moore, S.T.; Nakamura, T.; Nie, J.; Solivais, A.J.; Aristizábal-Ramírez, I.; Ueda, Y.; Manikandan, M.; Reddy, V.S.; Romano, D.R.; Hoffman, J.R.; et al. Generating High-Fidelity Cochlear Organoids from Human Pluripotent Stem Cells. *Cell Stem Cell* **2023**, *30*, 950–961.e7. [CrossRef]
21. Nie, J.; Ueda, Y.; Solivais, A.J.; Hashino, E. CHD7 Regulates Otic Lineage Specification and Hair Cell Differentiation in Human Inner Ear Organoids. *Nat. Commun.* **2022**, *13*, 7053. [CrossRef] [PubMed]
22. Steinhart, M.R.; van der Valk, W.H.; Osorio, D.; Serdy, S.A.; Zhang, J.; Nist-Lund, C.; Kim, J.; Moncada-Reid, C.; Sun, L.; Lee, J.; et al. Mapping Oto-Pharyngeal Development in a Human Inner Ear Organoid Model. *Development* **2023**, *150*, dev201871. [CrossRef] [PubMed]
23. Ueda, Y.; Nakamura, T.; Nie, J.; Solivais, A.J.; Hoffman, J.R.; Daye, B.J.; Hashino, E. Defining Developmental Trajectories of Prosensory Cells in Human Inner Ear Organoids at Single-Cell Resolution. *Development* **2023**, *150*, dev201071. [CrossRef] [PubMed]
24. van der Valk, W.H.; van Beelen, E.S.A.; Steinhart, M.R.; Nist-Lund, C.; Osorio, D.; de Groot, J.C.M.J.; Sun, L.; van Benthem, P.P.G.; Koehler, K.R.; Locher, H. A Single-Cell Level Comparison of Human Inner Ear Organoids with the Human Cochlea and Vestibular Organs. *Cell Rep.* **2023**, *42*, 112623. [CrossRef]
25. Urist, M.R.; Strates, B.S. Bone Morphogenetic Protein. *J. Dent. Res.* **1971**, *50*, 1392–1406. [CrossRef]
26. Britton, G.; Heemskerk, I.; Hodge, R.; Qutub, A.A.; Warmflash, A. A Novel Self-Organizing Embryonic Stem Cell System Reveals Signaling Logic Underlying the Patterning of Human Ectoderm. *Development* **2019**, *1*, 169–191. [CrossRef]
27. Camacho-Aguilar, E.; Yoon, S.T.; Ortiz-Salazar, M.A.; Du, S.; Guerra, M.C.; Warmflash, A. A Combinatorial Interpretation of BMP and WNT Controls the Decision between Primitive Streak and Extraembryonic Fates. *Cell Syst.* **2024**, *15*, 445–461.e4. [CrossRef]
28. Yan, Y.; Wang, Q. BMP Signaling: Lighting up the Way for Embryonic Dorsoventral Patterning. *Front. Cell Dev. Biol.* **2021**, *9*, 799772. [CrossRef]
29. Kwon, H.-J.; Bhat, N.; Sweet, E.M.; Cornell, R.A.; Riley, B.B. Identification of Early Requirements for Preplacodal Ectoderm and Sensory Organ Development. *PLoS Genet.* **2010**, *6*, e1001133. [CrossRef]
30. Leung, A.W.; Kent Morest, D.; Li, J.Y.H. Differential BMP Signaling Controls Formation and Differentiation of Multipotent Preplacodal Ectoderm Progenitors from Human Embryonic Stem Cells. *Dev. Biol.* **2013**, *379*, 208–220. [CrossRef]
31. Li, L.; Liu, C.; Biechele, S.; Zhu, Q.; Song, L.; Lanner, F.; Jing, N.; Rossant, J. Location of Transient Ectodermal Progenitor Potential in Mouse Development. *Development* **2013**, *140*, 4533–4543. [CrossRef] [PubMed]
32. Reichert, S.; Randall, R.A.; Hill, C.S. A BMP Regulatory Network Controls Ectodermal Cell Fate Decisions at the Neural Plate Border. *Development* **2013**, *140*, 4435–4444. [CrossRef] [PubMed]
33. Kattman, S.J.; Witty, A.D.; Gagliardi, M.; Dubois, N.C.; Niapour, M.; Hotta, A.; Ellis, J.; Keller, G. Stage-Specific Optimization of Activin/Nodal and BMP Signaling Promotes Cardiac Differentiation of Mouse and Human Pluripotent Stem Cell Lines. *Cell Stem Cell* **2011**, *8*, 228–240. [CrossRef] [PubMed]
34. Sa, S.; McCloskey, K.E. Activin A and BMP4 Signaling for Efficient Cardiac Differentiation of H7 and H9 Human Embryonic Stem Cells. *J. Stem Cells Regen. Med.* **2012**, *8*, 198–202. [CrossRef]
35. Teague, S.; Primavera, G.; Chen, B.; Liu, Z.-Y.; Yao, L.; Freeburne, E.; Khan, H.; Jo, K.; Johnson, C.; Heemskerk, I. Time-Integrated BMP Signaling Determines Fate in a Stem Cell Model for Early Human Development. *Nat. Commun.* **2024**, *15*, 1471. [CrossRef]
36. Kishimoto, Y.; Lee, K.-H.; Zon, L.; Hammerschmidt, M.; Schulte-Merker, S. The Molecular Nature of Zebrafish Swirl: BMP2 Function Is Essential during Early Dorsoventral Patterning. *Development* **1997**, *124*, 4457–4466. [CrossRef]
37. Wang, B.; Zhao, Q.; Gong, X.; Wang, C.; Bai, Y.; Wang, H.; Zhou, J.; Rong, X. Transmembrane Anterior Posterior Transformation 1 Regulates BMP Signaling and Modulates the Protein Stability of SMAD1/5. *J. Biol. Chem.* **2022**, *298*, 102684. [CrossRef]
38. Yanagita, M.; Oka, M.; Watabe, T.; Iguchi, H.; Niida, A.; Takahashi, S.; Akiyama, T.; Miyazono, K.; Yanagisawa, M.; Sakurai, T. USAG-1: A Bone Morphogenetic Protein Antagonist Abundantly Expressed in the Kidney. *Biochem. Biophys. Res. Commun.* **2004**, *316*, 490–500. [CrossRef]
39. Lee, H.; Seidl, C.; Sun, R.; Glinka, A.; Niehrs, C. R-Spondins Are BMP Receptor Antagonists in Xenopus Early Embryonic Development. *Nat. Commun.* **2020**, *11*, 5570. [CrossRef]
40. Lee, H.; Sun, R.; Niehrs, C. Uncoupling the BMP Receptor Antagonist Function from the WNT Agonist Function of R-Spondin 2 Using the Inhibitory Peptide Dendrimer RWd. *J. Biol. Chem.* **2022**, *298*, 101586. [CrossRef]

41. Suzuki, A.; Kaneko, E.; Ueno, N.; Hemmati-Brivanlou, A. Regulation of epidermal induction by BMP2 and BMP7 signaling. *Dev. Biol.* **1997**, *189*, 112–122. [CrossRef] [PubMed]
42. Wilson, P.A.; Hemmati-Brivanlou, A. Induction of epidermis and inhibition of neural fate by Bmp-4. *Nature* **1995**, *376*, 331–333. [CrossRef] [PubMed]
43. Wilson, P.A.; Lagna, G.; Suzuki, A.; Hemmati-Brivanlou, A. Concentration-Dependent Patterning of the Xenopus Ectoderm by BMP4 and Its Signal Transducer Smad1. *Development* **1997**, *124*, 3177–3184. [CrossRef] [PubMed]
44. Tchieu, J.; Zimmer, B.; Fattahi, F.; Amin, S.; Zeltner, N.; Chen, S.; Studer, L. A Modular Platform for Differentiation of Human PSCs into All Major Ectodermal Lineages. *Cell Stem Cell* **2017**, *21*, 399–410.e7. [CrossRef] [PubMed]
45. Lee, H.-K.; Lee, H.-S.; Moody, S.A. Neural Transcription Factors: From Embryos to Neural Stem Cells. *Mol. Cells* **2014**, *37*, 705–712. [CrossRef] [PubMed]
46. Zine, A.; Fritzsch, B. Early Steps towards Hearing: Placodes and Sensory Development. *Int. J. Mol. Sci.* **2023**, *24*, 6994. [CrossRef]
47. Metallo, C.M.; Ji, L.; de Pablo, J.J.; Palecek, S.P. Retinoic Acid and Bone Morphogenetic Protein Signaling Synergize to Efficiently Direct Epithelial Differentiation of Human Embryonic Stem Cells. *Stem Cells* **2008**, *26*, 372–380. [CrossRef]
48. Bakkers, J.; Hild, M.; Kramer, C.; Furutani-Seiki, M.; Hammerschmidt, M. Zebrafish ΔNp63 Is a Direct Target of Bmp Signaling and Encodes a Transcriptional Repressor Blocking Neural Specification in the Ventral Ectoderm. *Dev. Cell* **2002**, *2*, 617–627. [CrossRef]
49. Conti, E.; Harschnitz, O. Human Stem Cell Models to Study Placode Development, Function and Pathology. *Development* **2022**, *149*, dev200831. [CrossRef]
50. Ahrens, K.; Schlosser, G. Tissues and Signals Involved in the Induction of Placodal Six1 Expression in Xenopus Laevis. *Dev. Biol.* **2005**, *288*, 40–59. [CrossRef]
51. Pieper, M.; Ahrens, K.; Rink, E.; Peter, A.; Schlosser, G. Differential distribution of competence for panplacodal and neural crest induction to non-neural and neural ectoderm. *Development* **2012**, *139*, 1175–1187. [CrossRef] [PubMed]
52. Pandit, T.; Jidigam, V.K.; Gunhaga, L. BMP-induced L-Maf regulates subsequent BMP-independent differentiation of primary lens fibre cells. *Dev. Dyn.* **2011**, *240*, 1917–1928. [CrossRef] [PubMed]
53. Reza, H.M.; Ogino, H.; Yasuda, K. L-Maf, a downstream target of Pax6, is essential for chick lens development. *Mech. Dev.* **2002**, *116*, 61–73. [CrossRef] [PubMed]
54. Bailey, A.P.; Bhattacharyya, S.; Bronner-Fraser, M.; Streit, A. Lens specification is the ground state of all sensory placodes, from which FGF promotes olfactory identity. *Dev. Cell* **2006**, *11*, 505–517. [CrossRef] [PubMed]
55. Ito, A.; Miller, C.; Imamura, F. Suppression of BMP Signaling Restores Mitral Cell Development Impaired by FGF Signaling Deficits in Mouse Olfactory Bulb. *Mol. Cell. Neurosci.* **2024**, *128*, 103913. [CrossRef]
56. Panaliappan, T.K.; Wittmann, W.; Jidigam, V.K.; Mercurio, S.; Bertolini, J.A.; Sghari, S.; Bose, R.; Patthey, C.; Nicolis, S.K.; Gunhaga, L. Sox2 Is Required for Olfactory Pit Formation and Olfactory Neurogenesis through BMP Restriction and Hes5 Upregulation. *Development* **2018**, *145*, dev153791. [CrossRef]
57. Peretto, P.; Cummings, D.; Modena, C.; Behrens, M.; Venkatraman, G.; Fasolo, A.; Margolis, F.L. BMP MRNA and Protein Expression in the Developing Mouse Olfactory System. *J. Comp. Neurol.* **2002**, *451*, 267–278. [CrossRef]
58. Kikuta, H.; Tanaka, H.; Ozaki, T.; Ito, J.; Ma, J.; Moribe, S.; Hirano, M. Spontaneous Differentiation of Human Induced Pluripotent Stem Cells to Odorant-Responsive Olfactory Sensory Neurons. *Biochem. Biophys. Res. Commun.* **2024**, *719*, 150062. [CrossRef]
59. Sun, L.; Ping, L.; Gao, R.; Zhang, B.; Chen, X. Lmo4a Contributes to Zebrafish Inner Ear and Vestibular Development via Regulation of the Bmp Pathway. *Genes* **2023**, *14*, 1371. [CrossRef]
60. Pujades, C.; Kamaid, A.; Alsina, B.; Giraldez, F. BMP-Signaling Regulates the Generation of Hair-Cells. *Dev. Biol.* **2006**, *292*, 55–67. [CrossRef]
61. Lewis, R.M.; Keller, J.J.; Wan, L.; Stone, J.S. Bone Morphogenetic Protein 4 Antagonizes Hair Cell Regeneration in the Avian Auditory Epithelium. *Hear. Res.* **2018**, *364*, 1–11. [CrossRef] [PubMed]
62. Li, H.; Corrales, C.E.; Wang, Z.; Zhao, Y.; Wang, Y.; Liu, H.; Heller, S. BMP4 Signaling Is Involved in the Generation of Inner Ear Sensory Epithelia. *BMC Dev. Biol.* **2005**, *5*, 16. [CrossRef] [PubMed]
63. Ohyama, T.; Basch, M.L.; Mishina, Y.; Lyons, K.M.; Segil, N.; Groves, A.K. BMP Signaling Is Necessary for Patterning the Sensory and Nonsensory Regions of the Developing Mammalian Cochlea. *J. Neurosci.* **2010**, *30*, 15044–15051. [CrossRef] [PubMed]
64. Washausen, S.; Knabe, W. Responses of Epibranchial Placodes to Disruptions of the FGF and BMP Signaling Pathways in Embryonic Mice. *Front. Cell Dev. Biol.* **2021**, *9*, 712522. [CrossRef] [PubMed]
65. Engelhard, C.; Sarsfield, S.; Merte, J.; Wang, Q.; Li, P.; Beppu, H.; Kolodkin, A.L.; Sucov, H.M.; Ginty, D.D. MEGF8 is a modifier of BMP signaling in trigeminal sensory neurons. *Elife* **2013**, *17*, e01160. [CrossRef]
66. Zimmer, B.; Ewaleifoh, O.; Harschnitz, O.; Lee, Y.-S.; Peneau, C.; McAlpine, J.L.; Liu, B.; Tchieu, J.; Steinbeck, J.A.; Lafaille, F.; et al. Human IPSC-Derived Trigeminal Neurons Lack Constitutive TLR3-Dependent Immunity That Protects Cortical Neurons from HSV-1 Infection. *Proc. Natl. Acad. Sci. USA* **2018**, *115*, E8775–E8782. [CrossRef]
67. Thesleff, I. Epithelial-Mesenchymal Signalling Regulating Tooth Morphogenesis. *J. Cell Sci.* **2003**, *116*, 1647–1648. [CrossRef]
68. Li, J.; Feng, J.; Liu, Y.; Ho, T.-V.; Grimes, W.; Ho, H.A.; Park, S.; Wang, S.; Chai, Y. BMP-SHH Signaling Network Controls Epithelial Stem Cell Fate via Regulation of Its Niche in the Developing Tooth. *Dev. Cell* **2015**, *33*, 125–135. [CrossRef]
69. Yuan, G.; Yang, G.; Zheng, Y.; Zhu, X.; Chen, Z.; Zhang, Z.; Chen, Y. The Non-Canonical BMP and Wnt/β-Catenin Signaling Pathways Orchestrate Early Tooth Development. *Development* **2015**, *142*, 128–139. [CrossRef]

70. Kiso, H.; Takahashi, K.; Saito, K.; Togo, Y.; Tsukamoto, H.; Huang, B.; Sugai, M.; Shimizu, A.; Tabata, Y.; Economides, A.N.; et al. Interactions between BMP-7 and USAG-1 (Uterine Sensitization-Associated Gene-1) Regulate Supernumerary Organ Formations. *PLoS ONE* **2014**, *9*, e96938. [CrossRef]
71. Murashima-Suginami, A.; Takahashi, K.; Sakata, T.; Tsukamoto, H.; Sugai, M.; Yanagita, M.; Shimizu, A.; Sakurai, T.; Slavkin, H.C.; Bessho, K. Enhanced BMP Signaling Results in Supernumerary Tooth Formation in USAG-1 Deficient Mouse. *Biochem. Biophys. Res. Commun.* **2008**, *369*, 1012–1016. [CrossRef] [PubMed]
72. Murashima-Suginami, A.; Takahashi, K.; Kawabata, T.; Sakata, T.; Tsukamoto, H.; Sugai, M.; Yanagita, M.; Shimizu, A.; Sakurai, T.; Slavkin, H.C.; et al. Rudiment Incisors Survive and Erupt as Supernumerary Teeth as a Result of USAG-1 Abrogation. *Biochem. Biophys. Res. Commun.* **2007**, *359*, 549–555. [CrossRef] [PubMed]
73. Murashima-Suginami, A.; Kiso, H.; Tokita, Y.; Mihara, E.; Nambu, Y.; Uozumi, R.; Tabata, Y.; Bessho, K.; Takagi, J.; Sugai, M.; et al. Anti-USAG-1 Therapy for Tooth Regeneration through Enhanced BMP Signaling. *Sci. Adv.* **2021**, *7*, eabf1798. [CrossRef] [PubMed]
74. Li, Q.; Zhang, S.; Sui, Y.; Fu, X.; Li, Y.; Wei, S. Sequential Stimulation with Different Concentrations of BMP4 Promotes the Differentiation of Human Embryonic Stem Cells into Dental Epithelium with Potential for Tooth Formation. *Stem Cell Res. Ther.* **2019**, *10*, 276. [CrossRef]
75. Zhu, X.; Li, Y.; Dong, Q.; Tian, C.; Gong, J.; Bai, X.; Ruan, J.; Gao, J. Small Molecules Promote the Rapid Generation of Dental Epithelial Cells from Human-Induced Pluripotent Stem Cells. *Int. J. Mol. Sci.* **2024**, *25*, 4138. [CrossRef]
76. LaBonne, C.; Bronner-Fraser, M. Neural crest induction in Xenopus: Evidence for a two-signal model. *Development* **1998**, *125*, 2403–2414. [CrossRef]
77. Raible, D.W.; Ragland, J.W. Reiterated Wnt and BMP Signals in Neural Crest Development. *Semin. Cell Dev. Biol.* **2005**, *16*, 673–682. [CrossRef]
78. Steventon, B.; Araya, C.; Linker, C.; Kuriyama, S.; Mayor, R. Differential requirements of BMP and Wnt signalling during gastrulation and neurulation define two steps in neural crest induction. *Development* **2009**, *136*, 771–779. [CrossRef]
79. Villanueva, S.; Glavic, A.; Ruiz, P.; Mayor, R. Posteriorization by FGF, Wnt, and retinoic acid is required for neural crest induction. *Dev. Biol.* **2002**, *241*, 289–301. [CrossRef]
80. Mehrotra, P.; Ikhapoh, I.; Lei, P.; Tseropoulos, G.; Zhang, Y.; Wang, J.; Liu, S.; Bronner, M.E.; Andreadis, S.T. Wnt/BMP Mediated Metabolic Reprogramming Preserves Multipotency of Neural Crest-Like Stem Cells. *Stem Cells* **2023**, *41*, 287–305. [CrossRef]
81. Pegge, J.; Tatsinkam, A.J.; Rider, C.C.; Bell, E. Heparan sulfate proteoglycans regulate BMP signalling during neural crest induction. *Dev. Biol.* **2020**, *460*, 108–114. [CrossRef] [PubMed]
82. Galdos, F.X.; Guo, Y.; Paige, S.L.; VanDusen, N.J.; Wu, S.M.; Pu, W.T. Cardiac Regeneration. *Circ. Res.* **2017**, *120*, 941–959. [CrossRef] [PubMed]
83. Schultheiss, T.M.; Burch, J.B.; Lassar, A.B. A Role for Bone Morphogenetic Proteins in the Induction of Cardiac Myogenesis. *Genes Dev.* **1997**, *11*, 451–462. [CrossRef] [PubMed]
84. Yamagishi, H. Cardiac Neural Crest. *Cold Spring Harb. Perspect. Biol.* **2021**, *13*, a036715. [CrossRef] [PubMed]
85. Sande-Melón, M.; Marques, I.J.; Galardi-Castilla, M.; Langa, X.; Pérez-López, M.; Botos, M.-A.; Sánchez-Iranzo, H.; Guzmán-Martínez, G.; Ferreira Francisco, D.M.; Pavlinic, D.; et al. Adult Sox10+ Cardiomyocytes Contribute to Myocardial Regeneration in the Zebrafish. *Cell Rep.* **2019**, *29*, 1041–1054.e5. [CrossRef] [PubMed]
86. Tamura, Y.; Matsumura, K.; Sano, M.; Tabata, H.; Kimura, K.; Ieda, M.; Arai, T.; Ohno, Y.; Kanazawa, H.; Yuasa, S.; et al. Neural Crest–Derived Stem Cells Migrate and Differentiate into Cardiomyocytes After Myocardial Infarction. *Arterioscler. Thromb. Vasc. Biol.* **2011**, *31*, 582–589. [CrossRef] [PubMed]
87. Tang, W.; Martik, M.L.; Li, Y.; Bronner, M.E. Cardiac Neural Crest Contributes to Cardiomyocytes in Amniotes and Heart Regeneration in Zebrafish. *Elife* **2019**, *8*, e47929. [CrossRef]
88. Hatzistergos, K.E.; Takeuchi, L.M.; Saur, D.; Seidler, B.; Dymecki, S.M.; Mai, J.J.; White, I.A.; Balkan, W.; Kanashiro-Takeuchi, R.M.; Schally, A.V.; et al. CKit + Cardiac Progenitors of Neural Crest Origin. *Proc. Natl. Acad. Sci. USA* **2015**, *112*, 13051–13056. [CrossRef]
89. Arai, H.N.; Sato, F.; Yamamoto, T.; Woltjen, K.; Kiyonari, H.; Yoshimoto, Y.; Shukunami, C.; Akiyama, H.; Kist, R.; Sehara-Fujisawa, A. Metalloprotease-Dependent Attenuation of BMP Signaling Restricts Cardiac Neural Crest Cell Fate. *Cell Rep.* **2019**, *29*, 603–616.e5. [CrossRef]
90. Sela-Donenfeld, D.; Kalcheim, C. Regulation of the Onset of Neural Crest Migration by Coordinated Activity of BMP4 and Noggin in the Dorsal Neural Tube. *Development* **1999**, *126*, 4749–4762. [CrossRef]
91. Burstyn-Cohen, T.; Stanleigh, J.; Sela-Donenfeld, D.; Kalcheim, C. Canonical Wnt Activity Regulates Trunk Neural Crest Delamination Linking BMP/Noggin Signaling with G1/S Transition. *Development* **2004**, *131*, 5327–5339. [CrossRef] [PubMed]
92. Shoval, I.; Ludwig, A.; Kalcheim, C. Antagonistic Roles of Full-Length N-Cadherin and Its Soluble BMP Cleavage Product in Neural Crest Delamination. *Development* **2007**, *134*, 491–501. [CrossRef] [PubMed]
93. Lowery, J.W.; Rosen, V. The BMP Pathway and Its Inhibitors in the Skeleton. *Physiol. Rev.* **2018**, *98*, 2431–2452. [CrossRef] [PubMed]
94. Wu, M.; Wu, S.; Chen, W.; Li, Y.-P. The Roles and Regulatory Mechanisms of TGF-β and BMP Signaling in Bone and Cartilage Development, Homeostasis and Disease. *Cell Res.* **2024**, *34*, 101–123. [CrossRef]

95. Gultian, K.A.; Gandhi, R.; DeCesari, K.; Romiyo, V.; Kleinbart, E.P.; Martin, K.; Gentile, P.M.; Kim, T.W.B.; Vega, S.L. Injectable Hydrogel with Immobilized BMP-2 Mimetic Peptide for Local Bone Regeneration. *Front. Biomater. Sci.* **2022**, *1*, 948493. [CrossRef]
96. Hanada, K.; Dennis, J.E.; Caplan, A.I. Stimulatory Effects of Basic Fibroblast Growth Factor and Bone Morphogenetic Protein-2 on Osteogenic Differentiation of Rat Bone Marrow-Derived Mesenchymal Stem Cells. *J. Bone Miner. Res.* **1997**, *12*, 1606–1614. [CrossRef]
97. Love, S.A.; Gultian, K.A.; Jalloh, U.S.; Stevens, A.; Kim, T.W.B.; Vega, S.L. Mesenchymal Stem Cells Enhance Targeted Bone Growth from Injectable Hydrogels with BMP-2 Peptides. *J. Orthop. Res.* **2024**, *42*, 1599–1607. [CrossRef]
98. Moutsatsos, I.K.; Turgeman, G.; Zhou, S.; Kurkalli, B.G.; Pelled, G.; Tzur, L.; Kelley, P.; Stumm, N.; Mi, S.; Müller, R.; et al. Exogenously Regulated Stem Cell-Mediated Gene Therapy for Bone Regeneration. *Mol. Ther.* **2001**, *3*, 449–461. [CrossRef]
99. Freitas, G.P.; Lopes, H.B.; Souza, A.T.P.; Gomes, M.P.O.; Quiles, G.K.; Gordon, J.; Tye, C.; Stein, J.L.; Stein, G.S.; Lian, J.B.; et al. Mesenchymal Stem Cells Overexpressing BMP-9 by CRISPR-Cas9 Present High In Vitro Osteogenic Potential and Enhance in Vivo Bone Formation. *Gene Ther.* **2021**, *28*, 748–759. [CrossRef]
100. Cui, J.; Zhang, W.; Huang, E.; Wang, J.; Liao, J.; Li, R.; Yu, X.; Zhao, C.; Zeng, Z.; Shu, Y.; et al. BMP9-Induced Osteoblastic Differentiation Requires Functional Notch Signaling in Mesenchymal Stem Cells. *Lab. Investig.* **2019**, *99*, 58–71. [CrossRef]
101. Calixto, R.D.; Freitas, G.P.; Souza, P.G.; Ramos, J.I.R.; Santos, I.C.; de Oliveira, F.S.; Almeida, A.L.G.; Rosa, A.L.; Beloti, M.M. Effect of the Secretome of Mesenchymal Stem Cells Overexpressing BMP-9 on Osteoblast Differentiation and Bone Repair. *J. Cell. Physiol.* **2023**, *238*, 2625–2637. [CrossRef] [PubMed]
102. Lee, S.-B.; Lee, H.-J.; Park, J.-B. Bone Morphogenetic Protein-9 Promotes Osteogenic Differentiation and Mineralization in Human Stem-Cell-Derived Spheroids. *Medicina* **2023**, *59*, 1315. [CrossRef] [PubMed]
103. Kawai, S.; Yoshitomi, H.; Sunaga, J.; Alev, C.; Nagata, S.; Nishio, M.; Hada, M.; Koyama, Y.; Uemura, M.; Sekiguchi, K.; et al. In Vitro Bone-like Nodules Generated from Patient-Derived IPSCs Recapitulate Pathological Bone Phenotypes. *Nat. Biomed. Eng.* **2019**, *3*, 558–570. [CrossRef] [PubMed]
104. Oudina, K.; Paquet, J.; Moya, A.; Massourides, E.; Bensidhoum, M.; Larochette, N.; Deschepper, M.; Pinset, C.; Petite, H. The Paracrine Effects of Human Induced Pluripotent Stem Cells Promote Bone-like Structures via the Upregulation of BMP Expression in a Mouse Ectopic Model. *Sci. Rep.* **2018**, *8*, 17106. [CrossRef]
105. Graf, D.; Malik, Z.; Hayano, S.; Mishina, Y. Common Mechanisms in Development and Disease: BMP Signaling in Craniofacial Development. *Cytokine Growth Factor. Rev.* **2016**, *27*, 129–139. [CrossRef]
106. Mimura, S.; Suga, M.; Okada, K.; Kinehara, M.; Nikawa, H.; Furue, M.K. Bone Morphogenetic Protein 4 Promotes Craniofacial Neural Crest Induction from Human Pluripotent Stem Cells. *Int. J. Dev. Biol.* **2016**, *60*, 21–28. [CrossRef]
107. Komatsu, Y.; Yu, P.B.; Kamiya, N.; Pan, H.; Fukuda, T.; Scott, G.J.; Ray, M.K.; Yamamura, K.; Mishina, Y. Augmentation of Smad-Dependent BMP Signaling in Neural Crest Cells Causes Craniosynostosis in Mice. *J. Bone Miner. Res.* **2013**, *28*, 1422–1433. [CrossRef]
108. Ueharu, H.; Pan, H.; Liu, X.; Ishii, M.; Pongetti, J.; Kulkarni, A.K.; Adegbenro, F.E.; Wurn, J.; Maxson, R.E.; Sun, H.; et al. Augmentation of BMP Signaling in Cranial Neural Crest Cells Leads to Premature Cranial Sutures Fusion through Endochondral Ossification in Mice. *JBMR Plus* **2023**, *7*, e10716. [CrossRef]
109. Ueharu, H.; Pan, H.; Hayano, S.; Zapien-Guerra, K.; Yang, J.; Mishina, Y. Augmentation of Bone Morphogenetic Protein Signaling in Cranial Neural Crest Cells in Mice Deforms Skull Base Due to Premature Fusion of Intersphenoidal Synchondrosis. *Genesis* **2023**, *61*, e23509. [CrossRef]
110. Akintoye, S.O.; Lam, T.; Shi, S.; Brahim, J.; Collins, M.T.; Robey, P.G. Skeletal Site-Specific Characterization of Orofacial and Iliac Crest Human Bone Marrow Stromal Cells in Same Individuals. *Bone* **2006**, *38*, 758–768. [CrossRef]
111. Srinivasan, A.; Teo, N.; Poon, K.J.; Tiwari, P.; Ravichandran, A.; Wen, F.; Teoh, S.H.; Lim, T.C.; Toh, Y.-C. Comparative Craniofacial Bone Regeneration Capacities of Mesenchymal Stem Cells Derived from Human Neural Crest Stem Cells and Bone Marrow. *ACS Biomater. Sci. Eng.* **2021**, *7*, 207–221. [CrossRef] [PubMed]
112. Coucouvanis, E.; Martin, G.R. BMP Signaling Plays a Role in Visceral Endoderm Differentiation and Cavitation in the Early Mouse Embryo. *Development* **1999**, *126*, 535–546. [CrossRef] [PubMed]
113. Wang, R.N.; Green, J.; Wang, Z.; Deng, Y.; Qiao, M.; Peabody, M.; Zhang, Q.; Ye, J.; Yan, Z.; Denduluri, S.; et al. Bone Morphogenetic Protein (BMP) Signaling in Development and Human Diseases. *Genes Dis.* **2014**, *1*, 87–105. [CrossRef] [PubMed]
114. Oh, S.-H.; Johnson, R.; Wu, D.K. Differential Expression of Bone Morphogenetic Proteins in the Developing Vestibular and Auditory Sensory Organs. *J. Neurosci.* **1996**, *16*, 6463–6475. [CrossRef] [PubMed]
115. Solloway, M.J.; Robertson, E.J. Early Embryonic Lethality in Bmp5;Bmp7 Double Mutant Mice Suggests Functional Redundancy within the 60A Subgroup. *Development* **1999**, *126*, 1753–1768. [CrossRef]
116. Wu, M.Y.; Hill, C.S. TGF-β Superfamily Signaling in Embryonic Development and Homeostasis. *Dev. Cell* **2009**, *16*, 329–343. [CrossRef]
117. Morrison, S.J.; Perez, S.E.; Qiao, Z.; Verdi, J.M.; Hicks, C.; Weinmaster, G.; Anderson, D.J. Transient Notch Activation Initiates an Irreversible Switch from Neurogenesis to Gliogenesis by Neural Crest Stem Cells. *Cell* **2000**, *101*, 499–510. [CrossRef]
118. Lim, D.A.; Tramontin, A.D.; Trevejo, J.M.; Herrera, D.G.; García-Verdugo, J.M.; Alvarez-Buylla, A. Noggin Antagonizes BMP Signaling to Create a Niche for Adult Neurogenesis. *Neuron* **2000**, *28*, 713–726. [CrossRef]
119. Gomes, W.A.; Mehler, M.F.; Kessler, J.A. Transgenic Overexpression of BMP4 Increases Astroglial and Decreases Oligodendroglial Lineage Commitment. *Dev. Biol.* **2003**, *255*, 164–177. [CrossRef]

120. Winnier, G.; Blessing, M.; Labosky, P.A.; Hogan, B.L. Bone Morphogenetic Protein-4 Is Required for Mesoderm Formation and Patterning in the Mouse. *Genes Dev.* **1995**, *9*, 2105–2116. [CrossRef]
121. Zhang, H.; Bradley, A. Mice Deficient for BMP2 Are Nonviable and Have Defects in Amnion/Chorion and Cardiac Development. *Development* **1996**, *122*, 2977–2986. [CrossRef] [PubMed]
122. Dudley, A.T.; Lyons, K.M.; Robertson, E.J. A Requirement for Bone Morphogenetic Protein-7 during Development of the Mammalian Kidney and Eye. *Genes Dev.* **1995**, *9*, 2795–2807. [CrossRef] [PubMed]
123. Luo, G.; Hofmann, C.; Bronckers, A.L.; Sohocki, M.; Bradley, A.; Karsenty, G. BMP-7 Is an Inducer of Nephrogenesis, and Is Also Required for Eye Development and Skeletal Patterning. *Genes Dev.* **1995**, *9*, 2808–2820. [CrossRef] [PubMed]
124. Suzuki, K.; Adachi, Y.; Numata, T.; Nakada, S.; Yanagita, M.; Nakagata, N.; Evans, S.M.; Graf, D.; Economides, A.; Haraguchi, R.; et al. Reduced BMP Signaling Results in Hindlimb Fusion with Lethal Pelvic/Urogenital Organ Aplasia: A New Mouse Model of Sirenomelia. *PLoS ONE* **2012**, *7*, e43453. [CrossRef] [PubMed]
125. Correns, A.; Zimmermann, L.M.A.; Baldock, C.; Sengle, G. BMP Antagonists in Tissue Development and Disease. *Matrix Biol. Plus* **2021**, *11*, 100071. [CrossRef]
126. Gomez-Puerto, M.C.; Iyengar, P.V.; García de Vinuesa, A.; ten Dijke, P.; Sanchez-Duffhues, G. Bone Morphogenetic Protein Receptor Signal Transduction in Human Disease. *J. Pathol.* **2019**, *247*, 9–20. [CrossRef]
127. Sánchez-Duffhues, G.; Hiepen, C. Human IPSCs as Model Systems for BMP-Related Rare Diseases. *Cells* **2023**, *12*, 2200. [CrossRef]
128. Tang, J.; Tan, M.; Liao, S.; Pang, M.; Li, J. Recent Progress in the Biology and Physiology of BMP-8a. *Connect. Tissue Res.* **2023**, *64*, 219–228. [CrossRef]
129. Zhang, Y.; Que, J. BMP Signaling in Development, Stem Cells, and Diseases of the Gastrointestinal Tract. *Annu. Rev. Physiol.* **2020**, *82*, 251–273. [CrossRef]
130. Chang, W.; Lin, Z.; Kulessa, H.; Hebert, J.; Hogan, B.L.M.; Wu, D.K. Bmp4 Is Essential for the Formation of the Vestibular Apparatus That Detects Angular Head Movements. *PLoS Genet.* **2008**, *4*, e1000050. [CrossRef]
131. Morikawa, M.; Koinuma, D.; Mizutani, A.; Kawasaki, N.; Holmborn, K.; Sundqvist, A.; Tsutsumi, S.; Watabe, T.; Aburatani, H.; Heldin, C.-H.; et al. BMP Sustains Embryonic Stem Cell Self-Renewal through Distinct Functions of Different Krüppel-like Factors. *Stem Cell Rep.* **2016**, *6*, 64–73. [CrossRef] [PubMed]
132. Hirai, H.; Karian, P.; Kikyo, N. Regulation of Embryonic Stem Cell Self-Renewal and Pluripotency by Leukaemia Inhibitory Factor. *Biochem. J.* **2011**, *438*, 11–23. [CrossRef] [PubMed]
133. Tomizawa, M.; Shinozaki, F.; Sugiyama, T.; Yamamoto, S.; Sueishi, M.; Yoshida, T. Activin A Maintains Pluripotency Markers and Proliferative Potential of Human Induced Pluripotent Stem Cells. *Exp. Ther. Med.* **2011**, *2*, 405–408. [CrossRef] [PubMed]
134. Tomizawa, M.; Shinozaki, F.; Sugiyama, T.; Yamamoto, S.; Sueishi, M.; Yoshida, T. Activin A Is Essential for Feeder-free Culture of Human Induced Pluripotent Stem Cells. *J. Cell. Biochem.* **2013**, *114*, 584–588. [CrossRef] [PubMed]
135. Hayashi, Y.; Hsiao, E.C.; Sami, S.; Lancero, M.; Schlieve, C.R.; Nguyen, T.; Yano, K.; Nagahashi, A.; Ikeya, M.; Matsumoto, Y.; et al. BMP-SMAD-ID Promotes Reprogramming to Pluripotency by Inhibiting P16/INK4A-Dependent Senescence. *Proc. Natl. Acad. Sci. USA* **2016**, *113*, 13057–13062. [CrossRef] [PubMed]
136. Chowdhury, M.M.; Zimmerman, S.; Leeson, H.; Nefzger, C.M.; Mar, J.C.; Laslett, A.; Polo, J.M.; Wolvetang, E.; Cooper-White, J.J. Superior Induced Pluripotent Stem Cell Generation through Phactr3-Driven Mechanomodulation of Both Early and Late Phases of Cell Reprogramming. *Biomater. Res.* **2024**, *28*, 0025. [CrossRef]
137. Sagara, J.; Higuchi, T.; Hattori, Y.; Moriya, M.; Sarvotham, H.; Shima, H.; Shirato, H.; Kikuchi, K.; Taniguchi, S. Scapinin, a Putative Protein Phosphatase-1 Regulatory Subunit Associated with the Nuclear Nonchromatin Structure. *J. Biol. Chem.* **2003**, *278*, 45611–45619. [CrossRef]
138. Sagara, J.; Arata, T.; Taniguchi, S. Scapinin, the Protein Phosphatase 1 Binding Protein, Enhances Cell Spreading and Motility by Interacting with the Actin Cytoskeleton. *PLoS ONE* **2009**, *4*, e4247. [CrossRef]
139. Boog, H.; Medda, R.; Cavalcanti-Adam, E.A. Single Cell Center of Mass for the Analysis of BMP Receptor Heterodimers Distributions. *J. Imaging* **2021**, *7*, 219. [CrossRef]
140. Gabdoulline, R.; Kaisers, W.; Gaspar, A.; Meganathan, K.; Doss, M.X.; Jagtap, S.; Hescheler, J.; Sachinidis, A.; Schwender, H. Differences in the Early Development of Human and Mouse Embryonic Stem Cells. *PLoS ONE* **2015**, *10*, e0140803. [CrossRef]
141. Rossant, J. Mouse and Human Blastocyst-Derived Stem Cells: Vive Les Differences. *Development* **2015**, *142*, 9–12. [CrossRef] [PubMed]
142. Johnson Chacko, L.; Wertjanz, D.; Sergi, C.; Dudas, J.; Fischer, N.; Eberharter, T.; Hoermann, R.; Glueckert, R.; Fritsch, H.; Rask-Andersen, H.; et al. Growth and Cellular Patterning during Fetal Human Inner Ear Development Studied by a Correlative Imaging Approach. *BMC Dev. Biol.* **2019**, *19*, 11. [CrossRef] [PubMed]
143. Richard, C.; Courbon, G.; Laroche, N.; Prades, J.M.; Vico, L.; Malaval, L. Inner Ear Ossification and Mineralization Kinetics in Human Embryonic Development—Microtomographic and Histomorphological Study. *Sci. Rep.* **2017**, *7*, 4825. [CrossRef] [PubMed]
144. Kopecky, B.; Johnson, S.; Schmitz, H.; Santi, P.; Fritzsch, B. Scanning Thin-sheet Laser Imaging Microscopy Elucidates Details on Mouse Ear Development. *Dev. Dyn.* **2012**, *241*, 465–480. [CrossRef]
145. Shnerson, A.; Pujol, R. Age-Related Changes in the C57BL/6J Mouse Cochlea. I. Physiological Findings. *Dev. Brain Res.* **1981**, *2*, 65–75. [CrossRef]

146. Luo, Y.; Wu, K.; Zhang, X.; Wang, H.; Wang, Q. Genetic Correction of Induced Pluripotent Stem Cells from a DFNA36 Patient Results in Morphologic and Functional Recovery of Derived Hair Cell-like Cells. *Stem Cell Res. Ther.* **2024**, *15*, 4. [CrossRef]
147. Liu, X.; Lillywhite, J.; Zhu, W.; Huang, Z.; Clark, A.M.; Gosstola, N.; Maguire, C.T.; Dykxhoorn, D.; Chen, Z.-Y.; Yang, J. Generation and Genetic Correction of USH2A c.2299delG Mutation in Patient-Derived Induced Pluripotent Stem Cells. *Genes* **2021**, *12*, 805. [CrossRef]
148. Sanjurjo-Soriano, C.; Erkilic, N.; Baux, D.; Mamaeva, D.; Hamel, C.P.; Meunier, I.; Roux, A.-F.; Kalatzis, V. Genome Editing in Patient IPSCs Corrects the Most Prevalent USH2A Mutations and Reveals Intriguing Mutant MRNA Expression Profiles. *Mol. Ther.-Methods Clin. Dev.* **2020**, *17*, 156–173. [CrossRef]
149. Chen, C.; Guan, M.-X. Genetic Correction of TRMU Allele Restored the Mitochondrial Dysfunction-Induced Deficiencies in IPSCs-Derived Hair Cells of Hearing-Impaired Patients. *Hum. Mol. Genet.* **2022**, *31*, 3068–3082. [CrossRef]
150. Liu, X.; Wen, J.; Liu, X.; Chen, A.; Li, S.; Liu, J.; Sun, J.; Gong, W.; Kang, X.; Feng, Z.; et al. Gene Regulation Analysis of Patient-Derived IPSCs and Its CRISPR-Corrected Control Provides a New Tool for Studying Perturbations of ELMOD3 c.512A>G Mutation during the Development of Inherited Hearing Loss. *PLoS ONE* **2023**, *18*, e0288640. [CrossRef]
151. Tang, Z.-H.; Chen, J.-R.; Zheng, J.; Shi, H.-S.; Ding, J.; Qian, X.-D.; Zhang, C.; Chen, J.-L.; Wang, C.-C.; Li, L.; et al. Genetic Correction of Induced Pluripotent Stem Cells from a Deaf Patient with MYO7A Mutation Results in Morphologic and Functional Recovery of the Derived Hair Cell-Like Cells. *Stem Cells Transl. Med.* **2016**, *5*, 561–571. [CrossRef] [PubMed]
152. Qiu, Y.; Wang, H.; Fan, M.; Pan, H.; Guan, J.; Jiang, Y.; Jia, Z.; Wu, K.; Zhou, H.; Zhuang, Q.; et al. Impaired AIF-CHCHD4 Interaction and Mitochondrial Calcium Overload Contribute to Auditory Neuropathy Spectrum Disorder in Patient-IPSC-Derived Neurons with AIFM1 Variant. *Cell Death Dis.* **2023**, *14*, 375. [CrossRef] [PubMed]
153. Doetzlhofer, A.; White, P.M.; Johnson, J.E.; Segil, N.; Groves, A.K. In Vitro Growth and Differentiation of Mammalian Sensory Hair Cell Progenitors: A Requirement for EGF and Periotic Mesenchyme. *Dev. Biol.* **2004**, *272*, 432–447. [CrossRef] [PubMed]
154. Huh, S.-H.; Warchol, M.E.; Ornitz, D.M. Cochlear Progenitor Number Is Controlled through Mesenchymal FGF Receptor Signaling. *Elife* **2015**, *4*, e05921. [CrossRef] [PubMed]
155. Huang, J.; Zuo, N.; Wu, C.; Chen, P.; Ma, J.; Wang, C.; Li, W.; Liu, S. Role of the Periotic Mesenchyme in the Development of Sensory Cells in Early Mouse Cochlea. *J. Otol.* **2020**, *15*, 138–143. [CrossRef]
156. Rose, K.P.; Manilla, G.; Milon, B.; Zalzman, O.; Song, Y.; Coate, T.M.; Hertzano, R. Spatially Distinct Otic Mesenchyme Cells Show Molecular and Functional Heterogeneity Patterns before Hearing Onset. *iScience* **2023**, *26*, 107769. [CrossRef]
157. Moeinvaziri, F.; Shojaei, A.; Haghparast, N.; Yakhkeshi, S.; Nemati, S.; Hassani, S.-N.; Baharvand, H. Towards Maturation of Human Otic Hair Cell–like Cells in Pluripotent Stem Cell–Derived Organoid Transplants. *Cell Tissue Res.* **2021**, *386*, 321–333. [CrossRef]
158. Xia, M.; Ma, J.; Wu, M.; Guo, L.; Chen, Y.; Li, G.; Sun, S.; Chai, R.; Li, H.; Li, W. Generation of Innervated Cochlear Organoid Recapitulates Early Development of Auditory Unit. *Stem Cell Rep.* **2023**, *18*, 319–336. [CrossRef]
159. Lu, J.; Wang, M.; Meng, Y.; An, W.; Wang, X.; Sun, G.; Wang, H.; Liu, W. Current Advances in Biomaterials for Inner Ear Cell Regeneration. *Front. Neurosci.* **2024**, *17*, 1334162. [CrossRef]
160. Pressé, M.T.; Malgrange, B.; Delacroix, L. The Cochlear Matrisome: Importance in Hearing and Deafness. *Matrix Biol.* **2024**, *125*, 40–58. [CrossRef]
161. Ma, J.; You, D.; Li, W.; Lu, X.; Sun, S.; Li, H. Bone Morphogenetic Proteins and Inner Ear Development. *J. Zhejiang Univ. B* **2019**, *20*, 131–145. [CrossRef] [PubMed]
162. Saeki, T.; Yoshimatsu, S.; Ishikawa, M.; Hon, C.-C.; Koya, I.; Shibata, S.; Hosoya, M.; Saegusa, C.; Ogawa, K.; Shin, J.W.; et al. Critical Roles of FGF, RA, and WNT Signalling in the Development of the Human Otic Placode and Subsequent Lineages in a Dish. *Regen. Ther.* **2022**, *20*, 165–186. [CrossRef] [PubMed]
163. Maharana, S.K.; Saint-Jeannet, J.-P. Molecular Mechanisms of Hearing Loss in Nager Syndrome. *Dev. Biol.* **2021**, *476*, 200–208. [CrossRef] [PubMed]
164. Sher, G.; Naeem, M. A Novel CHSY1 Gene Mutation Underlies Temtamy Preaxial Brachydactyly Syndrome in a Pakistani Family. *Eur. J. Med. Genet.* **2014**, *57*, 21–24. [CrossRef] [PubMed]
165. Li, Y.; Laue, K.; Temtamy, S.; Aglan, M.; Kotan, L.D.; Yigit, G.; Canan, H.; Pawlik, B.; Nürnberg, G.; Wakeling, E.L.; et al. Temtamy Preaxial Brachydactyly Syndrome Is Caused by Loss-of-Function Mutations in Chondroitin Synthase 1, a Potential Target of BMP Signaling. *Am. J. Hum. Genet.* **2010**, *87*, 757–767. [CrossRef]
166. Lyu, Z.; Da, Y.; Liu, H.; Wang, Z.; Zhu, Y.; Tian, J. Chsy1 Deficiency Reduces Extracellular Matrix Productions and Aggravates Cartilage Injury in Osteoarthritis. *Gene* **2022**, *827*, 146466. [CrossRef]
167. Kaplan, F.S.; Xu, M.; Seemann, P.; Connor, J.M.; Glaser, D.L.; Carroll, L.; Delai, P.; Fastnacht-Urban, E.; Forman, S.J.; Gillessen-Kaesbach, G.; et al. Classic and Atypical Fibrodysplasia Ossificans Progressiva (FOP) Phenotypes Are Caused by Mutations in the Bone Morphogenetic Protein (BMP) Type I Receptor ACVR1. *Hum. Mutat.* **2009**, *30*, 379–390. [CrossRef]
168. Kaplan, F.S.; Kobori, J.A.; Orellana, C.; Calvo, I.; Rosello, M.; Martinez, F.; Lopez, B.; Xu, M.; Pignolo, R.J.; Shore, E.M.; et al. Multi-system Involvement in a Severe Variant of Fibrodysplasia Ossificans Progressiva (ACVR1 c.772G>A; R258G): A Report of Two Patients. *Am. J. Med. Genet. Part A* **2015**, *167*, 2265–2271. [CrossRef]
169. Levy, C.E.; Lash, A.T.; Janoff, H.B.; Kaplan, F.S. Conductive Hearing Loss in Individuals with Fibrodysplasia Ossificans Progressiva. *Am. J. Audiol.* **1999**, *8*, 29–33. [CrossRef]

170. Hasegawa, K.; Tanaka, H.; Futagawa, N.; Miyahara, H.; Tsukahara, H. Rapid Progression of Heterotopic Ossification in Severe Variant of Fibrodysplasia Ossificans Progressiva with p.Arg258Gly in ACVR1: A Case Report and Review of Clinical Phenotypes. *Case Rep. Genet.* **2022**, *2022*, 5021758. [CrossRef]
171. Ealy, M.; Meyer, N.C.; Corchado, J.C.; Schrauwen, I.; Bress, A.; Pfister, M.; Van Camp, G.; Smith, R.J.H. Rare Variants in BMP2 and BMP4 Found in Otosclerosis Patients Reduce Smad Signaling. *Otol. Neurotol.* **2014**, *35*, 395–400. [CrossRef] [PubMed]
172. Hansdah, K.; Singh, N.; Bouzid, A.; Priyadarshi, S.; Ray, C.S.; Desai, A.; Panda, K.C.; Choudhury, J.C.; Biswal, N.C.; Tekari, A.; et al. Evaluation of the Genetic Association and MRNA Expression of the COL1A1, BMP2, and BMP4 Genes in the Development of Otosclerosis. *Genet. Test. Mol. Biomark.* **2020**, *24*, 343–351. [CrossRef] [PubMed]
173. Priestley, J.R.C.; Deshwar, A.R.; Murthy, H.; D'Agostino, M.D.; Dupuis, L.; Gangaram, B.; Gray, C.; Jobling, R.; Pannia, E.; Platzer, K.; et al. Monoallelic Loss-of-Function BMP2 Variants Result in BMP2-Related Skeletal Dysplasia Spectrum. *Genet. Med.* **2023**, *25*, 100863. [CrossRef] [PubMed]
174. Schrauwen, I.; Thys, M.; Vanderstraeten, K.; Fransen, E.; Dieltjens, N.; Huyghe, J.R.; Ealy, M.; Claustres, M.; Cremers, C.R.; Dhooge, I.; et al. Association of Bone Morphogenetic Proteins with Otosclerosis. *J. Bone Miner. Res.* **2008**, *23*, 507–516. [CrossRef] [PubMed]
175. Tan, T.Y.; Gonzaga-Jauregui, C.; Bhoj, E.J.; Strauss, K.A.; Brigatti, K.; Puffenberger, E.; Li, D.; Xie, L.; Das, N.; Skubas, I.; et al. Monoallelic BMP2 Variants Predicted to Result in Haploinsufficiency Cause Craniofacial, Skeletal, and Cardiac Features Overlapping Those of 20p12 Deletions. *Am. J. Hum. Genet.* **2017**, *101*, 985–994. [CrossRef]
176. Nixon, T.R.W.; Richards, A.; Towns, L.K.; Fuller, G.; Abbs, S.; Alexander, P.; McNinch, A.; Sandford, R.N.; Snead, M.P. Bone Morphogenetic Protein 4 (BMP4) Loss-of-Function Variant Associated with Autosomal Dominant Stickler Syndrome and Renal Dysplasia. *Eur. J. Hum. Genet.* **2019**, *27*, 369–377. [CrossRef]
177. Wyatt, A.W.; Osborne, R.J.; Stewart, H.; Ragge, N.K. Bone Morphogenetic Protein 7 (BMP7) Mutations Are Associated with Variable Ocular, Brain, Ear, Palate, and Skeletal Anomalies. *Hum. Mutat.* **2010**, *31*, 781–787. [CrossRef]
178. Adeyemo, A.; Faridi, R.; Chattaraj, P.; Yousaf, R.; Tona, R.; Okorie, S.; Bharadwaj, T.; Nouel-Saied, L.M.; Acharya, A.; Schrauwen, I.; et al. Genomic Analysis of Childhood Hearing Loss in the Yoruba Population of Nigeria. *Eur. J. Hum. Genet.* **2022**, *30*, 42–52. [CrossRef]
179. Driesen, J.; Van Hoecke, H.; Maes, L.; Janssens, S.; Acke, F.; De Leenheer, E. CHD7 Disorder—Not CHARGE Syndrome—Presenting as Isolated Cochleovestibular Dysfunction. *Genes* **2024**, *15*, 643. [CrossRef]
180. Roux, I.; Fenollar-Ferrer, C.; Lee, H.J.; Chattaraj, P.; Lopez, I.A.; Han, K.; Honda, K.; Brewer, C.C.; Butman, J.A.; Morell, R.J.; et al. CHD7 Variants Associated with Hearing Loss and Enlargement of the Vestibular Aqueduct. *Hum. Genet.* **2023**, *142*, 1499–1517. [CrossRef]
181. Akahira-Azuma, M.; Enomoto, Y.; Nakamura, N.; Yokoi, T.; Minatogawa, M.; Harada, N.; Tsurusaki, Y.; Kurosawa, K. Novel COL2A1 Variants in Japanese Patients with Spondyloepiphyseal Dysplasia Congenita. *Hum. Genome Var.* **2022**, *9*, 16. [CrossRef] [PubMed]
182. Terhal, P.A.; Nievelstein, R.J.A.J.; Verver, E.J.J.; Topsakal, V.; van Dommelen, P.; Hoornaert, K.; Le Merrer, M.; Zankl, A.; Simon, M.E.H.; Smithson, S.F.; et al. A Study of the Clinical and Radiological Features in a Cohort of 93 Patients with a COL2A1 Mutation Causing Spondyloepiphyseal Dysplasia Congenita or a Related Phenotype. *Am. J. Med. Genet. Part A* **2015**, *167*, 461–475. [CrossRef] [PubMed]
183. Wu, K.; Li, Z.; Zhu, Y.; Wang, X.; Chen, G.; Hou, Z.; Zhang, Q. Discovery of Sensorineural Hearing Loss and Ossicle Deformity in a Chinese Li Nationality Family with Spondyloepiphyseal Dysplasia Congenita Caused by p.G504S Mutation of COL2A1. *BMC Med. Genom.* **2021**, *14*, 170. [CrossRef] [PubMed]
184. Ali, A.; Tabouni, M.; Kizhakkedath, P.; Baydoun, I.; Allam, M.; John, A.; Busafared, F.; Alnuaimi, A.; Al-Jasmi, F.; Alblooshi, H. Spectrum of Genetic Variants in Bilateral Sensorineural Hearing Loss. *Front. Genet.* **2024**, *15*, 1314535. [CrossRef]
185. Clarke, R.A.; Fang, Z.; Murrell, D.; Sheriff, T.; Eapen, V. GDF6 Knockdown in a Family with Multiple Synostosis Syndrome and Speech Impairment. *Genes* **2021**, *12*, 1354. [CrossRef]
186. Terhal, P.A.; Verbeek, N.E.; Knoers, N.; Nievelstein, R.J.A.J.; van den Ouweland, A.; Sakkers, R.J.; Speleman, L.; van Haaften, G. Further Delineation of the GDF6 Related Multiple Synostoses Syndrome. *Am. J. Med. Genet. Part A* **2018**, *176*, 225–229. [CrossRef]
187. Wang, J.; Yu, T.; Wang, Z.; Ohte, S.; Yao, R.; Zheng, Z.; Geng, J.; Cai, H.; Ge, Y.; Li, Y.; et al. A New Sub type of Multiple Synostoses Syndrome Is Caused by a Mutation in GDF6 That Decreases Its Sensitivity to Noggin and Enhances Its Potency as a BMP Signal. *J. Bone Miner. Res.* **2016**, *31*, 882–889. [CrossRef]
188. Carlson, R.J.; Quesnel, A.; Wells, D.; Brownstein, Z.; Gilony, D.; Gulsuner, S.; Leppig, K.A.; Avraham, K.B.; King, M.-C.; Walsh, T.; et al. Genetic Heterogeneity and Core Clinical Features of NOG-Related-Symphalangism Spectrum Disorder. *Otol. Neurotol.* **2021**, *42*, e1143–e1151. [CrossRef]
189. Hirshoren, N.; Gross, M.; Banin, E.; Sosna, J.; Bargal, R.; Raas-Rothschild, A. P35S Mutation in the NOG Gene Associated with Teunissen–Cremers Syndrome and Features of Multiple NOG Joint-Fusion Syndromes. *Eur. J. Med. Genet.* **2008**, *51*, 351–357. [CrossRef]
190. Ishino, T.; Takeno, S.; Hirakawa, K. Novel NOG Mutation in Japanese Patients with Stapes Ankylosis with Broad Thumbs and Toes. *Eur. J. Med. Genet.* **2015**, *58*, 427–432. [CrossRef]

191. Masuda, S.; Namba, K.; Mutai, H.; Usui, S.; Miyanaga, Y.; Kaneko, H.; Matsunaga, T. A Mutation in the Heparin-Binding Site of Noggin as a Novel Mechanism of Proximal Symphalangism and Conductive Hearing Loss. *Biochem. Biophys. Res. Commun.* **2014**, *447*, 496–502. [CrossRef] [PubMed]
192. Nakashima, T.; Ganaha, A.; Tsumagari, S.; Nakamura, T.; Yamada, Y.; Nakamura, E.; Usami, S.; Tono, T. Is the Conductive Hearing Loss in NOG-Related Symphalangism Spectrum Disorder Congenital? *ORL* **2021**, *83*, 196–202. [CrossRef] [PubMed]
193. Pang, X.; Wang, Z.; Chai, Y.; Chen, H.; Li, L.; Sun, L.; Jia, H.; Wu, H.; Yang, T. A Novel Missense Mutation of NOG Interferes with the Dimerization of NOG and Causes Proximal Symphalangism Syndrome in a Chinese Family. *Ann. Otol. Rhinol. Laryngol.* **2015**, *124*, 745–751. [CrossRef] [PubMed]
194. Sonoyama, T.; Ishino, T.; Ogawa, Y.; Oda, T.; Takeno, S. Identification of a Novel Nonsense NOG Mutation in a Patient with Stapes Ankylosis and Symphalangism Spectrum Disorder. *Hum. Genome Var.* **2023**, *10*, 12. [CrossRef] [PubMed]
195. Takano, K.; Ogasawara, N.; Matsunaga, T.; Mutai, H.; Sakurai, A.; Ishikawa, A.; Himi, T. A Novel Nonsense Mutation in the NOG Gene Causes Familial NOG-Related Symphalangism Spectrum Disorder. *Hum. Genome Var.* **2016**, *3*, 16023. [CrossRef]
196. Thomeer, H.G.X.M.; Admiraal, R.J.C.; Hoefsloot, L.; Kunst, H.P.M.; Cremers, C.W.R.J. Proximal Symphalangism, Hyperopia, Conductive Hearing Impairment, and the NOG Gene. *Otol. Neurotol.* **2011**, *32*, 632–638. [CrossRef]
197. Yu, R.; Jiang, H.; Liao, H.; Luo, W. Genetic and Clinical Phenotypic Analysis of Familial Stapes Sclerosis Caused by an NOG Mutation. *BMC Med. Genom.* **2020**, *13*, 187. [CrossRef]
198. Caputo, V.; Bocchinfuso, G.; Castori, M.; Traversa, A.; Pizzuti, A.; Stella, L.; Grammatico, P.; Tartaglia, M. Novel SMAD4 Mutation Causing Myhre Syndrome. *Am. J. Med. Genet. Part A* **2014**, *164*, 1835–1840. [CrossRef]
199. Cătană, A.; Simonescu-Colan, R.; Cuzmici-Barabaș, Z.; Militaru, D.; Iordănescu, I.; Militaru, M. First Documented Case of Myhre Syndrome in Romania: A Case Report. *Exp. Ther. Med.* **2022**, *23*, 323. [CrossRef]
200. Le Goff, C.; Mahaut, C.; Abhyankar, A.; Le Goff, W.; Serre, V.; Afenjar, A.; Destrée, A.; di Rocco, M.; Héron, D.; Jacquemont, S.; et al. Mutations at a Single Codon in Mad Homology 2 Domain of SMAD4 Cause Myhre Syndrome. *Nat. Genet.* **2012**, *44*, 85–88. [CrossRef]
201. Lin, A.E.; Alali, A.; Starr, L.J.; Shah, N.; Beavis, A.; Pereira, E.M.; Lindsay, M.E.; Klugman, S. Gain-of-function Pathogenic Variants in SMAD4 Are Associated with Neoplasia in Myhre Syndrome. *Am. J. Med. Genet. Part A* **2020**, *182*, 328–337. [CrossRef] [PubMed]
202. Michot, C.; Le Goff, C.; Mahaut, C.; Afenjar, A.; Brooks, A.S.; Campeau, P.M.; Destree, A.; Di Rocco, M.; Donnai, D.; Hennekam, R.; et al. Myhre and LAPS Syndromes: Clinical and Molecular Review of 32 Patients. *Eur. J. Hum. Genet.* **2014**, *22*, 1272–1277. [CrossRef] [PubMed]
203. Yang, K.; Wang, X.; Wang, W.; Han, M.; Hu, L.; Kang, D.; Yang, J.; Liu, M.; Gao, X.; Yuan, Y.; et al. A Newborn Male with Myhre Syndrome, Hearing Loss, and Complete Syndactyly of Fingers 3–4. *Mol. Genet. Genom. Med.* **2023**, *11*, e2103. [CrossRef] [PubMed]
204. Caputo, V.; Cianetti, L.; Niceta, M.; Carta, C.; Ciolfi, A.; Bocchinfuso, G.; Carrani, E.; Dentici, M.L.; Biamino, E.; Belligni, E.; et al. A Restricted Spectrum of Mutations in the SMAD4 Tumor-Suppressor Gene Underlies Myhre Syndrome. *Am. J. Hum. Genet.* **2012**, *90*, 161–169. [CrossRef] [PubMed]
205. Guo, L.; Iida, A.; Bhavani, G.S.; Gowrishankar, K.; Wang, Z.; Xue, J.; Wang, J.; Miyake, N.; Matsumoto, N.; Hasegawa, T.; et al. Deficiency of TMEM53 Causes a Previously Unknown Sclerosing Bone Disorder by Dysregulation of BMP-SMAD Signaling. *Nat. Commun.* **2021**, *12*, 2046. [CrossRef]
206. Whyte, M.P.; Weinstein, R.S.; Phillips, P.H.; McAlister, W.H.; Ramakrishnaiah, R.H.; Schaefer, G.B.; Cai, R.; Hutchison, M.R.; Duan, S.; Gottesman, G.S.; et al. Transmembrane Protein 53 Craniotubular Dysplasia (OMIM # 619727): The Skeletal Disease and Consequent Blindness of This New Disorder. *Bone* **2024**, *188*, 117218. [CrossRef]

Disclaimer/Publisher's Note: The statements, opinions and data contained in all publications are solely those of the individual author(s) and contributor(s) and not of MDPI and/or the editor(s). MDPI and/or the editor(s) disclaim responsibility for any injury to people or property resulting from any ideas, methods, instructions or products referred to in the content.

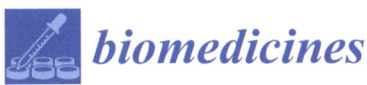

Review

Neuronal Cell Differentiation of iPSCs for the Clinical Treatment of Neurological Diseases

Dong-Hun Lee [1], Eun Chae Lee [2], Ji young Lee [3], Man Ryul Lee [4], Jae-won Shim [4,5,*] and Jae Sang Oh [3,*]

1. Industry-Academic Cooperation Foundation, The Catholic University of Korea, 222, Banpo-daro, Seocho-gu, Seoul 06591, Republic of Korea
2. Department of Medical Life Sciences, College of Medicine, The Catholic University of Korea, Seoul 06591, Republic of Korea
3. Department of Neurosurgery, Uijeongbu St. Mary's Hospital, College of Medicine, The Catholic University of Korea, Seoul 06591, Republic of Korea
4. Soonchunhyang Institute of Medi-Bio Science (SIMS), Soonchunhyang University, Cheonan-si 31151, Republic of Korea
5. Department of Integrated Biomedical Science, Soonchunhyang University, Cheonan-si 31151, Republic of Korea

* Correspondence: shimj@sch.ac.kr (J.-w.S.); metatron1324@hotmail.com (J.S.O.); Tel.: +82-41-413-5014 (J.-w.S.); +82-31-820-3024 (J.S.O.)

Abstract: Current chemical treatments for cerebrovascular disease and neurological disorders have limited efficacy in tissue repair and functional restoration. Induced pluripotent stem cells (iPSCs) present a promising avenue in regenerative medicine for addressing neurological conditions. iPSCs, which are capable of reprogramming adult cells to regain pluripotency, offer the potential for patient-specific, personalized therapies. The modulation of molecular mechanisms through specific growth factor inhibition and signaling pathways can direct iPSCs' differentiation into neural stem cells (NSCs). These include employing bone morphogenetic protein-4 (*BMP-4*), transforming growth factor-beta (*TGFβ*), and Sma-and Mad-related protein (SMAD) signaling. iPSC-derived NSCs can subsequently differentiate into various neuron types, each performing distinct functions. Cell transplantation underscores the potential of iPSC-derived NSCs to treat neurodegenerative diseases such as Parkinson's disease and points to future research directions for optimizing differentiation protocols and enhancing clinical applications.

Keywords: BMP-4 protein; induced pluripotent stem cells; neural stem cells; SMAD proteins; transforming growth factor beta; transplantation

1. Introduction

Neurological disorders, especially cerebrovascular diseases and strokes, are a significant global issue [1]. These conditions lead to irreversible neural damage, and currently, there are limited effective treatments available for repairing damaged tissue or restoring function [2–4]. To overcome this, regenerative medicine has begun to focus on the differentiation of neural cells from induced pluripotent stem cells (iPSCs) [5].

Stem cells inherently possess two key functions: the capacity for unlimited self-renewal and the ability to differentiate into one or more specialized cell types [6]. These characteristics play a fundamental role in exploring tissue repair and disease treatment methods through stem cells [7].

iPSCs are cells that have regained pluripotency through the reprogramming of already differentiated mature cells and are created by manipulating the expression of specific genes [8,9]. The technology of iPSCs, which restores pluripotency from mature cells, offers innovative potential for generating patient-specific disease models and developing personalized treatments [10]. Neural cells generated from iPSCs can be used to replace or repair damaged neural tissue [11]. Moreover, using neural cells differentiated from patient-derived iPSCs allows for effective testing of new drugs' efficacy or toxicity [12]. Transplanting these iPSC-derived neural cells could lead to functional recovery in neurodegenerative diseases such as Alzheimer's or Parkinson's disease.

Against this background, it is expected that the process of neuronal differentiation of iPSCs will be examined, and the mechanisms of neuronal differentiation will be elucidated, providing an important step in the development of regenerative medicine and disease therapies.

2. Inhibiting the SMAD Pathway in iPSCs for Neural Differentiation

The process of differentiating iPSCs into various cells includes several complex signaling pathways and molecular mechanisms. iPSCs have important advantages over embryonic stem cells (ESCs). iPSCs are derived from adult cells; they bypass the ethical issues of destroying embryos to derive ESCs [13,14]. iPSCs can be self-derived from the patient, allowing for the creation of patient-specific cell lines [12,15]. They can differentiate into multiple cell types, allowing drug testing to assess effectiveness and identify side effects safely and efficiently [16]. Furthermore, iPSCs retain the same pluripotency as that of ESCs [17]. Both iPSCs and ESCs exhibited equivalent neuronal differentiation potential, and both cells showed similar cholinergic motor neuron differentiation potential and the ability to induce the contraction of myotubes [18]. In another study, while iPSC-derived neural stem cells (NSCs) had decreased ATP production compared to that of ESC-derived NSCs, iPSC-derived astrocytes had increased ATP production compared to that of ESC-derived astrocytes [19].

Specifically, the differentiation of neuronal cells is induced by the dual inhibition of the Sma- and Mad-related protein (SMAD) pathway (Figure 1). Before understanding the SMAD pathway, it is necessary to understand the transforming growth factor-beta (*TGFβ*) signaling pathway, which includes SMAD.

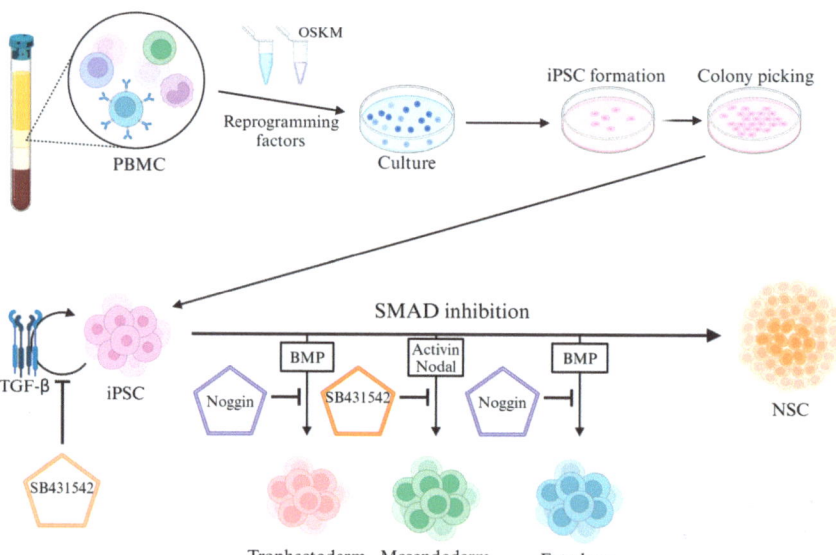

Figure 1. Adding reprogramming factors to PBMCs to induce their reverse differentiation into iPSCs. Reverse-differentiated iPSCs can be induced to undergo mesoderm or endoderm differentiation through the activation of the SMAD pathway. Inhibition of the SMAD pathway induces the neural stem cell differentiation of iPSCs. *BMP*: bone morphogenetic protein, *TGFβ*: transforming growth factor-beta, NSC: neural stem cell, iPSC: induced pluripotent stem cell, PBMC: peripheral blood mononuclear cell, OSKM: *Oct4/Sox2/Klf4/c-Myc*, SMAD: *Sma-* and *Mad*-related protein.

2.1. SMAD Pathway Inhibition

Inhibition of the SMAD pathway directs the fate of iPSCs towards the neuroectoderm and induces neural cell differentiation through the inhibition of *TGFβ* and *BMP-4* signaling, as mentioned above [20]. For the dual inhibition of the SMAD pathway, SB431542 is used to inhibit the *TGFβ* pathway and *Noggin* is used to inhibit the *BMP* pathway.

SB431542 inhibits the *Lefty/Activin/TGFβ* pathway by blocking the phosphorylation of *ALK4*, *ALK5*, and *ALK7* receptors. SB431542 also inhibits differentiation to the mesoderm by inhibiting *Activin/Nodal* signaling. *Noggin* inhibits differentiation to the ectoderm by inhibiting the *BMP* pathway. A combined treatment of SB431542 and *Noggin* induced the neural differentiation of stem cells with high efficiency [20]. The mechanisms by which *Noggin* and SB431542 induced neural cell differentiation include *Activin*- and *Nanog*-mediated network destabilization [21], *BMP*-induced inhibition of differentiation [22], and the inhibition of mesodermal and endodermal differentiation through the inhibition of endogenous *Activin* and *BMP* signaling [23,24]. Treatment with SB431542 decreases *Nanog* expression and significantly increases *CDX2* expression. The inhibition of *CDX2* in the presence of *Noggin* or SB431542 demonstrates that one of the key roles of *Noggin* is the inhibition of endogenous *BMP* signaling, which induces trophoblast fate during differentiation.

2.2. TGFβ Signaling Pathway

The *TGFβ* signaling pathway is a pathway that regulates cell growth, differentiation, migration, death, and homeostasis [25]. The superfamily of *TGFβ* includes bone morphogenetic protein (*BMP*), *Activin*, *Nodal*, and *TGFβ*. Signal transduction in this pathway begins with the binding of superfamily ligands of *TGFβ* to *TGFβ* receptor type II and *TGFβ* receptor type I [26]. Activated *TGFβ* receptors recruit *Smad2/3* for *TGFβ* and activation signaling [27] and form complexes of CoSmad and R-smad, such as *Smad4*, for *BMP* signaling [28]. Smad complexes accumulate in the nucleus and are directly involved in the transcriptional regulation of target genes [29].

2.3. BMP Signaling Pathway

BMPs are cytokines that belong to a group of growth factors [30]. *BMPs* have a role in early skeletal formation during embryonic development and were originally known to act as bone growth factors [31]. *BMPs* bind to a heteromeric receptor complex composed of type I and type II serine/threonine kinase receptors, which are received by different activin receptors and *BMP* receptors [32]. The two receptors are highly homologous and can activate both Smad and non-Smad signaling.

BMP-4 is a member of the *BMP* superfamily, which induces the ventral mesoderm to establish dorsal–ventral morphogenesis. *BMP4* signaling is found in the formation of early mesoderm and germ cells, and the development of the lungs and liver is attributed to *BMP4* signaling [33]. Inhibition of this *BMP-4* signaling induces neurogenesis and the formation of the neural plate. Indeed, the knockout of *BMP-4* in mice resulted in little mesodermal differentiation [34].

2.4. RA Pathway

Retinoic acid (RA) is a molecule that contributes to the development and homeostasis of the nervous system [35]. The RA signaling depends on cells having the ability to metabolize retinol. Transcription is regulated by the binding of RA to its receptor, RA receptor (*RAR*), which forms a complex with the retinoid X receptor (*RXR*) [36]. The RA is involved in the differentiation of NSCs into neurons, astrocytes, or oligodendrocytes [37]. RA activates the *Hox* gene, which is required for hindbrain development and regulates the head–trunk transition [38]. RA is required for the formation of primary neurons [39]. In an embryonal carcinoma cell line in vitro, RA promoted neurite outgrowth and stimulated the expression of neural differentiation markers [40].

Furthermore, RA is essential in embryonic development and is essential for the development of many organs, including the hindbrain, spinal cord, skeleton, heart, and brain [41].

2.5. BDNF, GDNF, and NGF Pathway Regulation

Brain-derived neurotrophic factor (BDNF) is a neurotrophic factor found primarily in the brain and central nervous system that regulates nerve cell survival, growth, and neurotransmission [42]. BDNF promotes neuronal survival and growth in dorsal root ganglion cells and in hippocampal and cortical neurons [43,44]. In in vitro experiments in which neural differentiation was induced in a variety of stem cells, neural differentiation was confirmed after treatment with BDNF [45,46].

Glial-cell-line-derived neurotrophic factor (GDNF) is a protein that promotes the survival of many different neurons [47]. GDNF can be secreted by neurons and peripheral cells during development, including astrocytes, and interacts with GDNF family receptor alpha 1 and 2 [48]. In particular, it has a protective effect on dopamine-producing nerve cells, making it an important target in neurodegenerative diseases such as Parkinson's disease [49].

Nerve growth factor (NGF) is a neuropeptide involved in regulating the growth, proliferation, and survival of neurons [50]. In vivo and in vitro studies, NGF has been shown to have an important role in the differentiation and survival of neurons, as well as in the protection of degenerating neurons.

3. Differentiation of Various Neural Cells from iPSCs

Through various mechanisms, neural cell differentiation from iPSCs can develop a diverse array of neurons (Figure 2, Table 1). It is possible to consider prior studies that successfully differentiated various neurons from iPSCs and the application of protocols used for the differentiation of human ESCs (hESCs) into iPSCs.

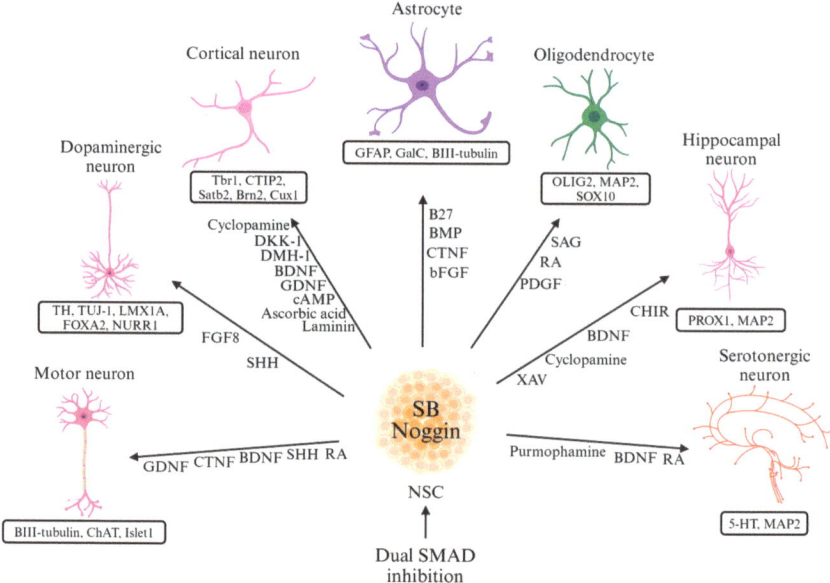

Figure 2. Different neural cells that can differentiate from neural stem cells. Cells induced to become neural stem cells due to the inhibition of the dual SMAD pathway with SB431542 and *Noggin* can be combined to add cytokines specific to each differentiation target. The cytokines described next to the black arrows indicate the fate of each neuron. Differentiated neurons are identified through the detection of the proteins listed under each neuron.

Table 1. Strategies for iPSCs differentiated into neural progenitor cells to become multifunctional neurons.

References	Type of Neuron	Differentiation Inducers	Specific Markers
[51,52]	Cortical Neurons	Cyclopamine, DKK-1, DMH-1, BDNF, GDNF, cAMP, Ascorbic acid, Laminin	Tbr1, CTIP2, Satb2, Brn2, Cux1
[53,54]	Dopaminergic Neurons	FGF8, SHH	TH, TUJ-1, LMX1A, FOXA2, NURR1
[55]	Motor Neurons	GDNF, CTNF, BDNF, SHH, RA	BIII-tubulin, ChAT, Islet1
[56]	Astrocytes	B27, BMP, CTNF, bFGF	GFAP, GalC, BIII-tubulin
[57]	Oligodendrocytes	PDGF, RA, SAG	OLIG2, MAP2, SOX10
[58]	Hippocampal Neurons	CHIR, BDNF, Cyclopamine, XAV	PROX1, MAP2
[59]	Serotonergic Neurons	Purmophamine, BDNF, RA	5-HT, MAP2

3.1. Differentiation into Cortical Neurons

iPSCs can differentiate into cortex neurons. The study by Kaveena Autar [51] induced an initial neural lineage in iPSCs using two small molecule inhibitors of the SMAD pathway, LDN193189 and SB431542, promoting neuroepithelial differentiation. Following the early neural induction, the neural epithelium was induced using *DKK-1*, a *Wnt/B* antagonist, and *DMH-1*, a *BMP* inhibitor, enhancing the development of rostral neuroepithelial cells. Finally, the application of cyclopamine, an *SHH* inhibitor, designated the cortex fate, while BDNF, GDNF, cAMP, ascorbic acid, and laminin improved the generation of cortical neurons.

In the research by Yichen Shi, cortical development was induced in both hESCs and iPSCs using dorsomorphin, an inhibitor of the SMAD pathway [52].

Cortical differentiation can be confirmed by the reduced expression of the pluripotency gene *Oct4* and the increased expression of the genes *Tbr1*, *CTIP2*, *Satb2*, *Brn2*, and *Cux1*.

3.2. Differentiation into Dopaminergic Neurons

Human iPSCs are capable of differentiating into midbrain dopaminergic neurons. In a study by Lixiang Ma, dopaminergic neurons were generated from iPSCs [53]. After inducing iPSCs into neural epithelial cells, applying *FGF8* and *SHH* efficiently produced dopaminergic neurons from midbrain precursors without the need for co-culture. Dopaminergic neurons can be identified by detecting markers such as *TH*, *TUJ-1*, *LMX1A*, *FOXA2*, and *NURR1*.

It is also possible to induce the dopaminergic neuronal differentiation of iPSCs without the use of pharmacological compounds for the inhibition of SMAD mechanisms [54]. Adeno-associated viral vectors were designed to upregulate *Lmx1a* through *SHH* and *Wnt* and then transfected into iPSCs. The iPSCs not only successfully generated dopaminergic neurons but also showed a consistent number of them.

3.3. Differentiation into Motor Neurons

iPSCs can differentiate into motor neurons [55]. After inducing iPSCs into embryonic bodies, treatment with RA and purmorphamine, an activator of the sonic hedgehog pathway, resulted in the expression of neural precursor markers. Cells forming neural rosettes were mechanically separated, plated in media containing RA and *Shh*, and cultured for a week. Following further culture with BDNF, CTNF, GDNF, and *Shh*, after 3–5 weeks, cells displayed motor neuron characteristics, and *BIII-tubulin*, *ChAT*, and *Islet1* were detected.

3.4. Differentiation into Astrocytes

iPSCs can differentiate into astrocytes [56]. iPSCs induced into NSCs were cultured in NSC media containing B27, *BMP*, CTNF, and *bFGF*. The differentiated astrocytes were co-cultured with the neuron layer. Throughout the culture, neurons were distinguished by their distinct cell bodies and measured along axons using fluorescence imaging. Neurons and astrocytes, as well as oligodendrocytes, were differentiated by expressing markers such as *BIII-tubulin*, *GFAP*, and *GalC*.

3.5. Differentiation into Oligodendrocytes

iPSCs can differentiate into oligodendrocytes [57]. Neural differentiation was induced through dual SMAD inhibition. After differentiation, adding *SAG* and RA promoted sphere aggregation, and using PDGF media encouraged OPC formation. The development of oligodendrocytes was confirmed through the detection of *OLIG2*, *MAP2*, and *SOX10*.

3.6. Differentiation into Hippocampal Neurons

NSCs derived from iPSCs can differentiate into the hippocampus [58]. Neural induction media composed of B27, N2, and *NEAA* were supplemented with LDN-193189, Cyclopamine, SB431542, and XAV-939 to induce differentiation, and CHIR-99021 and BDNF were added to promote hippocampal neuron development. The generation of hippocampal neurons was confirmed through the detection of *PROX1*.

3.7. Differentiation into Serotonergic Neurons

NSCs derived from iPSCs can differentiate into serotonergic neurons [59]. Human pluripotent stem cells (hPSCs) were cultured in an N2 medium combined with a knockout serum replacement medium and treated with SB431542, LDN193189, purmorphamine, and RA. After 11 days, the medium was switched to NB/B27 medium, and BDNF was added. Following differentiation, the presence of serotonergic neurons was confirmed through immunofluorescence staining for 5-HT, *MAP2*, *TUJ1*, *FEV*, and *TPH2* expression. Subsequent 3D culture also successfully yielded organoids, and the release of *5-HT* and its metabolites was observed.

4. Therapeutic Research Using Neural Cells Derived from iPSCs

Researchers are hopeful that the transplantation of neural cells derived from iPSCs can overcome neurodegenerative diseases. To treat Parkinson's disease, which has been identified as a disorder of dopaminergic neurons, the transplantation of iPSC-derived dopaminergic neurons is considered. If these transplanted neurons function normally, they could potentially cure Parkinson's disease. This anticipation has led to the execution of cell transplantation therapies targeting either cells or animals, and in some cases, applications have extended to clinical trials.

4.1. Dopaminergic Neuron Therapy in a Model of Parkinson's Disease

Dopaminergic neurons from PSCs may be a candidate for the treatment of Parkinson's disease. When dopaminergic neurons were transplanted into the nigrostriatal lesions of rats with Parkinson's disease, the neurons survived and interacted in the rats' brains for a long period of time [60]. After cell transplantation, the rats' motor function was restored.

4.2. In Vivo Transplantation and Survival of Astrocytes

Astrocytes derived from PSCs were transplanted into the striatum of mice to investigate their survival and function [56]. In the brains of mice obtained 2 weeks after astrocyte transplantation, *GFAP*-positive cells were still observed.

Furthermore, when iPSC-derived astrocyte progenitors were transplanted into the brain of an Alzheimer's disease model in mice and examined through immunostaining, they interacted and functionally integrated with other cells in vivo [61].

4.3. Survival of Oligodendrocytes after Transplantation in Mice

To investigate the function of iPSC-derived oligodendrocytes, cells were injected into the forebrain of immunocompromised mice. At 12 weeks after cell injection, the oligodendrocytes were detected through immunofluorescence staining of hNA+ and *OLIG2* protein in the corpus callosum.

4.4. Clinical Trials with iPSC Transplantation

There are very few studies in which iPSCs have been transplanted into humans. This is because questions about the safety, stability, and efficacy of iPSCs are constantly being raised. The first thing that researchers worry about is the ability to form tumors, which is a common concern in stem cell research [62]. iPSCs also have a theoretical risk of forming tumors, so safety considerations follow. In addition, treatments using iPSC technology may result in modifications to the human genome, which requires discussion of the long-term ethical implications. For example, concerns include human cloning or human–animal chimeras.

On the other side of the spectrum, there are also concerns related to the immune response. Even though iPSCs are self-derived cells, the immune system may recognize them as foreign and attack them [63,64]. This can happen mainly due to mismatches in human leukocyte antigens (HLAs), which is why it is important to select cells based on HLA matching. If iPSCs are generated from a donor with a specific HLA type, it is possible to use iPSCs from other people [63]. If an HLA is incompatible, one can also modulate HLA expression or use gene editing [64].

Finally, because iPSCs must undergo reverse differentiation from human-derived cells, it takes a significant amount of time just to generate the cells. This can make it difficult to use autologous cells to treat acute illnesses.

In 2020, a transplantation study of iPSC-derived dopamine progenitor cells for the treatment of Parkinson's disease patients was conducted [65]. After harvesting fibroblasts by skin biopsy, dopamine progenitor cells were characterized in vitro with dopamine-neuron-specific and other neuronal markers. Characterized dopamine progenitor cells were transplanted into patients with Parkinson's disease, and Parkinson's-disease-related measures were assessed at 1, 3, 6, 9, and 12 months and every 6 months thereafter. Transplanted cells survived for 2 years without side effects. F-DOPA PET-CT imaging from 0 to 24 months showed a modest increase in dopamine uptake in the posterior cingulate near the implantation site. They also showed improved quality of life in clinical assessments of motor signs in Parkinson's disease, although interpretation should be carried out with caution due to the lack of a control group comparison.

In 2021, there was a planned clinical study of the transplantation of iPSC-derived neural progenitor cells for the treatment of subacute complete spinal cord injury [66]. However, this was postponed due to the sudden onset of the COVID-19 pandemic. A clinical-grade iPSC line (YZWJs513) prepared at the GMP facility of Osaka National Hospital was induced to differentiate into neural progenitor cells (NPCs), and preclinical studies using mouse models confirmed its promotion of motor function recovery after spinal cord injury.

5. Conclusions

iPSCs can differentiate into a variety of neuronal cell types, including dopaminergic neurons, astrocytes, and microglia, which could be a revolutionary way to treat a variety of neurodegenerative diseases. Inhibition of TGFβ and the SMAD pathway induces neural progenitor cell differentiation of cells with restored pluripotency. The differentiated cells still survive and function in the body.

The chemical drugs used to treat neurodegenerative diseases have different susceptibilities in different patients and have short half-lives, meaning that they are quickly used up by the body. Drugs for neurodegenerative diseases such as Parkinson's disease and Alzheimer's disease can slow their progression by increasing the release of neurotransmitters, but they cannot reverse the course of the disease. In addition, unlike a body part such as an arm, it is very difficult to accurately deliver chemical drugs to the brain. Cell transplantation treatments using patient-derived iPSCs are entirely patient-derived, have a high degree of tolerance, and may be able to survive and function in the long term to reverse the progression of neurodegenerative diseases.

However, clinical experimental studies of iPSCs and neural progenitor cells differentiated from them are extremely rare and require careful handling. The response in experimental animals and humans may be different, and we do not yet fully understand the differentiation of iPSCs.

Future research should focus on optimizing protocols for iPSC-derived neural cell differentiation, ensuring long-term viability and the functional integration of transplanted cells in vivo and paving the way for clinical applications.

Author Contributions: Conceptualization: J.S.O.; Data curation: D.-H.L., E.C.L., J.y.L. and M.R.L.; Funding acquisition: J.S.O.; Project administration: J.S.O.; Visualization: D.-H.L.; Writing—original draft: D.-H.L., J.-w.S. and J.S.O.; Writing—review and editing: D.-H.L., J.-w.S. and J.S.O. All authors have read and agreed to the published version of the manuscript.

Funding: This research was supported by the Bio and Medical Technology Development Program of the National Research Foundation funded by the Korean government (2023RA1A2C100531), by a grant from the Patient-Centered Clinical Research Coordinating Center (PACEN) funded by the Ministry of Health and Welfare, Republic of Korea (HC22C0043), and by a grant from the Korean Fund for Regenerative Medicine (KFRM) funded by the Korean government (KFRM-2022-00070557). The authors wish to acknowledge the financial support of the Catholic University of Korea Uijeongbu and the St. Mary's Hospital Clinical Research Laboratory Foundation.

Institutional Review Board Statement: Not applicable.

Informed Consent Statement: Not applicable.

Conflicts of Interest: The authors declare no conflict of interest.

Abbreviations

BDNF	Brain-derived neurotrophic factor
BMP	Bone morphogenetic protein
ESC	Embryonic stem cell
GDNF	Glial-cell-line-derived neurotrophic factor
HLA	Human leukocyte antigen
iPSC	Induced pluripotent stem cell
NPC	Neural progenitor cell
NSC	Neural stem cell
PSC	Pluripotent stem cell
RA	Retinoic acid
RAR	Retinoic acid receptor
RXR	Retinoid X receptor
SMAD	Sma- and Mad-related protein
TGFβ	Transforming growth factor-beta

References

1. Tsao, C.W.; Aday, A.W.; Almarzooq, Z.I.; Anderson, C.A.M.; Arora, P.; Avery, C.L.; Baker-Smith, C.M.; Beaton, A.Z.; Boehme, A.K.; Buxton, A.E.; et al. Heart Disease and Stroke Statistics-2023 Update: A Report From the American Heart Association. *Circulation* **2023**, *147*, e93–e621. [CrossRef] [PubMed]
2. Zhang, X.; Shu, B.; Zhang, D.; Huang, L.; Fu, Q.; Du, G. The Efficacy and Safety of Pharmacological Treatments for Post-stroke Aphasia. *CNS Neurol. Disord. Drug Targets* **2018**, *17*, 509–521. [CrossRef] [PubMed]
3. Czlonkowska, A.; Lesniak, M. Pharmacotherapy in stroke rehabilitation. *Expert Opin. Pharmacother.* **2009**, *10*, 1249–1259. [CrossRef] [PubMed]
4. Chollet, F.; Cramer, S.C.; Stinear, C.; Kappelle, L.J.; Baron, J.C.; Weiller, C.; Azouvi, P.; Hommel, M.; Sabatini, U.; Moulin, T.; et al. Pharmacological therapies in post stroke recovery: Recommendations for future clinical trials. *J. Neurol.* **2014**, *261*, 1461–1468. [CrossRef]

5. Neaverson, A.; Andersson, M.H.L.; Arshad, O.A.; Foulser, L.; Goodwin-Trotman, M.; Hunter, A.; Newman, B.; Patel, M.; Roth, C.; Thwaites, T.; et al. Differentiation of human induced pluripotent stem cells into cortical neural stem cells. *Front. Cell Dev. Biol.* **2022**, *10*, 1023340. [CrossRef] [PubMed]
6. He, S.; Nakada, D.; Morrison, S.J. Mechanisms of stem cell self-renewal. *Annu. Rev. Cell Dev. Biol.* **2009**, *25*, 377–406. [CrossRef] [PubMed]
7. Biehl, J.K.; Russell, B. Introduction to stem cell therapy. *J. Cardiovasc. Nurs.* **2009**, *24*, 98–103. [CrossRef] [PubMed]
8. Zakrzewski, W.; Dobrzynski, M.; Szymonowicz, M.; Rybak, Z. Stem cells: Past, present, and future. *Stem Cell Res. Ther.* **2019**, *10*, 68. [CrossRef] [PubMed]
9. Chehelgerdi, M.; Behdarvand Dehkordi, F.; Chehelgerdi, M.; Kabiri, H.; Salehian-Dehkordi, H.; Abdolvand, M.; Salmanizadeh, S.; Rashidi, M.; Niazmand, A.; Ahmadi, S.; et al. Exploring the promising potential of induced pluripotent stem cells in cancer research and therapy. *Mol. Cancer* **2023**, *22*, 189. [CrossRef]
10. Adhya, D.; Swarup, V.; Nagy, R.; Dutan, L.; Shum, C.; Valencia-Alarcon, E.P.; Jozwik, K.M.; Mendez, M.A.; Horder, J.; Loth, E.; et al. Atypical Neurogenesis in Induced Pluripotent Stem Cells From Autistic Individuals. *Biol. Psychiatry* **2021**, *89*, 486–496. [CrossRef]
11. Liou, R.H.; Edwards, T.L.; Martin, K.R.; Wong, R.C. Neuronal Reprogramming for Tissue Repair and Neuroregeneration. *Int. J. Mol. Sci.* **2020**, *21*, 4273. [CrossRef] [PubMed]
12. Paik, D.T.; Chandy, M.; Wu, J.C. Patient and Disease-Specific Induced Pluripotent Stem Cells for Discovery of Personalized Cardiovascular Drugs and Therapeutics. *Pharmacol. Rev.* **2020**, *72*, 320–342. [CrossRef] [PubMed]
13. Thomson, J.A.; Itskovitz-Eldor, J.; Shapiro, S.S.; Waknitz, M.A.; Swiergiel, J.J.; Marshall, V.S.; Jones, J.M. Embryonic stem cell lines derived from human blastocysts. *Science* **1998**, *282*, 1145–1147. [CrossRef] [PubMed]
14. Baldwin, T. Morality and human embryo research. Introduction to the Talking Point on morality and human embryo research. *EMBO Rep.* **2009**, *10*, 299–300. [CrossRef] [PubMed]
15. Jang, J.; Yoo, J.E.; Lee, J.A.; Lee, D.R.; Kim, J.Y.; Huh, Y.J.; Kim, D.S.; Park, C.Y.; Hwang, D.Y.; Kim, H.S.; et al. Disease-specific induced pluripotent stem cells: A platform for human disease modeling and drug discovery. *Exp. Mol. Med.* **2012**, *44*, 202–213. [CrossRef] [PubMed]
16. Elitt, M.S.; Barbar, L.; Tesar, P.J. Drug screening for human genetic diseases using iPSC models. *Hum. Mol. Genet.* **2018**, *27*, R89–R98. [CrossRef] [PubMed]
17. Choi, J.; Lee, S.; Mallard, W.; Clement, K.; Tagliazucchi, G.M.; Lim, H.; Choi, I.Y.; Ferrari, F.; Tsankov, A.M.; Pop, R.; et al. A comparison of genetically matched cell lines reveals the equivalence of human iPSCs and ESCs. *Nat. Biotechnol.* **2015**, *33*, 1173–1181. [CrossRef]
18. Marei, H.E.; Althani, A.; Lashen, S.; Cenciarelli, C.; Hasan, A. Genetically unmatched human iPSC and ESC exhibit equivalent gene expression and neuronal differentiation potential. *Sci. Rep.* **2017**, *7*, 17504. [CrossRef]
19. Kristiansen, C.K.; Chen, A.; Hoyland, L.E.; Ziegler, M.; Sullivan, G.J.; Bindoff, L.A.; Liang, K.X. Comparing the mitochondrial signatures in ESCs and iPSCs and their neural derivations. *Cell Cycle* **2022**, *21*, 2206–2221. [CrossRef]
20. Chambers, S.M.; Fasano, C.A.; Papapetrou, E.P.; Tomishima, M.; Sadelain, M.; Studer, L. Highly efficient neural conversion of human ES and iPS cells by dual inhibition of SMAD signaling. *Nat. Biotechnol.* **2009**, *27*, 275–280. [CrossRef]
21. Xu, R.H.; Sampsell-Barron, T.L.; Gu, F.; Root, S.; Peck, R.M.; Pan, G.; Yu, J.; Antosiewicz-Bourget, J.; Tian, S.; Stewart, R.; et al. NANOG is a direct target of TGFbeta/activin-mediated SMAD signaling in human ESCs. *Cell Stem Cell* **2008**, *3*, 196–206. [CrossRef] [PubMed]
22. Xu, R.H.; Chen, X.; Li, D.S.; Li, R.; Addicks, G.C.; Glennon, C.; Zwaka, T.P.; Thomson, J.A. BMP4 initiates human embryonic stem cell differentiation to trophoblast. *Nat. Biotechnol.* **2002**, *20*, 1261–1264. [CrossRef]
23. D'Amour, K.A.; Agulnick, A.D.; Eliazer, S.; Kelly, O.G.; Kroon, E.; Baetge, E.E. Efficient differentiation of human embryonic stem cells to definitive endoderm. *Nat. Biotechnol.* **2005**, *23*, 1534–1541. [CrossRef]
24. Laflamme, M.A.; Chen, K.Y.; Naumova, A.V.; Muskheli, V.; Fugate, J.A.; Dupras, S.K.; Reinecke, H.; Xu, C.; Hassanipour, M.; Police, S.; et al. Cardiomyocytes derived from human embryonic stem cells in pro-survival factors enhance function of infarcted rat hearts. *Nat. Biotechnol.* **2007**, *25*, 1015–1024. [CrossRef]
25. Massague, J. The transforming growth factor-beta family. *Annu. Rev. Cell Biol.* **1990**, *6*, 597–641. [CrossRef] [PubMed]
26. Massague, J.; Chen, Y.G. Controlling TGF-beta signaling. *Genes Dev.* **2000**, *14*, 627–644. [CrossRef] [PubMed]
27. Chen, X.; Xu, L. Mechanism and regulation of nucleocytoplasmic trafficking of smad. *Cell Biosci.* **2011**, *1*, 40. [CrossRef]
28. Tang, L.Y.; Zhang, Y.E. Non-degradative ubiquitination in Smad-dependent TGF-beta signaling. *Cell Biosci.* **2011**, *1*, 43. [CrossRef]
29. Schmierer, B.; Hill, C.S. TGFbeta-SMAD signal transduction: Molecular specificity and functional flexibility. *Nat. Rev. Mol. Cell Biol.* **2007**, *8*, 970–982. [CrossRef]
30. Reddi, A.H.; Reddi, A. Bone morphogenetic proteins (BMPs): From morphogens to metabologens. *Cytokine Growth Factor Rev.* **2009**, *20*, 341–342. [CrossRef]
31. Sieber, C.; Kopf, J.; Hiepen, C.; Knaus, P. Recent advances in BMP receptor signaling. *Cytokine Growth Factor Rev.* **2009**, *20*, 343–355. [CrossRef]
32. Miyazono, K.; Maeda, S.; Imamura, T. Coordinate regulation of cell growth and differentiation by TGF-beta superfamily and Runx proteins. *Oncogene* **2004**, *23*, 4232–4237. [CrossRef] [PubMed]

33. Nilsson, E.E.; Skinner, M.K. Bone morphogenetic protein-4 acts as an ovarian follicle survival factor and promotes primordial follicle development. *Biol. Reprod.* **2003**, *69*, 1265–1272. [CrossRef]
34. Winnier, G.; Blessing, M.; Labosky, P.A.; Hogan, B.L. Bone morphogenetic protein-4 is required for mesoderm formation and patterning in the mouse. *Genes Dev.* **1995**, *9*, 2105–2116. [CrossRef]
35. Tan, B.T.; Wang, L.; Li, S.; Long, Z.Y.; Wu, Y.M.; Liu, Y. Retinoic acid induced the differentiation of neural stem cells from embryonic spinal cord into functional neurons in vitro. *Int. J. Clin. Exp. Pathol.* **2015**, *8*, 8129–8135.
36. Kurokawa, R.; Soderstrom, M.; Horlein, A.; Halachmi, S.; Brown, M.; Rosenfeld, M.G.; Glass, C.K. Polarity-specific activities of retinoic acid receptors determined by a co-repressor. *Nature* **1995**, *377*, 451–454. [CrossRef]
37. Mosher, K.I.; Schaffer, D.V. Proliferation versus Differentiation: Redefining Retinoic Acid's Role. *Stem Cell Rep.* **2018**, *10*, 1673–1675. [CrossRef] [PubMed]
38. Lee, K.; Skromne, I. Retinoic acid regulates size, pattern and alignment of tissues at the head-trunk transition. *Development* **2014**, *141*, 4375–4384. [CrossRef] [PubMed]
39. Sharpe, C.; Goldstone, K. The control of Xenopus embryonic primary neurogenesis is mediated by retinoid signalling in the neurectoderm. *Mech. Dev.* **2000**, *91*, 69–80. [CrossRef]
40. Maden, M.; Holder, N. Retinoic acid and development of the central nervous system. *Bioessays* **1992**, *14*, 431–438. [CrossRef]
41. Clagett-Dame, M.; DeLuca, H.F. The role of vitamin A in mammalian reproduction and embryonic development. *Annu. Rev. Nutr.* **2002**, *22*, 347–381. [CrossRef] [PubMed]
42. Binder, D.K.; Scharfman, H.E. Brain-derived neurotrophic factor. *Growth Factors* **2004**, *22*, 123–131. [CrossRef] [PubMed]
43. Acheson, A.; Conover, J.C.; Fandl, J.P.; DeChiara, T.M.; Russell, M.; Thadani, A.; Squinto, S.P.; Yancopoulos, G.D.; Lindsay, R.M. A BDNF autocrine loop in adult sensory neurons prevents cell death. *Nature* **1995**, *374*, 450–453. [CrossRef] [PubMed]
44. Huang, E.J.; Reichardt, L.F. Neurotrophins: Roles in neuronal development and function. *Annu. Rev. Neurosci.* **2001**, *24*, 677–736. [CrossRef] [PubMed]
45. Ahmed, S.; Reynolds, B.A.; Weiss, S. BDNF enhances the differentiation but not the survival of CNS stem cell-derived neuronal precursors. *J. Neurosci.* **1995**, *15*, 5765–5778. [CrossRef]
46. Lim, J.Y.; Park, S.I.; Oh, J.H.; Kim, S.M.; Jeong, C.H.; Jun, J.A.; Lee, K.S.; Oh, W.; Lee, J.K.; Jeun, S.S. Brain-derived neurotrophic factor stimulates the neural differentiation of human umbilical cord blood-derived mesenchymal stem cells and survival of differentiated cells through MAPK/ERK and PI3K/Akt-dependent signaling pathways. *J. Neurosci. Res.* **2008**, *86*, 2168–2178. [CrossRef]
47. Airaksinen, M.S.; Saarma, M. The GDNF family: Signalling, biological functions and therapeutic value. *Nat. Rev. Neurosci.* **2002**, *3*, 383–394. [CrossRef] [PubMed]
48. Cik, M.; Masure, S.; Lesage, A.S.; Van Der Linden, I.; Van Gompel, P.; Pangalos, M.N.; Gordon, R.D.; Leysen, J.E. Binding of GDNF and neurturin to human GDNF family receptor alpha 1 and 2. Influence of cRET and cooperative interactions. *J. Biol. Chem.* **2000**, *275*, 27505–27512. [CrossRef] [PubMed]
49. Matlik, K.; Garton, D.R.; Montano-Rodriguez, A.R.; Olfat, S.; Eren, F.; Casserly, L.; Damdimopoulos, A.; Panhelainen, A.; Porokuokka, L.L.; Kopra, J.J.; et al. Elevated endogenous GDNF induces altered dopamine signalling in mice and correlates with clinical severity in schizophrenia. *Mol. Psychiatry* **2022**, *27*, 3247–3261. [CrossRef]
50. Aloe, L.; Rocco, M.L.; Balzamino, B.O.; Micera, A. Nerve Growth Factor: A Focus on Neuroscience and Therapy. *Curr. Neuropharmacol.* **2015**, *13*, 294–303. [CrossRef]
51. Autar, K.; Guo, X.; Rumsey, J.W.; Long, C.J.; Akanda, N.; Jackson, M.; Narasimhan, N.S.; Caneus, J.; Morgan, D.; Hickman, J.J. A functional hiPSC-cortical neuron differentiation and maturation model and its application to neurological disorders. *Stem Cell Rep.* **2022**, *17*, 96–109. [CrossRef]
52. Shi, Y.; Kirwan, P.; Livesey, F.J. Directed differentiation of human pluripotent stem cells to cerebral cortex neurons and neural networks. *Nat. Protoc.* **2012**, *7*, 1836–1846. [CrossRef]
53. Ma, L.; Liu, Y.; Zhang, S.C. Directed differentiation of dopamine neurons from human pluripotent stem cells. *Methods Mol. Biol.* **2011**, *767*, 411–418. [CrossRef] [PubMed]
54. Mahajani, S.; Raina, A.; Fokken, C.; Kugler, S.; Bahr, M. Homogenous generation of dopaminergic neurons from multiple hiPSC lines by transient expression of transcription factors. *Cell Death Dis.* **2019**, *10*, 898. [CrossRef] [PubMed]
55. Karumbayaram, S.; Novitch, B.G.; Patterson, M.; Umbach, J.A.; Richter, L.; Lindgren, A.; Conway, A.E.; Clark, A.T.; Goldman, S.A.; Plath, K.; et al. Directed differentiation of human-induced pluripotent stem cells generates active motor neurons. *Stem Cells* **2009**, *27*, 806–811. [CrossRef] [PubMed]
56. Shaltouki, A.; Peng, J.; Liu, Q.; Rao, M.S.; Zeng, X. Efficient generation of astrocytes from human pluripotent stem cells in defined conditions. *Stem Cells* **2013**, *31*, 941–952. [CrossRef]
57. Douvaras, P.; Wang, J.; Zimmer, M.; Hanchuk, S.; O'Bara, M.A.; Sadiq, S.; Sim, F.J.; Goldman, J.; Fossati, V. Efficient generation of myelinating oligodendrocytes from primary progressive multiple sclerosis patients by induced pluripotent stem cells. *Stem Cell Rep.* **2014**, *3*, 250–259. [CrossRef]
58. Pomeshchik, Y.; Klementieva, O.; Gil, J.; Martinsson, I.; Hansen, M.G.; de Vries, T.; Sancho-Balsells, A.; Russ, K.; Savchenko, E.; Collin, A.; et al. Human iPSC-Derived Hippocampal Spheroids: An Innovative Tool for Stratifying Alzheimer Disease Patient-Specific Cellular Phenotypes and Developing Therapies. *Stem Cell Rep.* **2020**, *15*, 256–273. [CrossRef]

59. Valiulahi, P.; Vidyawan, V.; Puspita, L.; Oh, Y.; Juwono, V.B.; Sittipo, P.; Friedlander, G.; Yahalomi, D.; Sohn, J.W.; Lee, Y.K.; et al. Generation of caudal-type serotonin neurons and hindbrain-fate organoids from hPSCs. *Stem Cell Rep.* **2021**, *16*, 1938–1952. [CrossRef]
60. Yang, D.; Zhang, Z.J.; Oldenburg, M.; Ayala, M.; Zhang, S.C. Human embryonic stem cell-derived dopaminergic neurons reverse functional deficit in parkinsonian rats. *Stem Cells* **2008**, *26*, 55–63. [CrossRef]
61. Preman, P.; Tcw, J.; Calafate, S.; Snellinx, A.; Alfonso-Triguero, M.; Corthout, N.; Munck, S.; Thal, D.R.; Goate, A.M.; De Strooper, B.; et al. Human iPSC-derived astrocytes transplanted into the mouse brain undergo morphological changes in response to amyloid-beta plaques. *Mol. Neurodegener.* **2021**, *16*, 68. [CrossRef]
62. Moradi, S.; Mahdizadeh, H.; Saric, T.; Kim, J.; Harati, J.; Shahsavarani, H.; Greber, B.; Moore, J.B.t. Research and therapy with induced pluripotent stem cells (iPSCs): Social, legal, and ethical considerations. *Stem Cell Res. Ther.* **2019**, *10*, 341. [CrossRef] [PubMed]
63. Flahou, C.; Morishima, T.; Takizawa, H.; Sugimoto, N. Fit-For-All iPSC-Derived Cell Therapies and Their Evaluation in Humanized Mice with NK Cell Immunity. *Front. Immunol.* **2021**, *12*, 662360. [CrossRef] [PubMed]
64. Otsuka, R.; Wada, H.; Murata, T.; Seino, K.I. Immune reaction and regulation in transplantation based on pluripotent stem cell technology. *Inflamm. Regen.* **2020**, *40*, 12. [CrossRef] [PubMed]
65. Schweitzer, J.S.; Song, B.; Herrington, T.M.; Park, T.Y.; Lee, N.; Ko, S.; Jeon, J.; Cha, Y.; Kim, K.; Li, Q.; et al. Personalized iPSC-Derived Dopamine Progenitor Cells for Parkinson's Disease. *N. Engl. J. Med.* **2020**, *382*, 1926–1932. [CrossRef]
66. Sugai, K.; Sumida, M.; Shofuda, T.; Yamaguchi, R.; Tamura, T.; Kohzuki, T.; Abe, T.; Shibata, R.; Kamata, Y.; Ito, S.; et al. First-in-human clinical trial of transplantation of iPSC-derived NS/PCs in subacute complete spinal cord injury: Study protocol. *Regen. Ther.* **2021**, *18*, 321–333. [CrossRef]

Disclaimer/Publisher's Note: The statements, opinions and data contained in all publications are solely those of the individual author(s) and contributor(s) and not of MDPI and/or the editor(s). MDPI and/or the editor(s) disclaim responsibility for any injury to people or property resulting from any ideas, methods, instructions or products referred to in the content.

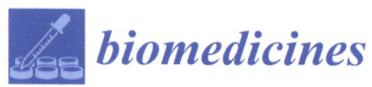

Review

Cell-Based Therapy for Urethral Regeneration: A Narrative Review and Future Perspectives

Yangwang Jin [1], Weixin Zhao [2], Ming Yang [1], Wenzhuo Fang [1], Guo Gao [3], Ying Wang [1,*] and Qiang Fu [1,*]

[1] Department of Urology, Shanghai Sixth People's Hospital Affiliated to Shanghai Jiao Tong University School of Medicine, Shanghai Eastern Institute of Urologic Reconstruction, Shanghai Jiao Tong University, Shanghai 200233, China; jinyw_med@163.com (Y.J.)
[2] Wake Forest Institute for Regenerative Medicine, Winston Salem, NC 27157, USA
[3] Key Laboratory for Thin Film and Micro Fabrication of the Ministry of Education, School of Sensing Science and Engineering, School of Electronic Information and Electrical Engineering, Shanghai Jiao Tong University, Shanghai 200240, China
* Correspondence: sdzbbswangying@alumni.sjtu.edu.cn (Y.W.); jamesqfu@aliyun.com (Q.F.)

Abstract: Urethral stricture is a common urological disease that seriously affects quality of life. Urethroplasty with grafts is the primary treatment, but the autografts used in clinical practice have unavoidable disadvantages, which have contributed to the development of urethral tissue engineering. Using various types of seed cells in combination with biomaterials to construct a tissue-engineered urethra provides a new treatment method to repair long-segment urethral strictures. To date, various cell types have been explored and applied in the field of urethral regeneration. However, no optimal strategy for the source, selection, and application conditions of the cells is available. This review systematically summarizes the use of various cell types in urethral regeneration and their characteristics in recent years and discusses possible future directions of cell-based therapies.

Keywords: cell therapy; stem cell; urethral regeneration; tissue engineering

Citation: Jin, Y.; Zhao, W.; Yang, M.; Fang, W.; Gao, G.; Wang, Y.; Fu, Q. Cell-Based Therapy for Urethral Regeneration: A Narrative Review and Future Perspectives. *Biomedicines* 2023, 11, 2366. https://doi.org/10.3390/biomedicines11092366

Academic Editors: Aline Yen Ling Wang and Shaker A. Mousa

Received: 4 June 2023
Revised: 29 July 2023
Accepted: 16 August 2023
Published: 24 August 2023

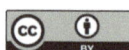

Copyright: © 2023 by the authors. Licensee MDPI, Basel, Switzerland. This article is an open access article distributed under the terms and conditions of the Creative Commons Attribution (CC BY) license (https://creativecommons.org/licenses/by/4.0/).

1. Introduction

Urethral stricture is a pathological narrowing of the urethral lumen associated with excessive fibrosis of the epithelium and surrounding tissues [1]. As a common urological disease, urethral stricture can be caused by various factors such as trauma, inflammation, congenital malformation, and medically induced injury [2]. Urethral stricture can lead to urinary retention, bladder stones, fistula formation, urinary tract infection, hydronephrosis, and, in severe cases, renal failure, thus affecting quality of life, while treatment of urethral stricture also puts considerable pressure on the healthcare system [3,4]. Treatment of urethral strictures usually employs different repair strategies depending on the length, location, and cause of the injury [5]. Currently, urethroplasty is usually performed clinically using a graft in patients with long-segment urethral strictures/defects, recurrent strictures, or penile urethral strictures [6]. Grafts are usually autologous tissues, such as buccal mucosa, penile flap, and bladder mucosa, but they are limited in number and difficult to obtain. This treatment mode of sacrificing healthy tissues to repair lesions is also controversial because of the numerous complications associated with the donor site [7]. Therefore, reconstructive repair of the injured urethra remains challenging for urologists.

Tissue engineering is a derivative of regenerative medicine, which aims to create organs using cells, biomaterials, and engineering techniques [8]. Tissue-engineered grafts avoid the complications of autologous tissue collection and reduce patient pain. Over the past 30 years, using tissue engineering techniques to construct a tissue-engineered urethra has made great strides and is gradually being incorporated into urological practice. Single biomaterial scaffolds were first applied to urethral reconstruction, which provide good mechanical support and spatial structure for the migration of host cells and facilitate remodeling of the urethral tissue structure, achieving a certain degree of success in urethral repair. Some classical tissue engineering materials, such as small intestinal submucosa (SIS), bladder acellular matrix (BAM), and acellular dermal matrix, have been evaluated in several clinical trials. However, successful repair with a single scaffold is very dependent on a healthy urethral bed at the injury, adequate vascular distribution, and the absence of spongy fibrosis, which otherwise predisposes to chronic immune reactions, fibrosis formation and calcification, and graft shrinkage or restriction, for which a single scaffold is often inadequate to treat long defects [9]. A research shows that the maximum distance to repair the urethra using tubular acellular matrix grafts appears to be only 0.5 cm [10].

The natural healing process of the urethra involves interactions between multiple factors, such as intercellular contacts, secretions from resident and migrating cells, growth factors, cytokines, and various signaling pathways [11]. Therefore, many investigators have begun to explore cell-based regeneration strategies for long-segment urethral repair. A systematic evaluation showed that the long-term success rate of cell–scaffold material complex grafts inoculated with cells was 5.67 times higher than that of the scaffold material alone [12]. Transplanted cells promote rapid vascularization and re-epithelialization of the scaffold material at the graft repair site, reducing local inflammation and scar formation for better repair results [13–15]. Therefore, the involvement of cells is indispensable for urethral regeneration, particularly the repair of long-segment urethral defects.

To date, various cell types have been explored and applied in the field of urethral regeneration. However, no optimal strategy for the source, selection, and application conditions of the cells is available. This review systematically summarizes the use of various cell types in urethral regeneration and their characteristics in recent years and discusses possible future directions of cell-based therapies.

2. Non-Stem Cell-Based Regenerative Therapy

In most cases, the use of differentiated cells in urethral regeneration has been well established and includes mainly epithelial cells, smooth muscle cells, and endothelial cells.

2.1. Epithelial Cells

Epithelial cells are the key cells in urethra regeneration. A continuous layer of epithelial cells provides a barrier against corrosion effects and urinary fistula, thereby reducing inflammation and fibrous tissue deposition during the healing process [16].

Transitional epithelial cells of the bladder mucosa, mainly obtained by bladder biopsy, are considered the best candidates to reconstruct the epithelial cell layer of the urethra. Although structurally different from the compound columnar epithelium in the urethra, both the transitional epithelium in the bladder and the urethral epithelium are formed by p63+ cells from the urogenital sinus of the fetus [17], and both function as a barrier to urine in the urinary tract. In one study, the bladder mucosa was isolated and digested, and the obtained epithelial cells were cultured in supplemented CnT-07 for proliferation or CnT-02 with 1.07 mM/L $CaCl_2$ for stratification [16]. The expanded autologous bladder epithelial cells were subsequently seeded on a type I collagen-based cell carrier, cultured in layers for 8 days, and labeled with PKH26. The collagen-based cell carrier grafts were then used to repair urethral strictures in minipigs. Immunofluorescence analysis confirmed the epithelial cell phenotype, junction formation, and differentiation at 2 weeks, and that the grafted cells were present at the repair site 6 months after surgery. No recurrence of the stricture was observed in the experimental animals at the final 6-month transplantation [16]. Another study using a rabbit model showed that scaffolds implanted with bladder epithelial cells supported epithelial integrity, stratification, and continuity with the normal urothelium [18]. Wang et al. [19] implanted bladder epithelial cells into human amniotic scaffolds to reduce rejection and improve the biocompatibility of the graft material. The results showed milder inflammatory cell infiltration, i.e., less accumulation of CD4 and CD8 cells, neutrophils, and other types of immune cells, in cell-seeded human amniotic scaffold grafts compared with the epithelial cell-free group.

The number of cells obtained by biopsy is limited, and the procedure requires general anesthesia and is invasive. Bladder washing is a feasible alternative to harvesting viable autologous bladder epithelial cells in a non-invasive manner [20]. Amesty et al. [21] obtained autologous epithelial cells by bladder washing and seeded the submucosal matrix of acellular porcine small intestines to construct a tissue-engineered urethra. They found that the epithelial cell seeding group formed multilayered urothelial cells and successfully repaired urethral defects in rabbits. Epithelial cells collected by the bladder washing procedure have the same effect as biopsy acquisition, and it avoids donor site damage caused by biopsy, providing the possibility of obtaining cells several times for repeat procedures if needed [20].

Autologous urethral epithelial cells cannot, however, be obtained from patients with chronic inflammation of the urinary tract [22]. Oral mucosal cells exist in a humid physiological environment similar to the urinary tract and are resistant to a wet environment and infection because of the expression of beta-defensins and interleukin-8 in their membranes [23]. The differences between oral and urethral mucosae are minimal [24], and the collection of oral mucosal epithelial cells can be performed under local anesthesia in a simple and well-tolerated procedure. Therefore, autologous oral-derived epithelial cells are also an effective cell source for urethral regeneration. Huang et al. [25] used lingual keratinocytes seeded in a bacterial cellulose (BC) scaffold to treat rabbit urethral injuries. The cell–scaffold material composite group exhibited faster and more complete epithelial regeneration compared with the BC alone group. Lv et al. [26] cultured autologous lingual keratinocytes and seeded them on a novel three-dimensional (3D) scaffold composed of a combination of silk fibroin (SF) and BC and observed good regeneration of the urothelial cells in a dog urethral repair model. Oral mucosal epithelial cells have been developed to construct a tissue-engineered buccal mucosa for urethral repair and reconstruction, with encouraging results [2,27]. However, a potential limitation of oral mucosal epithelial cells is their low proliferative capacity and clonogenicity, hindering their large-scale expansion in vitro, which is required for clinical use.

Epidermal cells can also be isolated and expanded by minimally invasive methods from hairless skin, such as foreskin, and cultured to form a thick barrier that isolates urine. A study has demonstrated successful repair of rabbit urethral defects using a tubular acellular collagen matrix seeded with foreskin epithelial cells [28]. However, because of complications and malformations at the harvest site associated with a foreskin biopsy, recent studies have begun to explore the use of epidermal cells from other sites for urethral repair procedures. Rogovaya et al. [29] collected rabbit ear epithelial cells and cultured them to prepare cell sheets for rabbit urethral repair. The rabbits regained voluntary urinary function at 4–7 days postoperatively with no scarring or abnormal fistula formation in the urethra. Complete recovery of rabbit urothelial cells was observed at 45 days postoperatively in the grafted area, and the presence of a multilayered migrating epithelium was observed. In another study, Zhang et al. [30] obtained skin epidermal cells (SEC) from rabbit abdominal skin and constructed cryopreserved SEC-AM (amniotic membrane) urethral scaffolds for rabbit urethra repair, which also achieved good results.

2.2. Mesothelial Cells

Epithelial cells have a low proliferative capacity and often require long culture cycles. Additionally, epithelial cells are unavailable under malignant conditions, a history of lichen sclerosis, or oral disease. Mesothelial cells have a higher proliferative capacity and plasticity than urothelial cells [31]. Studies have reported the successful use of mesothelial cell-lined grafts as urethral grafts, including peritoneal [32] and vaginal endografts [33]. Thus, mesothelial cells may be a suitable alternative to epithelial cells. Jiang et al. [34] seeded mesothelial cells onto autogenous granulation tissue to construct a mesothelium-lined compound graft for tubularized urethroplasty in male rabbits. Histologically, urothelial layers surrounded by increasingly organized smooth muscles were observed in seeded grafts. Conversely, myofibroblast accumulation and extensive scarring occurred in unseeded grafts. Although mesothelial cells of large omentum origin may have some advantages, long-term culture of mesothelial cells appears to be difficult because of early senescence. Thus, further studies on mesothelial cells are needed.

2.3. Smooth Muscle Cells

The well-developed smooth muscle layer enhances the mechanical properties of the urethra and maintains structural stability during stretching and urination, to some extent avoiding the occurrence of urethral strictures. Therefore, seeding smooth muscle cells (SMCs) for remuscularization of a tissue-engineered urethra is an effective method to possibly repair urethral injury while avoiding strictures. A bladder biopsy is the most common source of SMCs in urethral repair and reconstruction. In one study, bladder muscle tissue was clipped and digested, and a composite SMC scaffold was used to repair urethral defects in rabbits [35]. After 3 months, immunohistochemical examination showed a higher and well-arranged smooth muscle content in the SMC group compared with that in the control group, which resulted in a significantly lower rate of tubular obstruction and complications, including stone formation, urinary fistula, and urethral stricture incidence, in the SMC group. In a report by Lv et al. [36], earlier muscle regeneration was observed in the SMC-seeded scaffold group compared with the unseeded cell group. In another preclinical study, Niu et al. [37] seeded SMCs into a synthetic scaffold for rabbit urethral repair reconstruction and found that it promoted the regeneration of multilayered smooth muscle tissue, obtaining grafting results similar to those of autologous tissue. Similar success was subsequently achieved by their group in a dog model [38]. Ultimately, SMC composite scaffolds result in earlier, more mature muscle regeneration, thereby facilitating the avoidance of urethral strictures.

SMCs may also help support epithelial–mesenchymal interactions required for normal maturation of the urothelium [22,39]. In a preclinical study [14], autologous epithelial and smooth muscle cells were seeded in a tubular collagen scaffold and used for urethroplasty in 15 dogs. After up to 12 months of follow-up, computed tomography urethrograms showed a wide urethral caliber in animals treated with seeded cell grafts. Conversely, six control animals treated with unseeded scaffolds had blocked urethras. The seeded group showed superior epithelial tissue and muscle fiber formation, whereas the unseeded group showed fibrosis and few muscle fibers. In another study, autologous bladder epithelial and smooth muscle cells from nine male rabbits were expanded and seeded onto preconfigured tubular matrices constructed from acellular bladder matrices obtained from the lamina propria. Urethroplasties were performed with tubularized matrices seeded with cells in nine animals and matrices without cells in six animals. The urethrograms showed that animals implanted with cell-seeded matrices maintained a wide urethral caliber without strictures. Conversely, urethras with unseeded scaffolds collapsed and developed strictures [40]. Similarly, Lv et al. [26] successfully repaired urethral defects in dogs using a composite bilayer scaffold of lingual keratinocytes and lingual muscle cells. However, the low proliferative potential of smooth muscle cells and the relatively high trauma during primary cell collection make it difficult to obtain sufficient seeded smooth muscle cells.

2.4. Endothelial Cells

Blood vessels provide oxygen and nutrients to tissues and are necessary for tissue regeneration; therefore, vascularization of urethral grafts is an important step in the reconstruction of the urethra. Vascular endothelial cells have become a cell type of great interest. In one study, Heller and colleagues isolated human dermal microvascular endothelial cells from the foreskin to develop a pre-vascularized buccal mucosal substitute to repair urethral defects [41]. Their results showed successful pre-vascularization and the formation of dense capillary-like structures in the substitutes, which became functional vessels by anastomosis with host vessels after implantation into nude mice. Although endothelial cells have been shown to play a crucial role in promoting angiogenesis, harvesting primary endothelial cells remains challenging. Table 1 summarized the functions performed by differentiated cells in urethral regeneration.

Table 1. Summary of the functions performed by differentiated cells in urethral regeneration.

Cell Type	Source	Function in Urethral Regeneration	References
Mucosal epithelial cells	Bladder mucosa	Support epithelial integrity, stratification, and continuity with normal urothelium; reduce potential rejection reactions; and improve the biocompatibility of the graft material.	[16,18,19,21]
	Oral mucosa	Promotion of urethral epithelial regeneration; participation in the construction of tissue-engineered buccal mucosa (TEBM).	[2,25–27]
	Skin/foreskin	Form a thick barrier to isolate urine.	[19,30]
Mesothelial cells	Peritoneal/vaginal endothelial	Act as a substitute for epithelial cells.	[34]
Smooth muscle cells	Bladder	Promote earlier, more mature regeneration of urethral smooth muscle; enhance the mechanical properties of grafts; and support the epithelial–mesenchymal interactions required for normal maturation of the urothelium.	[14,22,26,35–40]
Endothelial cells	Foreskin	Promote tissue angiogenesis and graft vascularization.	[41]

3. Stem Cell-Based Regenerative Therapy

Stem cells are self-renewing and pluripotent, allowing them to differentiate into various cell types in the urothelial tissue in a specific microenvironment, and their paracrine secretion of various growth factors and bioactive cytokines stimulates the growth of nearby cells and has been shown to enhance angiogenesis and reduce fibrosis [42–44]. Therefore, stem cell therapy has great potential and has been a hot research topic in recent years [45,46]. Stem cells used for urethral regeneration mainly include bone marrow-derived stem cells (BMDSC), adipose-derived stem cells (ADSCs), and urine-derived stem cells (UDSC).

3.1. Pluripotent Stem Cells

Pluripotent stem cells include embryonic stem cells (ESCs) and induced pluripotent stem cells (iPSCs). ESCs are isolated from the inner cell mass of an embryonic blastocyst and have great clinical potential because they form cells of ectodermal, endodermal, and mesodermal origins. Blank et al. [47] established the first in vitro system to induce differentiation of mouse ESCs into SMCs by retinoic acid in 1995. Ottamasanthien et al. [48] described the differentiation of pluripotent stem cells towards the uroepithelium in a mouse model when ESCs were directed to the uroepithelial lineage through tissue reconstitution experiments with mouse embryonic bladder mesenchyme. However, ESCs have ethical restrictions because of embryo destruction for collection. iPSCs have similar regenerative and differentiation abilities to ESCs without the associated ethical controversies. Suzuki et al. [49] used a combination of PPAR (peroxisome proliferator-activated receptor)-γ agonists and EGFR (epidermal growth factor receptor) inhibitors, as well as FGF10 and transwell cultures, to demonstrate directed differentiation of iPSCs into mature stratified bladder epithelium. However, iPSCs have some concerns, including low reprogramming and differentiation efficiencies and potential tumorigenicity [22].

3.2. Bone Marrow-Derived Stem Cells

Mesenchymal stem cells differentiate into various cell and tissue types. As a type of mesenchymal stem cell, BMDSCs can differentiate into urothelial cells and bladder SMCs in vitro and in vivo, and initial success in urethral regeneration has been achieved. Demirel et al. [50] evaluated the effects of BMDSC injection in a rat model of posterior urethral injury and demonstrated that BMDSC treatment significantly reduced the development of fibrosis in a uroepithelial injury model. In addition to BMDSC injection alone, a composite scaffold may promote their further differentiation and improve pro-regenerative and tissue fusion effects. Zhang et al. [51] compared bladder regeneration of BMDSC-seeded and bladder SMC-seeded SIS scaffolds. Histological evaluation showed that SIS grafts implanted with BMDSCs showed solid smooth muscle bundle formation throughout the graft at 10 weeks after surgery, which was similar to the results achieved in the bladder SMC cell-seeded SIS group. Another study compared the therapeutic effects of a BMDSC composite scaffold and an autologous oral mucosa graft for urethral reconstruction [52]. To track BMDSCs in vivo, they were labeled with superparamagnetic iron oxide nanoparticles. Twelve weeks of follow-up revealed that the BMDSC composite scaffold formed good fusion with the surrounding urethral tissue, and histology showed less fibrosis and inflammatory cell infiltration of lymphocytes, histiocytes, and plasma cells in the experimental group compared with those in the autologous oral mucosa graft group. Interestingly, nanoparticle-labeled BMDSCs were detected in the urethral epithelium and muscle layer, which colocalized with uroepithelial cytokeratin markers AE1 and AE3, suggesting differentiation of inter-BMDSCs into new urethral epithelium.

Interactions of BMDSCs with other cells may further promote tissue regeneration. A study evaluated the effect of a cell/scaffold composite graft consisting of human BMDSCs with CD34+ hematopoietic stem/progenitor cells on modulating inflammation and wound healing in a rodent model of substitution urethroplasty [53]. The urethra of cell-seeded animals showed 1.3- and 1.7-fold reductions in levels of the inflammatory cytokine TNF (tumor necrosis factor)-α and neutrophil migration, respectively, within 2 days after surgery compared with unseeded animals. This early difference in the inflammatory response between seeded and unseeded animals became more pronounced over time, eventually leading to 4.6- and 8.8-fold reductions in the levels of TNF-α and neutrophil migration, respectively, at 4 weeks. Histologically, changes in vascular profiles were evident, with initially small and numerous vessels developing into larger, more mature vessels during the healing process in the seeded group. Conversely, the control group showed no such progression. On the basis of AM, Chen et al. [54] seeded BMDSCs and endothelial progenitor cells (EPCs) to successfully repair long-segment circumferential urethral defects in a canine model. The presence of BMDSCs promoted EC survival, proliferation, and migration and contributed to EPC recruitment for angiogenesis.

Despite these positive results, BMDSC acquisition requires bone marrow aspiration, and this highly invasive method of acquisition limits their use.

3.3. Adipose-Derived Stem Cells

ADSCs that are widely distributed and abundant in the human body are readily available because >400,000 liposuction surgeries are performed annually for cosmetic or medical purposes, with up to 3 L of liposuction fluid discarded after each procedure [55]. Additionally, their proliferation efficiency and potential for multidirectional differentiation have been extensively studied. In an epithelial-specific microenvironment, ADSCs display a stratified epithelial-like morphology with increased expression of epithelial-specific proteins and eventually differentiate into uroepithelial-like cells [56–58]. Urethral reconstruction using post-epithelial induction ADSC composite BAM showed that post-induction ADSC composite BAM replantation formed epithelial-like structures at the replacement site in vivo and reduced scar contracture and stricture formation in the reconstructed urethral segment to some extent [59]. ADSCs can also differentiate towards smooth muscle in response to mechanical or specific microenvironmental stimuli [60,61]. Fu et al. [60] used mechanical stimulation to differentiate ADSCs towards smooth muscle cells and subsequently seeded the cells in a PGA (polyglycolic acid) scaffold that was applied with good results in a dog urethral repair model. The differentiated ADSCs constituted an engineered urethra that adapted to the mechanical extension generated by the urinary stream and helped to reduce the incidence of urethral strictures.

Prevention of fibrosis and reduction of scarring play a crucial role in urethral repair, and the anti-fibrotic effects of ADSCs have been widely explored in recent years. One study evaluated the anti-urethral fibrosis effect of ADSCs [62]. The urethral walls of rats were incised and injected with the fibrosis inducer transforming growth factor-β1. One day later, ADSCs were injected into the urethral walls of rats in the ADSCs group. After 4 weeks, the rats were evaluated histologically and functionally. Compared with the control group, the ADSCs-treated group showed a significant increase in single-void volume, urine flow rate, bladder compliance, and bladder volume with prolonged voiding intervals. Moreover, the overall structure of the spongious urethra, and the collagen and elastin contents of the penile shafts approximated the normal urethra. Because of the complex histopathological microenvironmental changes at the injury site, cell transplantation alone may not be sufficient. MiR-21 has been proven to assist stem cell differentiation and paracrine secretion. Recent studies have shown that miR-21 also plays a major role in skin fibrosis [63,64]. Feng et al. [65] explored whether miR-21 modification improved the efficacy of ADSCs against urethral fibrosis and thus limited the recurrence of urethral strictures. They established miR-21-modified ADSCs by lentivirus-mediated transfer of pre-miR-21 and GFP reporter genes. In vitro results showed that miR-21 modification increased angiogenic gene expression in ADSCs and enhanced their antioxidant effects against reactive oxygen species damage. In vivo results demonstrated that the miR-21 modification contributed to improved urodynamic parameters and better formation of epithelial and muscle layers compared with the group injected with ADSCs alone. This study validated the potential of miR-21 to improve the anti-urethral fibrosis of ADSCs, but further studies are needed to determine long-term efficacy. A recent study showed that human mesenchymal stem cells inhibit fibroblast activation and the associated inflammatory responses via miR-146a in exosomes, which may also contribute to the mechanism of ADSC-mediated inhibition of urethral fibrotic strictures [66]. Notably, however, because most human urethral fibrosis is in advanced and chronic stages, further evaluation of the effect of stem cell injection therapy on established and recurrent urethral fibroses is important to translate this therapy into the clinic.

ADSC composite scaffolds have also undergone significant improvements. In one study, autologous ADSCs from dogs were grown and seeded onto a premade acellular arterial matrix [67]. Seeded scaffolds were used to repair surgically produced urethral defects in six male dogs, and the results were compared with those of six control animals treated with the acellular arterial matrix. Serial urethrography was performed postoperatively at 1 and 3 months. All six animals in the experimental group had a wide urethral caliber without any signs of stricture. Conversely, three animals in the control group showed urethral strictures. Similar success was achieved in a rabbit urethroplasty model using an ADSC-seeded SF scaffold [68]. Compared with the application of SF alone, the composite group showed a milder inflammatory response and more vascular and smooth muscle tissue formation. Yang et al. [69] constructed a composite hydrogel patch accommodating ADSCs for rabbit urethral repair by multilayer 3D bioprinting. Compared with the unseeded ADSC control group, the seeded ADSC group showed reductions in bulk scarring and the urographic obstruction rate, and pathology showed that the introduction of ADSCs significantly reduced the collagen fiber content. Notably, evidence that the therapeutic advantage of ADSCs lies not only in their multipotency but also in their trophic and paracrine functions is growing [70]. Therefore, exploring methods to increase the paracrine activity of ADSCs may further promote tissue regeneration. Under hypoxic preconditioning, ADCSs have enhanced paracrine activity, proliferation, and survival [71,72]. Modulation of ADSC paracrine factors is also an effective method to enhance the pro-regenerative effect of ADSCs. As a protein that broadly affects the FGF signaling pathway, FGFR2 (Fibroblast growth factor receptors 2) is closely associated with the development and repair of the urinary tract. Therefore, targeted modification of ADSCs to overexpress FGFR2 may contribute to their secretory function and reparative effects. Zhu et al. [73] constructed a composite scaffold of ADSCs overexpressing FGFR2 (Figure 1a). The ADSC modification promoted the secretion of angiogenic factors and enhanced their proliferation and migration abilities, which promoted tissue angiogenesis and regeneration, resulting in excellent reparative effects in a rabbit urethral injury model. TIMP-1, which is highly expressed in urethral scar tissue, plays a crucial role in the urethra stricture [74–76]. Sa et al. [77] performed the first miRNA modification of epithelial differentiated adipose-derived stem cells (E-ADSCs) to reduce expression of the profibrotic factor TIMP-1 and evaluated their effectiveness for urethral repair. The modified E-ADSCs seeded in BAM inhibited fibrosis in urethral tissue, leading to a wider urethral caliber. In another study, hypoxia-treated ADSCs were seeded in porous nanofiber scaffolds and used to repair rabbit urethral defects (Figure 1b–d). The in vivo results showed that hypoxia-preconditioned ADSCs combined with scaffolds led to a larger urethral lumen diameter, preserved urethral morphology, and enhanced angiogenesis compared with normoxia-preconditioned ADSCs [78].

The extracellular matrix (ECM) of ADSCs retains its secreted biological factors, which facilitate tissue regeneration, and is a good alternative source of decellularized matrix [79]. In urethral repair and reconstruction, decellularized tissue matrices such as SIS and BAM have been used with some degree of success in preclinical and clinical studies. However, the limited amount of autologous tissue-derived ECM is prone to surgical complications at the donor site, and there is a risk of disease transmission and ethical issues [80,81]. Zhou et al. [82] fabricated an ADSC-ECM using a repeated freeze–thaw cycle, Triton X-100, and SDS decellularization. Oral mucosal epithelial cells had a higher survival rate on ADSC-ECM compared with SF and formed a continuous layer of epidermal cells. Compared with SIS, mononuclear macrophage infiltration was less in ADSC-ECM when implanted subcutaneously into rats. Additionally, mRNA expression of cytokines, such as IL-4 and IL-10, was significantly higher in ADSC-ECM than in SIS at 3 weeks post-implantation.

3.4. Urine-Derived Stem Cells

UDSCs are a subpopulation of stem cells isolated from human urine that differentiate into various cell types, including SMCs, epithelial cells, and endothelial cells [83–85]. UDSCs express smooth muscle-specific proteins, including α-smooth muscle action, desmin, and myosin when cultured under PDGF (platelet-derived growth factor)-BB and TGF (transforming growth factor)-β1 induction, and uroepithelial-specific proteins AE1, AE3, and E-cadherin when cultured under epidermal growth factor induction (Figure 1e,f) [86]. They share many biological properties with mesenchymal stem cells, such as potent paracrine effects and immunomodulatory capacity. However, compared with other stem cells, autologous UDSCs can be harvested by a simple, safe, low-cost, and non-invasive procedure [84,87]. Additionally, up to 75% of fresh UDSCs can be safely persevered in urine for 24 h and retain their original stem cell properties [88]. Interest in UDSCs has increased over the past decade because of their great potential for regenerative medicine applications.

In one study [89], human UDSCs were extracted, and five induction methods were used to optimize their differentiation towards the uroepithelium. Induced cells were assessed for expression of gene and protein markers of urothelial cells by RT-PCR, Western blotting, and immunofluorescence staining. The barrier function and ultrastructure of tight junctions were assessed by permeability assays and transmission electron microscopy. Phenotypic and functional characteristics similar to those of native urothelial cells were observed in induced UDSCs. Additionally, multilayered urothelial tissue had formed 2 weeks after the inoculation of induced UDSCs on the intestinal submucosal matrix. Liu et al. [87] obtained rabbit autologous UDSCs from urine and bladder washings and seeded them on SIS to repair urethral defects in a rabbit model. It was found that autologous UDSCs differentiated into urothelial cells and SMCs in the natural urethral environment and performed corresponding functions. Compared with the unseeded cell group, the urethral caliber, urethral regeneration rate, smooth muscle content, and vascular density were significantly improved in the autologous UDSC-seeded SIS group.

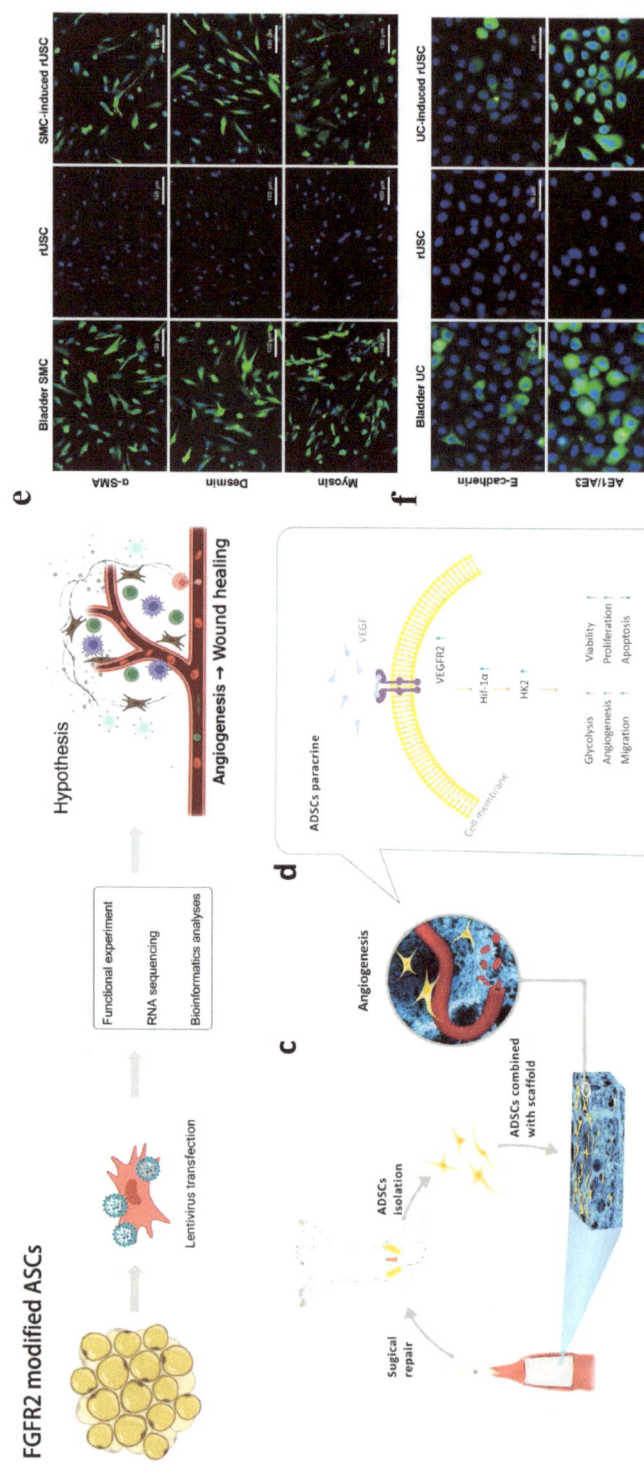

Figure 1. Methods to promote paracrine secretion in ADSCs and differentiation of UDSCs. (**a**) ADSCs overexpressing FGFR2. Reprinted (adapted) with permission from Ref. [73]. Copyright ©2022, Springer Nature. (**b**) ADSCs isolated from bilateral inguinal adipose tissues and then seeded on a scaffold to repair a urethral defect. (**c**) Hypoxia-preconditioned ADSCs grow in macropores and promote angiogenesis. (**d**) Mechanism of hypoxia-preconditioned ADSCs secreting more VEGFA to promote expression of VEGFR2, HIF-1α, and HK2 to upregulate glycolysis. Reprinted (adapted) with permission from Ref. [78]. Copyright ©2020, Springer Nature. (**e**) UDSCs expressing smooth muscle-specific markers desmin, myosin, and α-SMA assessed by immunofluorescence after culture in myogenic differentiation medium containing TGF-β (2.5 ng/mL) and PDGF (5 ng/mL) for 14 days. (**f**) UDSCs expressing urothelial-specific markers AE1 and AE3 assessed by immunofluorescence were significantly increased at 14 days after culture in uroepithelial differentiation medium with epidermal growth factor (30 ng/mL) compared with non-induced rUSCs. Reprinted (adapted) with permission from Ref. [86]. Copyright ©2018, Springer Nature.

UDSCs are innate to the urinary tract and thus have better histocompatibility and can survive in urine similarly to healthy urothelial cells. Therefore, UDSCs have great application potential and are a good source of tissue-engineered urothelial seed cells. However, the current literature concerning UDSC applications is limited, and further studies are needed.

3.5. Other Stem Cell Types

EPCs participate in vascular remodeling and angiogenesis by migrating to sites where blood vessels are needed [90]. Chen et al. [54] isolated EPCs from bone marrow, seeded them into AM, and successfully repaired a 3 cm long segmental circumferential urethral defect in a canine model. Complete vasculature development was observed in animals that received scaffolds seeded with EPCs, in contrast to those that received unseeded scaffolds or a sham operation [54]. In another preclinical study, more pronounced angiogenesis was observed in the EPC-seeded group compared with the control group [91].

Human amniotic fluid stem cells (HAFSCs) are multipotent stem cells of mesenchymal origin extracted from amniotic fluid [92]. HAFSCs can differentiate into various tissue types, such as skin, cartilage, and kidneys. Because stem cell extraction does not require the destruction of human embryos, the use of HAFSCs is less controversial. Kang et al. [93] demonstrated that microenvironmental changes induced by bladder-specific culture medium were sufficient to induce differentiation of HAFSCs into urothelial cells. Therefore, HAFSCs may be an effective alternative source of urothelial cells. However, further in vivo studies are needed to verify their effectiveness in urethral regeneration.

Recently, human amniotic mesenchymal stem cells (hAMSCs) derived from the amniotic membrane have attracted attention [94]. Similar to BMSCs and ADSCs, hAMSCs are multipotent, highly proliferative, and immunotolerant [95,96]. A major advantage of hAMSCs is that they are readily available, which eliminates the invasive procedures and ethical issues of cell harvesting [94]. Lv et al. [97] used hAMSC composite scaffolds to repair urethral defects in rabbits. The results showed a significantly lower incidence of urethral stricture, urinary fistula, and complications compared with the unseeded cell group. The seeded cell group formed a multilayered mucosa similar to normal urethral tissue after 12 weeks. Table 2 summarized the functions performed by stem cells in urethral regeneration.

Table 2. Summary of the functions performed by stem cells in urethral regeneration.

Cell Type	Source	Function in Urethral Regeneration	References
Pluripotent stem cells	Human embryos Reprogrammed cells from adult tissues	Differentiate to any cell type in the urethra.	[47–49]
BMDSCs	Bone marrow	Differentiate into urothelial cells and bladder SMCs; reduce fibrosis and inflammation; and interact with other cells to further promote tissue regeneration.	[50–54]
ADSCs	Adipose tissue	Differentiate into urothelial cells and SMCs; prevent fibrosis and reduce scarring; promote regeneration of vascular and smooth muscle tissues; and reduce the inflammatory response. Paracrine function promotes regeneration.	[56–73,77,78]
UDSCs	Urine	Differentiate into urothelial cells, SMCs, and endothelial cells; promote regeneration of vascular and smooth muscle tissues; secrete various growth factors; and promote vascularization.	[83–89]
EPCs	Venous blood and bone marrow	Involved in vascular remodeling and angiogenesis.	[54,90,91]
hAFSCs	Amniotic fluid	Differentiate into urothelial cells.	[92,93]
AMSCs	Amniotic membrane	Promotes regeneration of the urethral epithelium.	[97]

4. Cell Sheet Technology

The cell sheet technique may be a promising novel approach in the field of urethral regeneration. A cell sheet retains the extracellular matrix with active factors, which facilitates local cell proliferation and regeneration [98]. It does not require enzymatic digestion and has a higher cell viability rate. A study compared the effectiveness of the cell sheet technique with the cellular perfusion technique for recellularization of the urethral decellularized stroma and found that the cell sheet technique achieved more effective recellularization as assessed by histopathology [99]. Alternatively, a cell sheet retains tight junctions between cells, and its dense structure restores the smooth and watertight properties of the urethral mucosa, ensuring unobstructed urination and preventing urine leakage, mimicking the native urethral epithelium. Liang et al. [100] successfully repaired rabbit urethral mucosal defects using autologous ADSC sheets (Figure 2a). The cell sheets were labeled with indocyanine green, and second near-infrared fluorescence imaging was performed to track ADSC sheets in vivo. Histological analysis showed that, in the ADSC sheet group, continuous epithelial cells covered the urethra at the graft site, and a large number of vascular endothelial cells were seen. In the cell sheet-free group, there was no continuous epithelial cell coverage at the urethral repair site, and expression of the proinflammatory factor TNF-α was increased. Similar success was achieved with transplanted skin epithelial cell membranes in a rabbit urethral injury model [29]. Cell sheets are more manipulable and can be arranged and compounded in accordance with the tissue anatomy and cellular composition to form a biomimetic material scaffold with a 3D structure. Mikami et al. [101] collected oral tissues by biopsy, isolated mucosal and muscle cells, and cultured epithelial and muscle cell sheets, respectively. After 2 weeks, the two cell sheets were ligated and tubularized to construct two layers of tissue-engineered urethra and transplanted into urethral defects in dogs (Figure 2b). Histological analysis at 12 weeks after grafting demonstrated that urethras in the cell sheets group had formed stratified epithelia, and a well-vascularized submucosa was observed under the epithelial layers with cells. The urethrogram at 12 weeks revealed maintenance of a wide urethral caliber without stricture, leakage, or dilatation in the cell sheet group. The urethral histological structure consists of mucosa, submucosa, and muscles from the inside to the outside. Guided by the histological features of the urethra, Zhou et al. [102] chose various seed cells (oral mucosal epithelial cells, oral mucosal fibroblasts, and ADSCs) to construct the corresponding cell sheets and labeled the cells with ultrasmall superparamagnetic iron oxide at optimized concentrations (Figure 2b). Biomimetic urethral subcutaneous grafts significantly increased the urethral vascular density after 3 weeks and were subsequently used to repair urethral defects in dogs. After 3 months of urethral replacement, the biomimetic urethra maintained a three-layer structure and functions in a manner similar to the natural urethra. In another study, ADSC sheet self-assembled scaffolds supported the adhesion and growth of urothelial cells and SMCs. Seeding with both cell types is expected to lead to the development of a fully functional human urethra [103]. Notably, however, cell sheets tend to have long culture cycles and poor mechanical properties. To overcome these limitations, Zhang et al. [30] explored the possibility of using cryopreserved epithelial cell sheets combined with AM for rabbit urethral repair. The addition of AM enhanced the mechanical properties of epithelial cell sheets and reduced cell damage caused by cryopreservation. Histological examinations after 1 month showed that the urethral epithelium had completely regenerated with slight collagen deposition and adequate vascular regeneration under the mucosal layer.

The advantage of cell sheet technology is that it removes the influence of scaffold material degradation [98]. Notably, however, the current cost required to produce patient-derived cell sheets limits their widespread use.

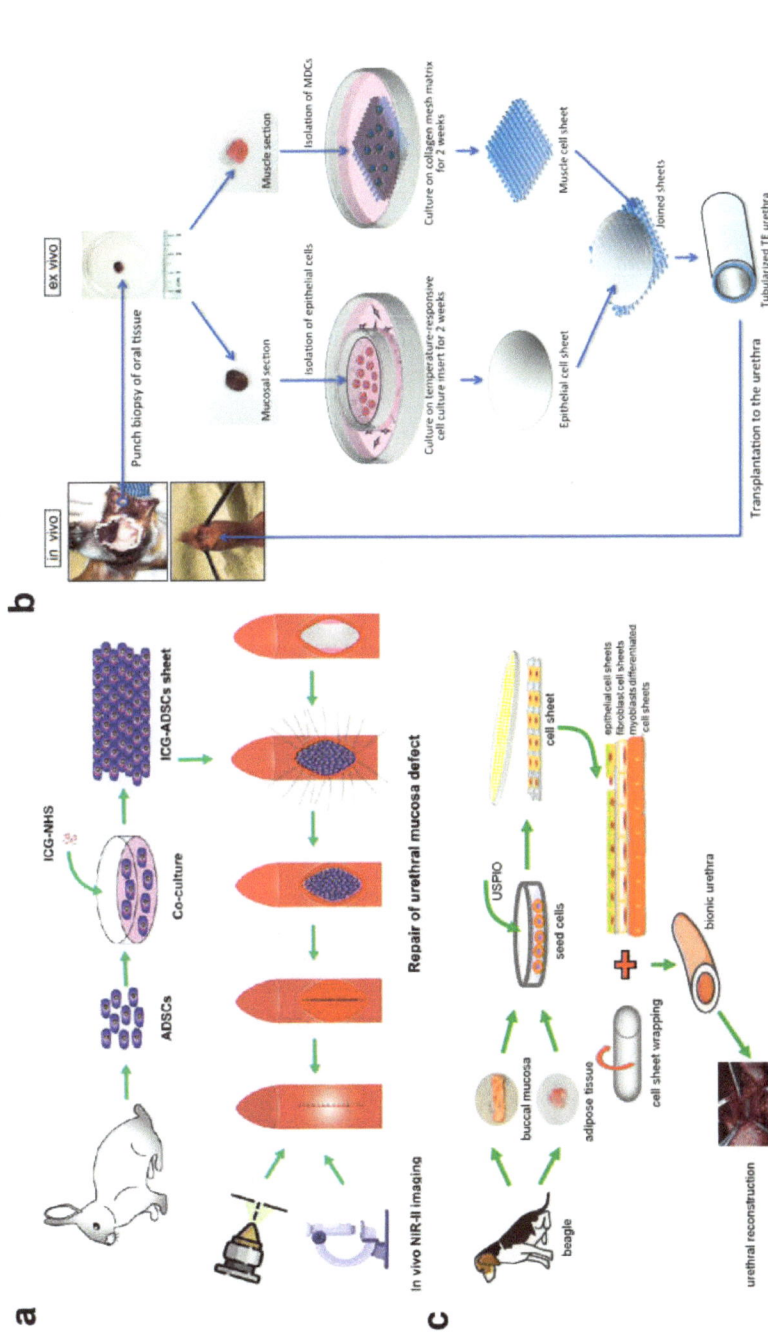

Figure 2. Cell sheet technology. (**a**) Repairing rabbit urethral mucosal defects using autologous ADSC sheets. ADSC sheets were labeled with indocyanine green (ICG), and second near-infrared (NIR-II) fluorescence imaging was performed to track ADSC sheets. Reprinted (adapted) with permission from Ref. [100]. Copyright © 2022, American Chemical Society. (**b**) Epithelial and muscle cell sheets were ligated and tubularized to construct two layers of tissue-engineered urethra and transplanted into urethral defects in dogs. Reprinted (adapted) with permission from Ref. [101]. Copyright © 2023 American Urological Association Education and Research, Inc. (**c**) Three types of cell sheets (oral mucosal epithelial cells, oral mucosal fibroblasts, and ADSCs) were cultured to construct a biomimetic urethra. Reproduced under terms of the CC-BY license [102]. Copyright © 2023 Ivyspring International Publisher.

5. Clinical Studies

Urethroplasty is the standard treatment for long-segment urethral strictures [104], which has a high success rate and long-term durability, but it is highly invasive, technically demanding, and has a steep learning curve [105,106]. Patients undergo endoscopic treatment several times before urethroplasty. Therefore, researchers have tried to improve endoscopic treatment to further improve the results of urethrotomy or dilation. Although treatments by injection of various drugs have been proposed, no benefit has been shown in clinical trials [107]. However, cell-based therapies offer promising directions that have shown initial success. Vaddi et al. [108] reported BEES-HAUS (buccal epithelium expanded and encapsulated in a scaffold-hybrid approach to urethral stricture). Autologous cultured buccal epithelial cells that are expanded and encapsulated in TGP scaffolds are implanted at the stricture site after a wide endoscopic urethrotomy to form an epithelial layer. The procedure was successful in four of six patients, yielding more than a 3-year recurrence-free interval. The subsequent use of this method in a rabbit model confirmed the success of buccal mucosal epithelial cell transplantation [109,110]. Recently, Scott et al. [107] proposed a novel method of urethral stricture treatment using liquid buccal mucosal grafts to augment direct vision internal urethrotomy. The results showed a 67% transplantation rate in the treatment group, but its treatment success rate was not statistically significant compared with the control group. In another prospective human study, encouraging results were obtained by buccal mucosal epithelial cell transplantation. Kulkarni et al. [111] evaluated the safety and efficacy of AALBECs (autologous adult living cultured buccal epithelial cells) in the treatment of male bulbar urethral strictures. Approximately 1×1.5 cm of oral mucosal tissue was collected from the inner cheek under local anesthesia, from which the epithelial layer was isolated and cultured, expanded in vitro, tested, and prepared as a suspension of 2.5 million cells/0.4 mL DMEM (Dulbecco's modified Eagle's medium) per vial, which was then injected into the stricture site after cystoscopic dissection of the stricture. After AALBEC treatment, patients showed a decrease in voiding time and urinary flow time ($p < 0.05$) and a 90.5% reduction in the mean AUA (American Urological Association) symptom index, and no patient required surgery within 24 weeks after treatment. These results demonstrate that buccal epithelial cell transplantation may be an effective alternative to urethrotomy and dilatation and may be a novel treatment option for urethral reconstruction. However, the results need to be further substantiated in large, well-designed studies.

Buccal mucosa is one of the most widely used grafts to repair urethral strictures. However, it is limited in number and prone to donor site complications [112,113]. The development of tissue-engineered buccal mucosa (TEBM) may overcome the limitations of autologous oral mucosa grafts. In 2008, Bhargava et al. [114] first reported the results of TEBM in a clinical trial. Keratinocytes and fibroblasts were isolated and cultured, seeded on a sterilized donor's de-epidermized dermis, and maintained at the air–liquid interface for 7–10 days to obtain TEBM grafts. Five patients with urethral strictures secondary to lichen sclerosus underwent TEBM urethroplasty. At a mean follow-up of 33.6 months, three of the five patients had a patent urethra, while the other two developed fibrosis and constriction. This study demonstrated the potential of TEBM for the treatment of urethral strictures. MukoCell is a commercial tissue-engineered graft containing autologous oral epithelial cells on a collagen matrix [115]. Ram-Liebig et al. [27] reported the results of a multicenter, prospective, observational trial using an industrial tissue-engineered oral mucosa graft with market authorization in Germany (MukoCell) in 99 men. Using conservative Kaplan–Meier assessment, no stricture recurrence was observed in 67.3% (95% CI 57.6–77.0) of men at 12 months after the operation or in 58.2% (95% CI 47.7–68.7) of men at 24 months. These results were broadly similar to buccal mucosal urethroplasty [113]. In another retrospective multicenter study, 38 patients with recurrent strictures (median stricture length of 5 cm) underwent MukoCell urethroplasty with a median follow-up of 55 months, resulting in 32 (84.2%) successful treatments. No local or systemic adverse effects due to the engineered material were observed [116]. TEBM offers a safe and effective treatment opportunity for patients with urethral strictures, but it needs to be validated in long-term clinical trials with large samples. At present, regulatory, legal, and financial issues are major factors that restrict and impede the widespread use of these technologies in many countries [117].

6. Future Perspectives

In the past decades, urethral tissue engineering has made great strides, and the development of biomaterials has been gradually integrated into urological practice. However, the use of biomaterials alone has many shortcomings in practical use, especially for long segments of urethral strictures. Using various types of seed cells in combination with biomaterials to construct a tissue-engineered urethra provides a new treatment method to repair long-segment urethral strictures.

Differentiated cells were first explored for application in the field of urethral regeneration, and many researchers have attempted to apply them in clinical studies. One of the most popular is epithelial cells because the continuous epithelial layer plays an important role in resisting urine, effectively avoiding wound erosion and urethral fistula. Clinical studies have shown that buccal mucosal epithelial cell injection alone effectively prevents urethral fibrosis, and TEBM constructed with buccal mucosal epithelial cells has also produced good results. In addition to epithelial cells, SMCs and endothelial cells also play an important role in urethral wound healing, but these two cell types are more difficult to be obtained and have low cell proliferation potential. Thus, they are unsuitable for clinical research and practice until these issues are resolved.

Stem cells have been a hot research topic in recent years and, in many respects, have advantages over differentiated cells. Stem cells expand in vitro and are highly plastic, differentiating into specific cell types in urethral tissue in a specific microenvironment. In addition to secreting paracrine growth factors to enhance angiogenesis and reduce fibrosis, stem cells promote tissue regeneration by secreting active factors to recruit endogenous cells [118,119]. More importantly, they possess immune escape properties while allowing the use of allogeneic sources [120], which eliminates the need for autologous cell harvesting and expansion, thereby reducing the overall cost and duration of treatment [121]. Among them, pluripotent stem cells have received great attention in the field of regenerative medicine, but moral and ethical issues have limited their application. Most current studies have favored MSCs, especially ADSCs, which are a good cell source for urethral regeneration because of their abundance, easy access, and high proliferation efficiency, and promising results have been obtained in many studies. UDSCs of urinary tract origin are also very attractive. Unlike other stem cells, UDSCs can be obtained non-invasively (i.e., from urine). One study [122] has compared the stem cell properties and differentiated abilities of UDSCs and ADSCs collected from the same patient. Population-doubling time colony formation assays showed that UDSCs possessed a greater growth capacity. Additionally, analysis of multipotent differentiation (myogenic, neurogenic, and endothelial cells) showed that UDSCs were better than ADSCs. However, the current conditions for stem cell differentiation are stringent and need to be further optimized to achieve more stable and mature differentiation. Moreover, because stem cells are affected by the microenvironment, the effects of microenvironmental stimuli, such as mechanical forces, pH, signaling molecules, and oxygen levels, in the urethra on stem cells should be fully studied and considered before proceeding to human trials.

In tissue engineering, the biological microenvironment affects cell survival, colonization, and differentiation. Therefore, cell culture conditions, delivery methods, and biomaterial types and structures are also very important factors that need to be further explored. A reasonable combination of these factors may facilitate the full utilization of cells to construct a structurally and functionally complete biomimetic urethra more precisely and further improve the urethral reparative effect. An important direction in the field of urethral regeneration in the future may be cell sheet technology. Cell sheet technology achieves more effective recellularization of biological materials or damaged tissues. It also preserves the tight connections between cells and is more conducive to constructing a biomimetic urethra. Notably, however, the fabrication time and cost of cell sheets are obstacles that need to be overcome.

7. Conclusions

Cell-based therapies are promising in the field of urethral regeneration. To date, several cell types have been explored and applied in the field of urethral regeneration, but there is no optimal strategy for the source, selection, and application conditions of the cells. In this review, we summarized the various cell types applied to urethral regeneration and discussed their characteristics and conditions of application. We suggest that stem cells are a promising option for the future and that ADSCs and urinary tract-derived UDSCs may be the best cell sources for cell-based therapies. However, the differentiation conditions of stem cells need to be further optimized. The key to successful urethral regeneration lies in the construction of well-organized and functional biomimetic urethral grafts, which cannot be achieved without a rational combination of cell and tissue engineering technologies, including scaffolds and cell delivery techniques.

Author Contributions: Conceptualization, Q.F. and Y.W.; Original draft preparation, Y.J., W.Z. and Y.W.; Review and editing, M.Y., W.F., G.G. and Y.J.; supervision, Q.F., Y.W. and G.G.; funding acquisition, Q.F. and Y.W. All authors have read and agreed to the published version of the manuscript.

Funding: This research was founded by the National Natural Science Foundation of China (Nos. 82100714 and 82170694), the Shanghai Outstanding Academic Leaders Plan (No. 17XD1403100), the Natural Science Foundation of Shanghai (No. 20ZR1442100), the Interdisciplinary Program of Shanghai Jiao Tong University (Nos. YG2021QN102 and YG2022ZD020), the Shanghai "Science and Technology Innovation Action Plan" Medical Innovation Research Project (No. 22Y11905000), and the Program of Shanghai Sixth People's Hospital (No. ynts202004).

Institutional Review Board Statement: Not applicable.

Informed Consent Statement: Not applicable.

Data Availability Statement: As no new data were created in this article, data sharing is not applicable to this article.

Conflicts of Interest: The authors declare no conflict of interest.

References

1. Mundy, A.R.; Andrich, D.E. Urethral strictures. *BJU Int.* **2011**, *107*, 6–26. [CrossRef] [PubMed]
2. Simsek, A.; Bullock, A.J.; Roman, S.; Chapple, C.R.; Macneil, S. Developing improved tissue-engineered buccal mucosa grafts for urethral reconstruction. *Can. Urol. Assoc. J.* **2018**, *12*, E234–E242. [CrossRef] [PubMed]
3. Santucci, R.A.; Joyce, G.F.; Wise, M. Male Urethral Stricture Disease. *J. Urol.* **2007**, *177*, 1667–1674. [CrossRef] [PubMed]
4. Davis, N.F.; Quinlan, M.R.; Bhatt, N.R.; Browne, C.; MacCraith, E.; Manecksha, R.; Walsh, M.T.; Thornhill, J.A.; Mulvin, D. Incidence, Cost, Complications and Clinical Outcomes of Iatrogenic Urethral Catheterization Injuries: A Prospective Multi-Institutional Study. *J. Urol.* **2016**, *196*, 1473–1477. [CrossRef] [PubMed]
5. Marshall, S.D.; Raup, V.T.; Brandes, S.B. Dorsal inlay buccal mucosal graft (Asopa) urethroplasty for anterior urethral stricture. *Transl. Androl. Urol.* **2015**, *4*, 10–15. [CrossRef] [PubMed]
6. Atala, A.; Danilevskiy, M.; Lyundup, A.; Glybochko, P.; Butnaru, D.; Vinarov, A.; Yoo, J.J. The potential role of tissue-engineered urethral substitution: Clinical and preclinical studies. *J. Tissue Eng. Regen. Med.* **2017**, *11*, 3–19. [CrossRef] [PubMed]
7. Lumen, N.; Vierstraete-Verlinde, S.; Oosterlinck, W.; Hoebeke, P.; Palminteri, E.; Goes, C.; Maes, H.; Spinoit, A.F. Buccal Versus Lingual Mucosa Graft in Anterior Urethroplasty: A Prospective Comparison of Surgical Outcome and Donor Site Morbidity. *J. Urol.* **2016**, *195*, 112–117. [CrossRef] [PubMed]
8. Atala, A. Engineering organs. *Curr. Opin. Biotechnol.* **2009**, *20*, 575–592. [CrossRef]
9. Liu, Y.; Bharadwaj, S.; Lee, S.J.; Atala, A.; Zhang, Y. Optimization of a natural collagen scaffold to aid cell-matrix penetration for urologic tissue engineering. *Biomaterials* **2009**, *30*, 3865–3873. [CrossRef]
10. Dorin, R.P.; Pohl, H.G.; De Filippo, R.E.; Yoo, J.J.; Atala, A. Tubularized urethral replacement with unseeded matrices: What is the maximum distance for normal tissue regeneration? *World J. Urol.* **2008**, *26*, 323–326. [CrossRef]
11. Farzamfar, S.; Elia, E.; Chabaud, S.; Naji, M.; Bolduc, S. Prospects and Challenges of Electrospun Cell and Drug Delivery Vehicles to Correct Urethral Stricture. *Int. J. Mol. Sci.* **2022**, *23*, 10519. [CrossRef] [PubMed]
12. Xue, J.D.; Gao, J.; Fu, Q.; Feng, C.; Xie, H. Seeding cell approach for tissue-engineered urethral reconstruction in animal study: A systematic review and meta-analysis. *Exp. Biol. Med.* **2016**, *241*, 1416–1428. [CrossRef] [PubMed]

13. Fu, Q.; Cao, Y.L. Tissue engineering and stem cell application of urethroplasty: From bench to bedside. *Urology* **2012**, *79*, 246–253. [CrossRef] [PubMed]
14. Orabi, H.; AbouShwareb, T.; Zhang, Y.; Yoo, J.J.; Atala, A. Cell-seeded tubularized scaffolds for reconstruction of long urethral defects: A preclinical study. *Eur. Urol.* **2013**, *63*, 531–538. [CrossRef]
15. Chan, Y.Y.; Bury, M.I.; Yura, E.M.; Hofer, M.D.; Cheng, E.Y.; Sharma, A.K. The current state of tissue engineering in the management of hypospadias. *Nat. Rev. Urol.* **2020**, *17*, 162–175. [CrossRef] [PubMed]
16. Sievert, K.D.; Daum, L.; Maurer, S.; Toomey, P.; Vaegler, M.; Aufderklamm, S.; Amend, B. Urethroplasty performed with an autologous urothelium-vegetated collagen fleece to treat urethral stricture in the minipig model. *World J. Urol.* **2020**, *38*, 2123–2131. [CrossRef] [PubMed]
17. De Graaf, P.; van der Linde, E.M.; Rosier, P.; Izeta, A.; Sievert, K.D.; Bosch, J.; de Kort, L.M.O. Systematic Review to Compare Urothelium Differentiation with Urethral Epithelium Differentiation in Fetal Development, as a Basis for Tissue Engineering of the Male Urethra. *Tissue Eng. Part. B Rev.* **2017**, *23*, 257–267. [CrossRef] [PubMed]
18. Liu, G.; Fu, M.; Li, F.; Fu, W.; Zhao, Z.; Xia, H.; Niu, Y. Tissue-engineered PLLA/gelatine nanofibrous scaffold promoting the phenotypic expression of epithelial and smooth muscle cells for urethral reconstruction. *Mater. Sci. Eng. C Mater. Biol. Appl.* **2020**, *111*, 110810. [CrossRef]
19. Wang, F.; Liu, T.; Yang, L.; Zhang, G.; Liu, H.; Yi, X.; Yang, X.; Lin, T.Y.; Qin, W.; Yuan, J. Urethral reconstruction with tissue-engineered human amniotic scaffold in rabbit urethral injury models. *Med. Sci. Monit.* **2014**, *20*, 2430–2438. [CrossRef]
20. Fossum, M.; Gustafson, C.J.; Nordenskjöld, A.; Kratz, G. Isolation and in vitro cultivation of human urothelial cells from bladder washings of adult patients and children. *Scand. J. Plast. Reconstr. Surg. Hand Surg.* **2003**, *37*, 41–45. [CrossRef]
21. Amesty, M.V.; Chamorro, C.I.; López-Pereira, P.; Martínez-Urrutia, M.J.; Sanz, B.; Rivas, S.; Lobato, R.; Fossum, M. Creation of Tissue-Engineered Urethras for Large Urethral Defect Repair in a Rabbit Experimental Model. *Front. Pediatr.* **2021**, *9*, 691131. [CrossRef] [PubMed]
22. Xuan, Z.; Zachar, V.; Pennisi, C.P. Sources, Selection, and Microenvironmental Preconditioning of Cells for Urethral Tissue Engineering. *Int. J. Mol. Sci.* **2022**, *23*, 14074. [CrossRef] [PubMed]
23. Kimball, J.R.; Nittayananta, W.; Klausner, M.; Chung, W.O.; Dale, B.A. Antimicrobial barrier of an in vitro oral epithelial model. *Arch. Oral. Biol.* **2006**, *51*, 775–783. [CrossRef] [PubMed]
24. Corradini, F.; Zattoni, M.; Barbagli, G.; Bianchi, G.; Giovanardi, M.; Serafini, C.; Genna, V.G.; Ribbene, A.; Balò, S.; Fidanza, F.; et al. Comparative Assessment of Cultures from Oral and Urethral Stem Cells for Urethral Regeneration. *Curr. Stem Cell Res. Ther.* **2016**, *11*, 643–651. [CrossRef] [PubMed]
25. Huang, J.W.; Lv, X.G.; Li, Z.; Song, L.J.; Feng, C.; Xie, M.K.; Li, C.; Li, H.B.; Wang, J.H.; Zhu, W.D.; et al. Urethral reconstruction with a 3D porous bacterial cellulose scaffold seeded with lingual keratinocytes in a rabbit model. *Biomed. Mater.* **2015**, *10*, 055005. [CrossRef] [PubMed]
26. Lv, X.; Feng, C.; Liu, Y.; Peng, X.; Chen, S.; Xiao, D.; Wang, H.; Li, Z.; Xu, Y.; Lu, M. A smart bilayered scaffold supporting keratinocytes and muscle cells in micro/nano-scale for urethral reconstruction. *Theranostics* **2018**, *8*, 3153–3163. [CrossRef] [PubMed]
27. Ram-Liebig, G.; Barbagli, G.; Heidenreich, A.; Fahlenkamp, D.; Romano, G.; Rebmann, U.; Standhaft, D.; van Ahlen, H.; Schakaki, S.; Balsmeyer, U.; et al. Results of Use of Tissue-Engineered Autologous Oral Mucosa Graft for Urethral Reconstruction: A Multicenter, Prospective, Observational Trial. *EBioMedicine* **2017**, *23*, 185–192. [CrossRef] [PubMed]
28. Fu, Q.; Deng, C.L.; Liu, W.; Cao, Y.L. Urethral replacement using epidermal cell-seeded tubular acellular bladder collagen matrix. *BJU Int.* **2007**, *99*, 1162–1165. [CrossRef]
29. Rogovaya, O.S.; Fayzulin, A.K.; Vasiliev, A.V.; Kononov, A.V.; Terskikh, V.V. Reconstruction of rabbit urethral epithelium with skin keratinocytes. *Acta Nat.* **2015**, *7*, 70–77. [CrossRef]
30. Zhang, D.; Hou, J.; Gu, Y.; Shao, J.; Zhou, S.; Zhuang, J.; Song, L.; Wang, X. Cryopreserved skin epithelial cell sheet combined with acellular amniotic membrane as an off-the-shelf scaffold for urethral regeneration. *Mater. Sci. Eng. C Mater. Biol. Appl.* **2021**, *122*, 111926. [CrossRef]
31. Dauleh, S.; Santeramo, I.; Fielding, C.; Ward, K.; Herrmann, A.; Murray, P.; Wilm, B. Characterisation of Cultured Mesothelial Cells Derived from the Murine Adult Omentum. *PLoS ONE* **2016**, *11*, e0158997. [CrossRef] [PubMed]
32. Nanni, L.; Vallasciani, S.; Fadda, G.; Perrelli, L. Free peritoneal grafts for patch urethroplasty in male rabbits. *J. Urol.* **2001**, *165*, 578–580. [CrossRef] [PubMed]
33. Kajbafzadeh, A.M.; Arshadi, H.; Payabvash, S.; Salmasi, A.H.; Najjaran-Tousi, V.; Sahebpor, A.R. Proximal hypospadias with severe chordee: Single stage repair using corporeal tunica vaginalis free graft. *J. Urol.* **2007**, *178*, 1036–1042, discussion 1042. [CrossRef] [PubMed]
34. Jiang, S.; Xu, Z.; Zhao, Y.; Yan, L.; Zhou, Z.; Gu, G. Urethral Reconstruction Using Mesothelial Cell-Seeded Autogenous Granulation Tissue Tube: An Experimental Study in Male Rabbits. *Biomed. Res. Int.* **2017**, *2017*, 1850256. [CrossRef]
35. Wang, C.; Chen, C.; Guo, M.; Li, B.; Han, F.; Chen, W. Stretchable collagen-coated polyurethane-urea hydrogel seeded with bladder smooth muscle cells for urethral defect repair in a rabbit model. *J. Mater. Sci. Mater. Med.* **2019**, *30*, 135. [CrossRef] [PubMed]

36. Lv, X.; Yang, J.; Feng, C.; Li, Z.; Chen, S.; Xie, M.; Huang, J.; Li, H.; Wang, H.; Xu, Y. Bacterial Cellulose-Based Biomimetic Nanofibrous Scaffold with Muscle Cells for Hollow Organ Tissue Engineering. *ACS Biomater. Sci. Eng.* **2016**, *2*, 19–29. [CrossRef] [PubMed]
37. Niu, Y.; Liu, G.; Fu, M.; Chen, C.; Fu, W.; Zhang, Z.; Xia, H.; Stadler, F.J. Designing a multifaceted bio-interface nanofiber tissue-engineered tubular scaffold graft to promote neo-vascularization for urethral regeneration. *J. Mater. Chem. B* **2020**, *8*, 1748–1758. [CrossRef]
38. Niu, Y.; Liu, G.; Chen, C.; Fu, M.; Fu, W.; Zhao, Z.; Xia, H.; Stadler, F.J. Urethral reconstruction using an amphiphilic tissue-engineered autologous polyurethane nanofiber scaffold with rapid vascularization function. *Biomater. Sci.* **2020**, *8*, 2164–2174. [CrossRef]
39. Bouhout, S.; Chabaud, S.; Bolduc, S. Organ-specific matrix self-assembled by mesenchymal cells improves the normal urothelial differentiation in vitro. *World J. Urol.* **2016**, *34*, 121–130. [CrossRef]
40. De Filippo, R.E.; Kornitzer, B.S.; Yoo, J.J.; Atala, A. Penile urethra replacement with autologous cell-seeded tubularized collagen matrices. *J. Tissue Eng. Regen. Med.* **2015**, *9*, 257–264. [CrossRef]
41. Heller, M.; Frerick-Ochs, E.V.; Bauer, H.K.; Schiegnitz, E.; Flesch, D.; Brieger, J.; Stein, R.; Al-Nawas, B.; Brochhausen, C.; Thüroff, J.W.; et al. Tissue engineered pre-vascularized buccal mucosa equivalents utilizing a primary triculture of epithelial cells, endothelial cells and fibroblasts. *Biomaterials* **2016**, *77*, 207–215. [CrossRef] [PubMed]
42. Sharma, A.K.; Cheng, E.Y. Growth factor and small molecule influence on urological tissue regeneration utilizing cell seeded scaffolds. *Adv. Drug Deliv. Rev.* **2015**, *82–83*, 86–92. [CrossRef] [PubMed]
43. Caplan, A.I.; Correa, D. The MSC: An injury drugstore. *Cell Stem Cell* **2011**, *9*, 11–15. [CrossRef] [PubMed]
44. Beegle, J.; Lakatos, K.; Kalomoiris, S.; Stewart, H.; Isseroff, R.R.; Nolta, J.A.; Fierro, F.A. Hypoxic preconditioning of mesenchymal stromal cells induces metabolic changes, enhances survival, and promotes cell retention in vivo. *Stem Cells* **2015**, *33*, 1818–1828. [CrossRef]
45. Clément, F.; Grockowiak, E.; Zylbersztejn, F.; Fossard, G.; Gobert, S.; Maguer-Satta, V. Stem cell manipulation, gene therapy and the risk of cancer stem cell emergence. *Stem Cell Investig.* **2017**, *4*, 67. [CrossRef] [PubMed]
46. Pederzoli, F.; Joice, G.; Salonia, A.; Bivalacqua, T.J.; Sopko, N.A. Regenerative and engineered options for urethroplasty. *Nat. Rev. Urol.* **2019**, *16*, 453–464. [CrossRef]
47. Blank, R.S.; Swartz, E.A.; Thompson, M.M.; Olson, E.N.; Owens, G.K. A retinoic acid-induced clonal cell line derived from multipotential P19 embryonal carcinoma cells expresses smooth muscle characteristics. *Circ. Res.* **1995**, *76*, 742–749. [CrossRef] [PubMed]
48. Oottamasathien, S.; Wang, Y.; Williams, K.; Franco, O.E.; Wills, M.L.; Thomas, J.C.; Saba, K.; Sharif-Afshar, A.R.; Makari, J.H.; Bhowmick, N.A.; et al. Directed differentiation of embryonic stem cells into bladder tissue. *Dev. Biol.* **2007**, *304*, 556–566. [CrossRef]
49. Suzuki, K.; Koyanagi-Aoi, M.; Uehara, K.; Hinata, N.; Fujisawa, M.; Aoi, T. Directed differentiation of human induced pluripotent stem cells into mature stratified bladder urothelium. *Sci. Rep.* **2019**, *9*, 10506. [CrossRef]
50. Demirel, B.D.; Bıçakcı, Ü.; Rızalar, R.; Alpaslan Pınarlı, F.; Aydın, O. Histopathological effects of mesenchymal stem cells in rats with bladder and posterior urethral injuries. *Turk. J. Med. Sci.* **2017**, *47*, 1912–1919. [CrossRef]
51. Zhang, Y.; Lin, H.K.; Frimberger, D.; Epstein, R.B.; Kropp, B.P. Growth of bone marrow stromal cells on small intestinal submucosa: An alternative cell source for tissue engineered bladder. *BJU Int.* **2005**, *96*, 1120–1125. [CrossRef] [PubMed]
52. Yudintceva, N.M.; Nashchekina, Y.A.; Mikhailova, N.A.; Vinogradova, T.I.; Yablonsky, P.K.; Gorelova, A.A.; Muraviov, A.N.; Gorelov, A.V.; Samusenko, I.A.; Nikolaev, B.P.; et al. Urethroplasty with a bilayered poly-D,L-lactide-co-ε-caprolactone scaffold seeded with allogenic mesenchymal stem cells. *J. Biomed. Mater. Res. B Appl. Biomater.* **2020**, *108*, 1010–1021. [CrossRef] [PubMed]
53. Liu, J.S.; Bury, M.I.; Fuller, N.J.; Sturm, R.M.; Ahmad, N.; Sharma, A.K. Bone Marrow Stem/Progenitor Cells Attenuate the Inflammatory Milieu Following Substitution Urethroplasty. *Sci. Rep.* **2016**, *6*, 35638. [CrossRef] [PubMed]
54. Chen, C.; Zheng, S.; Zhang, X.; Dai, P.; Gao, Y.; Nan, L.; Zhang, Y. Transplantation of Amniotic Scaffold-Seeded Mesenchymal Stem Cells and/or Endothelial Progenitor Cells From Bone Marrow to Efficiently Repair 3-cm Circumferential Urethral Defect in Model Dogs. *Tissue Eng. Part A* **2018**, *24*, 47–56. [CrossRef] [PubMed]
55. Katz, A.J.; Llull, R.; Hedrick, M.H.; Futrell, J.W. Emerging approaches to the tissue engineering of fat. *Clin. Plast. Surg.* **1999**, *26*, 587–603. [CrossRef] [PubMed]
56. Li, H.; Xu, Y.; Fu, Q.; Li, C. Effects of multiple agents on epithelial differentiation of rabbit adipose-derived stem cells in 3D culture. *Tissue Eng. Part A* **2012**, *18*, 1760–1770. [CrossRef] [PubMed]
57. Zhang, M.; Xu, M.X.; Zhou, Z.; Zhang, K.; Zhou, J.; Zhao, Y.; Wang, Z.; Lu, M.J. The differentiation of human adipose-derived stem cells towards a urothelium-like phenotype in vitro and the dynamic temporal changes of related cytokines by both paracrine and autocrine signal regulation. *PLoS ONE* **2014**, *9*, e95583. [CrossRef]
58. Zhang, M.; Peng, Y.; Zhou, Z.; Zhou, J.; Wang, Z.; Lu, M. Differentiation of human adipose-derived stem cells co-cultured with urothelium cell line toward a urothelium-like phenotype in a nude murine model. *Urology* **2013**, *81*, 465.e15–465.e22. [CrossRef]
59. Li, H.; Xu, Y.; Xie, H.; Li, C.; Song, L.; Feng, C.; Zhang, Q.; Xie, M.; Wang, Y.; Lv, X. Epithelial-differentiated adipose-derived stem cells seeded bladder acellular matrix grafts for urethral reconstruction: An animal model. *Tissue Eng. Part A* **2014**, *20*, 774–784. [CrossRef]

60. Fu, Q.; Deng, C.L.; Zhao, R.Y.; Wang, Y.; Cao, Y. The effect of mechanical extension stimulation combined with epithelial cell sorting on outcomes of implanted tissue-engineered muscular urethras. *Biomaterials* **2014**, *35*, 105–112. [CrossRef]
61. Zhang, R.; Jack, G.S.; Rao, N.; Zuk, P.; Ignarro, L.J.; Wu, B.; Rodríguez, L.V. Nuclear fusion-independent smooth muscle differentiation of human adipose-derived stem cells induced by a smooth muscle environment. *Stem Cells* **2012**, *30*, 481–490. [CrossRef]
62. Castiglione, F.; Dewulf, K.; Hakim, L.; Weyne, E.; Montorsi, F.; Russo, A.; Boeri, L.; Bivalacqua, T.J.; De Ridder, D.; Joniau, S.; et al. Adipose-derived Stem Cells Counteract Urethral Stricture Formation in Rats. *Eur. Urol.* **2016**, *70*, 1032–1041. [CrossRef] [PubMed]
63. Huang, Y.; He, Y.; Li, J. MicroRNA-21: A central regulator of fibrotic diseases via various targets. *Curr. Pharm. Des.* **2015**, *21*, 2236–2242. [CrossRef] [PubMed]
64. Meng, F.; Henson, R.; Wehbe-Janek, H.; Ghoshal, K.; Jacob, S.T.; Patel, T. MicroRNA-21 regulates expression of the PTEN tumor suppressor gene in human hepatocellular cancer. *Gastroenterology* **2007**, *133*, 647–658. [CrossRef] [PubMed]
65. Feng, Z.; Chen, H.; Fu, T.; Zhang, L.; Liu, Y. miR-21 modification enhances the performance of adipose tissue-derived mesenchymal stem cells for counteracting urethral stricture formation. *J. Cell. Mol. Med.* **2018**, *22*, 5607–5616. [CrossRef] [PubMed]
66. Liang, Y.C.; Wu, Y.P.; Li, X.D.; Chen, S.H.; Ye, X.J.; Xue, X.Y.; Xu, N. TNF-α-induced exosomal miR-146a mediates mesenchymal stem cell-dependent suppression of urethral stricture. *J. Cell. Physiol.* **2019**, *234*, 23243–23255. [CrossRef] [PubMed]
67. Zhong, H.; Shen, Y.; Zhao, D.; Yan, G.; Wu, C.; Huang, G.; Liu, Z.; Zhai, J.; Han, Q. Cell-Seeded Acellular Artery for Reconstruction of Long Urethral Defects in a Canine Model. *Stem Cells Int.* **2021**, *2021*, 8854479. [CrossRef]
68. Tian, B.; Song, L.; Liang, T.; Li, Z.; Ye, X.; Fu, Q.; Li, Y. Repair of urethral defects by an adipose mesenchymal stem cell-porous silk fibroin material. *Mol. Med. Rep.* **2018**, *18*, 209–215. [CrossRef]
69. Yang, M.; Zhang, Y.; Fang, C.; Song, L.; Wang, Y.; Lu, L.; Yang, R.; Bu, Z.; Liang, X.; Zhang, K.; et al. Urine-Microenvironment-Initiated Composite Hydrogel Patch Reconfiguration Propels Scarless Memory Repair and Reinvigoration of the Urethra. *Adv. Mater.* **2022**, *34*, e2109522. [CrossRef]
70. Qazi, T.H.; Mooney, D.J.; Duda, G.N.; Geissler, S. Biomaterials that promote cell-cell interactions enhance the paracrine function of MSCs. *Biomaterials* **2017**, *140*, 103–114. [CrossRef]
71. Przybyt, E.; Krenning, G.; Brinker, M.G.; Harmsen, M.C. Adipose stromal cells primed with hypoxia and inflammation enhance cardiomyocyte proliferation rate in vitro through STAT3 and Erk1/2. *J. Transl. Med.* **2013**, *11*, 39. [CrossRef] [PubMed]
72. Kang, S.; Kim, S.M.; Sung, J.H. Cellular and molecular stimulation of adipose-derived stem cells under hypoxia. *Cell Biol. Int.* **2014**, *38*, 553–562. [CrossRef] [PubMed]
73. Zhu, Z.; Yang, J.; Ji, X.; Wang, Z.; Dai, C.; Li, S.; Li, X.; Xie, Y.; Zheng, Y.; Lin, J.; et al. Clinical application of a double-modified sulfated bacterial cellulose scaffold material loaded with FGFR2-modified adipose-derived stem cells in urethral reconstruction. *Stem Cell Res. Ther.* **2022**, *13*, 463. [CrossRef] [PubMed]
74. Chen, B.; Wen, Y.; Zhang, Z.; Wang, H.; Warrington, J.A.; Polan, M.L. Menstrual phase-dependent gene expression differences in periurethral vaginal tissue from women with stress incontinence. *Am. J. Obstet. Gynecol.* **2003**, *189*, 89–97. [CrossRef] [PubMed]
75. Gobet, R.; Bleakley, J.; Cisek, L.; Kaefer, M.; Moses, M.A.; Fernandez, C.A.; Peters, C.A. Fetal partial urethral obstruction causes renal fibrosis and is associated with proteolytic imbalance. *J. Urol.* **1999**, *162*, 854–860. [CrossRef] [PubMed]
76. Chen, B.; Wen, Y.; Wang, H.; Polan, M.L. Differences in estrogen modulation of tissue inhibitor of matrix metalloproteinase-1 and matrix metalloproteinase-1 expression in cultured fibroblasts from continent and incontinent women. *Am. J. Obstet. Gynecol.* **2003**, *189*, 59–65. [CrossRef] [PubMed]
77. Sa, Y.; Wang, L.; Shu, H.; Gu, J. Post-transcriptional suppression of TIMP-1 in epithelial-differentiated adipose-derived stem cells seeded bladder acellular matrix grafts reduces urethral scar formation. *Artif. Cells Nanomed. Biotechnol.* **2018**, *46*, 306–313. [CrossRef] [PubMed]
78. Wan, X.; Xie, M.K.; Xu, H.; Wei, Z.W.; Yao, H.J.; Wang, Z.; Zheng, D.C. Hypoxia-preconditioned adipose-derived stem cells combined with scaffold promote urethral reconstruction by upregulation of angiogenesis and glycolysis. *Stem Cell Res. Ther.* **2020**, *11*, 535. [CrossRef]
79. Riis, S.; Hansen, A.C.; Johansen, L.; Lund, K.; Pedersen, C.; Pitsa, A.; Hyldig, K.; Zachar, V.; Fink, T.; Pennisi, C.P. Fabrication and characterization of extracellular matrix scaffolds obtained from adipose-derived stem cells. *Methods* **2020**, *171*, 68–76. [CrossRef]
80. Orabi, H.; Bouhout, S.; Morissette, A.; Rousseau, A.; Chabaud, S.; Bolduc, S. Tissue engineering of urinary bladder and urethra: Advances from bench to patients. *Sci. World J.* **2013**, *2013*, 154564. [CrossRef]
81. Anisimova, N.Y.; Kiselevsky, M.V.; Sukhorukova, I.V.; Shvindina, N.V.; Shtansky, D.V. Fabrication method, structure, mechanical and biological properties of decellularized extracellular matrix for replacement of wide bone tissue defects. *J. Mech. Behav. Biomed. Mater.* **2015**, *49*, 255–268. [CrossRef] [PubMed]
82. Zhou, Y.; Wang, Y.; Zhang, K.; Cao, N.; Yang, R.; Huang, J.; Zhao, W.; Rahman, M.; Liao, H.; Fu, Q. The Fabrication and Evaluation of a Potential Biomaterial Produced with Stem Cell Sheet Technology for Future Regenerative Medicine. *Stem Cells Int.* **2020**, *2020*, 9567362. [CrossRef] [PubMed]
83. Bharadwaj, S.; Liu, G.; Shi, Y.; Wu, R.; Yang, B.; He, T.; Fan, Y.; Lu, X.; Zhou, X.; Liu, H.; et al. Multipotential differentiation of human urine-derived stem cells: Potential for therapeutic applications in urology. *Stem Cells.* **2013**, *31*, 1840–1856. [CrossRef]
84. Zhang, D.; Wei, G.; Li, P.; Zhou, X.; Zhang, Y. Urine-derived stem cells: A novel and versatile progenitor source for cell-based therapy and regenerative medicine. *Genes Dis.* **2014**, *1*, 8–17. [CrossRef] [PubMed]

85. Wu, S.; Liu, Y.; Bharadwaj, S.; Atala, A.; Zhang, Y. Human urine-derived stem cells seeded in a modified 3D porous small intestinal submucosa scaffold for urethral tissue engineering. *Biomaterials* **2011**, *32*, 1317–1326. [CrossRef] [PubMed]
86. Yang, H.; Chen, B.; Deng, J.; Zhuang, G.; Wu, S.; Liu, G.; Deng, C.; Yang, G.; Qiu, X.; Wei, P.; et al. Characterization of rabbit urine-derived stem cells for potential application in lower urinary tract tissue regeneration. *Cell Tissue Res.* **2018**, *374*, 303–315. [CrossRef]
87. Liu, Y.; Ma, W.; Liu, B.; Wang, Y.; Chu, J.; Xiong, G.; Shen, L.; Long, C.; Lin, T.; He, D.; et al. Urethral reconstruction with autologous urine-derived stem cells seeded in three-dimensional porous small intestinal submucosa in a rabbit model. *Stem Cell Res. Ther.* **2017**, *8*, 63. [CrossRef]
88. Lang, R.; Liu, G.; Shi, Y.; Bharadwaj, S.; Leng, X.; Zhou, X.; Liu, H.; Atala, A.; Zhang, Y. Self-renewal and differentiation capacity of urine-derived stem cells after urine preservation for 24 hours. *PLoS ONE* **2013**, *8*, e53980. [CrossRef]
89. Wan, Q.; Xiong, G.; Liu, G.; Shupe, T.D.; Wei, G.; Zhang, D.; Liang, D.; Lu, X.; Atala, A.; Zhang, Y. Urothelium with barrier function differentiated from human urine-derived stem cells for potential use in urinary tract reconstruction. *Stem Cell Res. Ther.* **2018**, *9*, 304. [CrossRef]
90. Kirton, J.P.; Xu, Q. Endothelial precursors in vascular repair. *Microvasc. Res.* **2010**, *79*, 193–199. [CrossRef]
91. Li, Y.; Wu, J.; Feng, F.; Men, C.; Yang, D.; Gao, Z.; Zhu, Z.; Cui, Y.; Zhao, H. A Preclinical Study of Cell-seeded Tubularized Scaffolds Specially Secreting LL37 for Reconstruction of Long Urethral Defects. *Anticancer Res.* **2017**, *37*, 4295–4301. [CrossRef] [PubMed]
92. De Coppi, P.; Bartsch, G., Jr.; Siddiqui, M.M.; Xu, T.; Santos, C.C.; Perin, L.; Mostoslavsky, G.; Serre, A.C.; Snyder, E.Y.; Yoo, J.J.; et al. Isolation of amniotic stem cell lines with potential for therapy. *Nat. Biotechnol.* **2007**, *25*, 100–106. [CrossRef] [PubMed]
93. Kang, H.H.; Kang, J.J.; Kang, H.G.; Chung, S.S. Urothelial differentiation of human amniotic fluid stem cells by urothelium specific conditioned medium. *Cell Biol. Int.* **2014**, *38*, 531–537. [CrossRef] [PubMed]
94. Díaz-Prado, S.; Muiños-López, E.; Hermida-Gómez, T.; Cicione, C.; Rendal-Vázquez, M.E.; Fuentes-Boquete, I.; de Toro, F.J.; Blanco, F.J. Human amniotic membrane as an alternative source of stem cells for regenerative medicine. *Differentiation* **2011**, *81*, 162–171. [CrossRef] [PubMed]
95. Seo, M.S.; Park, S.B.; Kim, H.S.; Kang, J.G.; Chae, J.S.; Kang, K.S. Isolation and characterization of equine amniotic membrane-derived mesenchymal stem cells. *J. Vet. Sci.* **2013**, *14*, 151–159. [CrossRef] [PubMed]
96. Alviano, F.; Fossati, V.; Marchionni, C.; Arpinati, M.; Bonsi, L.; Franchina, M.; Lanzoni, G.; Cantoni, S.; Cavallini, C.; Bianchi, F.; et al. Term Amniotic membrane is a high throughput source for multipotent Mesenchymal Stem Cells with the ability to differentiate into endothelial cells in vitro. *BMC Dev. Biol.* **2007**, *7*, 11. [CrossRef] [PubMed]
97. Lv, X.; Guo, Q.; Han, F.; Chen, C.; Ling, C.; Chen, W.; Li, B. Electrospun Poly(l-lactide)/Poly(ethylene glycol) Scaffolds Seeded with Human Amniotic Mesenchymal Stem Cells for Urethral Epithelium Repair. *Int. J. Mol. Sci.* **2016**, *17*, 1262. [CrossRef] [PubMed]
98. Tan, Q.; Le, H.; Tang, C.; Zhang, M.; Yang, W.; Hong, Y.; Wang, X. Tailor-made natural and synthetic grafts for precise urethral reconstruction. *J. Nanobiotechnol.* **2022**, *20*, 392. [CrossRef]
99. Kajbafzadeh, A.M.; Abbasioun, R.; Sabetkish, S.; Sabetkish, N.; Rahmani, P.; Tavakkolitabassi, K.; Arshadi, H. Future Prospects for Human Tissue Engineered Urethra Transplantation: Decellularization and Recellularization-Based Urethra Regeneration. *Ann. Biomed. Eng.* **2017**, *45*, 1795–1806. [CrossRef]
100. Liang, Y.; Yang, C.; Ye, F.; Cheng, Z.; Li, W.; Hu, Y.; Hu, J.; Zou, L.; Jiang, H. Repair of the Urethral Mucosa Defect Model Using Adipose-Derived Stem Cell Sheets and Monitoring the Fate of Indocyanine Green-Labeled Sheets by Near Infrared-II. *ACS Biomater. Sci. Eng.* **2022**, *8*, 4909–4920. [CrossRef]
101. Mikami, H.; Kuwahara, G.; Nakamura, N.; Yamato, M.; Tanaka, M.; Kodama, S. Two-layer tissue engineered urethra using oral epithelial and muscle derived cells. *J. Urol.* **2012**, *187*, 1882–1889. [CrossRef] [PubMed]
102. Zhou, S.; Yang, R.; Zou, Q.; Zhang, K.; Yin, T.; Zhao, W.; Shapter, J.G.; Gao, G.; Fu, Q. Fabrication of Tissue-Engineered Bionic Urethra Using Cell Sheet Technology and Labeling By Ultrasmall Superparamagnetic Iron Oxide for Full-Thickness Urethral Reconstruction. *Theranostics* **2017**, *7*, 2509–2523. [CrossRef] [PubMed]
103. Rashidbenam, Z.; Jasman, M.H.; Tan, G.H.; Goh, E.H.; Fam, X.I.; Ho, C.C.K.; Zainuddin, Z.M.; Rajan, R.; Rani, R.A.; Nor, F.M.; et al. Fabrication of Adipose-Derived Stem Cell-Based Self-Assembled Scaffold under Hypoxia and Mechanical Stimulation for Urethral Tissue Engineering. *Int. J. Mol. Sci.* **2021**, *22*, 3350. [CrossRef] [PubMed]
104. Bhargava, S.; Chapple, C.R. Buccal mucosal urethroplasty: Is it the new gold standard? *BJU Int.* **2004**, *93*, 1191–1193. [CrossRef] [PubMed]
105. Barbagli, G.; Kulkarni, S.B.; Fossati, N.; Larcher, A.; Sansalone, S.; Guazzoni, G.; Romano, G.; Pankaj, J.M.; Dell'Acqua, V.; Lazzeri, M. Long-term followup and deterioration rate of anterior substitution urethroplasty. *J. Urol.* **2014**, *192*, 808–813. [CrossRef] [PubMed]
106. Al Taweel, W.; Seyam, R. Visual Internal Urethrotomy for Adult Male Urethral Stricture Has Poor Long-Term Results. *Adv. Urol.* **2015**, *2015*, 656459. [CrossRef] [PubMed]
107. Scott, K.A.; Li, G.; Manwaring, J.; Nikolavsky, D.A.; Fudym, Y.; Caza, T.; Badar, Z.; Taylor, N.; Bratslavsky, G.; Kotula, L.; et al. Liquid buccal mucosa graft endoscopic urethroplasty: A validation animal study. *World J. Urol.* **2020**, *38*, 2139–2145. [CrossRef]
108. Vaddi, S.P.; Reddy, V.B.; Abraham, S.J. Buccal epithelium Expanded and Encapsulated in Scaffold-Hybrid Approach to Urethral Stricture (BEES-HAUS) procedure: A novel cell therapy-based pilot study. *Int. J. Urol.* **2019**, *26*, 253–257. [CrossRef]

109. Horiguchi, A.; Ojima, K.; Shinchi, M.; Kushibiki, T.; Mayumi, Y.; Miyai, K.; Katoh, S.; Takeda, M.; Iwasaki, M.; Prakash, V.S.; et al. Successful engraftment of epithelial cells derived from autologous rabbit buccal mucosal tissue, encapsulated in a polymer scaffold in a rabbit model of a urethral stricture, transplanted using the transurethral approach. *Regen. Ther.* **2021**, *18*, 127–132. [CrossRef]
110. Horiguchi, A.; Shinchi, M.; Ojima, K.; Hirano, Y.; Kushibiki, T.; Mayumi, Y.; Miyai, K.; Miura, I.; Iwasaki, M.; Suryaprakash, V.; et al. Engraftment of Transplanted Buccal Epithelial Cells onto the Urethrotomy Site, Proven Immunohistochemically in Rabbit Model; a Feat to Prevent Urethral Stricture Recurrence. *Stem Cell Rev. Rep.* **2023**, *19*, 275–278. [CrossRef]
111. Kulkarni, S.B.; Pathak, H.; Khanna, S.; Choubey, S. A prospective, multi-center, open-label, single-arm phase 2b study of autologous adult live cultured buccal epithelial cells (AALBEC) in the treatment of bulbar urethral stricture. *World J. Urol.* **2021**, *39*, 2081–2087. [CrossRef] [PubMed]
112. Barbagli, G.; Sansalone, S.; Djinovic, R.; Romano, G.; Lazzeri, M. Current controversies in reconstructive surgery of the anterior urethra: A clinical overview. *Int. Braz. J. Urol.* **2012**, *38*, 307–316, discussion 316. [CrossRef] [PubMed]
113. Lumen, N.; Oosterlinck, W.; Hoebeke, P. Urethral reconstruction using buccal mucosa or penile skin grafts: Systematic review and meta-analysis. *Urol. Int.* **2012**, *89*, 387–394. [CrossRef] [PubMed]
114. Bhargava, S.; Patterson, J.M.; Inman, R.D.; MacNeil, S.; Chapple, C.R. Tissue-engineered buccal mucosa urethroplasty-clinical outcomes. *Eur. Urol.* **2008**, *53*, 1263–1269. [CrossRef] [PubMed]
115. Lazzeri, M.; Barbagli, G.; Fahlenkamp, D.; Romano, G.; Balsmeyer, U.; Knispel, H.; Spiegeler, M.E.; Stuerzebecher, B.; Ram-Liebig, G. MP9-04 preclinical and clinical examination of tissue-engineered graft for urethral reconstruction (mukocell) with regard to its safety. *J. Urol.* **2014**, *191*, e122–e123. [CrossRef]
116. Barbagli, G.; Akbarov, I.; Heidenreich, A.; Zugor, V.; Olianas, R.; Aragona, M.; Romano, G.; Balsmeyer, U.; Fahlenkamp, D.; Rebmann, U.; et al. Anterior Urethroplasty Using a New Tissue Engineered Oral Mucosa Graft: Surgical Techniques and Outcomes. *J. Urol.* **2018**, *200*, 448–456. [CrossRef] [PubMed]
117. Barbagli, G.; Heidenreich, A.; Zugor, V.; Karapanos, L.; Lazzeri, M. Urothelial or oral mucosa cells for tissue-engineered urethroplasty: A critical revision of the clinical outcome. *Asian J. Urol.* **2020**, *7*, 18–23. [CrossRef]
118. Roh, J.D.; Sawh-Martinez, R.; Brennan, M.P.; Jay, S.M.; Devine, L.; Rao, D.A.; Yi, T.; Mirensky, T.L.; Nalbandian, A.; Udelsman, B.; et al. Tissue-engineered vascular grafts transform into mature blood vessels via an inflammation-mediated process of vascular remodeling. *Proc. Natl. Acad. Sci. USA* **2010**, *107*, 4669–4674. [CrossRef]
119. Hibino, N.; Villalona, G.; Pietris, N.; Duncan, D.R.; Schoffner, A.; Roh, J.D.; Yi, T.; Dobrucki, L.W.; Mejias, D.; Sawh-Martinez, R.; et al. Tissue-engineered vascular grafts form neovessels that arise from regeneration of the adjacent blood vessel. *FASEB J.* **2011**, *25*, 2731–2739. [CrossRef]
120. Ankrum, J.A.; Ong, J.F.; Karp, J.M. Mesenchymal stem cells: Immune evasive, not immune privileged. *Nat. Biotechnol.* **2014**, *32*, 252–260. [CrossRef]
121. Davis, N.F.; Cunnane, E.M.; Mulvihill, J.J.; Quinlan, M.R.; Bolton, D.M.; Walsh, M.T.; Jack, G.S. The Role of Stem Cells for Reconstructing the Lower Urinary Tracts. *Curr. Stem Cell Res. Ther.* **2018**, *13*, 458–465. [CrossRef]
122. Kang, H.S.; Choi, S.H.; Kim, B.S.; Choi, J.Y.; Park, G.B.; Kwon, T.G.; Chun, S.Y. Advanced Properties of Urine Derived Stem Cells Compared to Adipose Tissue Derived Stem Cells in Terms of Cell Proliferation, Immune Modulation and Multi Differentiation. *J. Korean Med. Sci.* **2015**, *30*, 1764–1776. [CrossRef]

Disclaimer/Publisher's Note: The statements, opinions and data contained in all publications are solely those of the individual author(s) and contributor(s) and not of MDPI and/or the editor(s). MDPI and/or the editor(s) disclaim responsibility for any injury to people or property resulting from any ideas, methods, instructions or products referred to in the content.

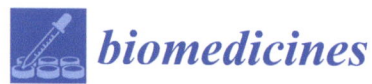

Review

Signaling Mechanisms of Stem Cell Therapy for Intervertebral Disc Degeneration

Xiaotian Du, Kejiong Liang, Shili Ding and Haifei Shi *

Department of Orthopedic Surgery, The First Affiliated Hospital, Zhejiang University School of Medicine, Hangzhou 310003, China; 21618580@zju.edu.cn (X.D.); lkj1020@zju.edu.cn (K.L.); 1515071@zju.edu.cn (S.D.)
* Correspondence: shihaifei@zju.edu.cn

Abstract: Low back pain is the leading cause of disability worldwide. Intervertebral disc degeneration (IDD) is the primary clinical risk factor for low back pain and the pathological cause of disc herniation, spinal stenosis, and spinal deformity. A possible approach to improve the clinical practice of IDD-related diseases is to incorporate biomarkers in diagnosis, therapeutic intervention, and prognosis prediction. IDD pathology is still unclear. Regarding molecular mechanisms, cellular signaling pathways constitute a complex network of signaling pathways that coordinate cell survival, proliferation, differentiation, and metabolism. Recently, stem cells have shown great potential in clinical applications for IDD. In this review, the roles of multiple signaling pathways and related stem cell treatment in IDD are summarized and described. This review seeks to investigate the mechanisms and potential therapeutic effects of stem cells in IDD and identify new therapeutic treatments for IDD-related disorders.

Keywords: intervertebral disc; tissue degeneration; signaling pathway; stem cell treatment

1. Background

Low back pain is the leading global disability [1]. To date, intervertebral disc degeneration (IDD) has become the primary clinical risk factor for low back pain and the pathological basis for developing disc herniation, spinal stenosis, and spinal deformities [2]. It is reported that ordinary populations have a 10% lifetime prevalence of sciatica-related low back pain [3]. While a number of approaches are used to treat symptomatic IDD-related diseases, there are marked heterogeneities in therapeutic efficacies. For instance, surgery is indicated for disc herniation patients who failed conservative treatments, but back pain and leg pain remained in approximately a third of surgical cases two years later [4]. Such heterogeneities in clinical outcomes reflect the need for early diagnosis and precise prognostic judgment.

Anatomically, the intervertebral disc (IVD) connects vertebral bodies in the spine with three compartments: nucleus pulposus (NP), annulus fibrosus (AF), and cartilaginous endplate (CEP). IDD causes decreased water content of the NP and AF, loss of elasticity of the NP, centripetal fissures, structural changes of collagen fibers in the AF, extensive damage in the CEP, subchondral osteosclerosis, angiogenesis, neoinnervation, significant reduction or even loss of IVD height, and IVD-related biomechanical changes. Degenerated IVD cells have fewer active cells, aberrant extracellular matrix metabolism, and pro-inflammatory chemicals [5].

To date, IDD pathology is unclear. Mechanical stress, trauma, infection, genetic vulnerability, and inflammation can increase IDD pathology [6]. Recent developments in gene microarray technology have yielded fresh insights into the molecular pathogenesis of IDD-related diseases. Using single-Cell RNA Sequencing technology, several cell types including chondrocyte 1–5, endothelial, macrophage, neutrophil, and T cells were delineated in IVD. Specifically, chondrocytes 5 expressing FN1, SESN2, and GDF15, and chondrocytes 4 expressing PTGES, TREM1, and TIMP1 may exacerbate IDD, while chondrocytes 2 expressing

Citation: Du, X.; Liang, K.; Ding, S.; Shi, H. Signaling Mechanisms of Stem Cell Therapy for Intervertebral Disc Degeneration. *Biomedicines* **2023**, *11*, 2467. https://doi.org/10.3390/biomedicines11092467

Academic Editors: Christian Morsczeck and Aline Yen Ling Wang

Received: 5 July 2023
Revised: 27 August 2023
Accepted: 28 August 2023
Published: 6 September 2023

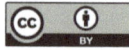

Copyright: © 2023 by the authors. Licensee MDPI, Basel, Switzerland. This article is an open access article distributed under the terms and conditions of the Creative Commons Attribution (CC BY) license (https://creativecommons.org/licenses/by/4.0/).

MGP, MT1G, and GPX3 may mitigate this degenerative process [7]. Regarding molecular mechanisms, cellular signaling pathways such as Wnt/β-catenin, NF-κB, mitogen-activated protein kinase (MAPK), lipoyl inositol-3 kinase (PI3K)/serine-threonine protein kinase (Akt), and transforming growth factor β (TGF-β)/Smads constituted a complex network of signaling pathways that coordinate the cell survival, proliferation, differentiation, and metabolism. Studying the molecular pathogenesis of IDD and delaying or correcting its pathological alterations is a key problem and research hotspot in orthopedics.

Stem cells are multipotent, self-renewing cells, and are implicated in various basic processes, such as cellular differentiation, proliferation, angiogenesis, oxidative stress response, inflammation, and extracellular matrix synthesis [8]. The potential of stem cell therapy has been investigated in the treatment of degenerative musculoskeletal diseases [9]. Recently, stem cells derived from NP, CEP, bone marrow, and adipose tissue have shown great potential in clinical applications for IDD by regulating signaling pathways in the IDD process. The present review was made to investigate the mechanisms and potential therapeutic effects of stem cells in IDD and identify new therapeutic treatments for IDD-related disorders. Recent advances in IDD-related signaling pathways and related stem cell treatment in IDD are summarized and described below.

2. Wnt/β-Catenin Signaling Pathway

The classical Wnt signaling pathway includes secreted Wnt family proteins, transmembrane receptor proteins of the Frizzled family (Dishevelled, GSK3, Axin, APC, and β-catenin), and downstream transcriptional regulators of the TCF/LEF family. This route involves embryonic development, stem cell proliferation, and degenerative disorder development [10]. For the skeletal system, the Wnt signaling pathway was crucial for developing craniofacial, limb, and joint structures, and mutations in members of this pathway would lead to skeletal malformations in mice and humans [11].

The Wnt signaling pathway's dynamic activity during IVD growth, maturation, and degeneration has been studied (Table 1). Excessive activation of this pathway, for example, may lead to severe structural malformations in IVD, as evidenced by disruption of the growth plate, excessive cellular proliferation, disruption of the lamellar structure in the AF, and reduction in proteoglycans in the NP. β-catenin deficiency also accelerates bone formation between the CEP and growth plate [12]. Moreover, for the degenerative process, the Wnt/β-catenin signaling pathway activation can accelerate this process by inducing the inflammatory factors production [10], promoting cellular apoptosis and senescence [13], and degradation of the extracellular matrix of IVD cells [14]. For example, conditional activation of β-catenin in mice can lead to severe structural defects in IVD [15]. Furthermore, the upregulation of β-catenin in the canine IVD can upregulate the Runx2 expression in the IVD and promote degenerative calcification in the IVD [14]. Additionally, in IVD, WNT/β-catenin pathway activation promotes cellular senescence, matrix disintegration, and IDD [13].

Various active substances can promote IDD by upregulating the Wnt/β-catenin pathway expression (Table 1). For example, lncRNA HOTAIR and circITCH can promote cellular senescence, apoptosis, and matrix degradation in IVD by activating the Wnt/β-catenin pathway [16]. In IVD cells, TNF-α and Wnt signaling can generate a positive feedback loop [17]. IDD may be alleviated by inhibiting this mechanism. For example, RBMS3 RBMS3 (RNA binding motif, single-stranded interacting protein 3) is a member of the c-myc single-strand binding protein family and encodes an RNA-binding protein [18]. In addition, by inhibiting the Wnt/β-catenin signaling pathway, RBMS3 can enhance the proliferative capacity of IVD cells and suppress apoptosis and inflammatory responses in IVD [19].

Table 1. Effects of signaling pathway activation for IDD and pathway activator.

Signaling Pathway	Wnt/β-Catenin Signaling Pathway	NF-κB Signaling Pathway	MAPK Signaling Pathway	PI3K/Akt Signaling Pathway	TGF-β1 Signaling Pathway
Effects of pathway activation for IDD	↑[10,13–15]	↑[20–29]	See details in Table 2	↓[30–38]	↑[39–41] ↓[42–51]
Activator	LncRNA HOTAIR [16], circRNA ITCH [52], TNF-α [17]	TREM2 [53], CGRP [28], Ca²⁺ [24], IL-1β [25], HMGB1 [20], N-Ac-PGP [21], ROS [22], S100A9 [26], ARG2 [27]	CHI3L1 [54], ROS [22,55], MALAT1 [56], Resistin [57], Syndecan-4 [58], IL-17A [59], IAPP [60], Glucose [61], Visfatin [62]	17Beta-estradiol [34], BMP2 [33], Apelin-13/APJ [35], Resveratrol [63]	Smad3 [43], ASIC3 [42], caveolin-1 [46], Parathyroid hormone [50]

↑: Deteriorating effect. ↓: Mitigating effect.

As mentioned, the Wnt/β-catenin signaling pathway plays a crucial role in IDD and may function as a potential therapeutic target for stem-cell-related treatment. For example, the aberrant apoptosis of NP cells is one of the most remarkable pathological changes in IDD development. The compression leads to an increase in apoptosis and Wnt-related gene expression, which can both be suppressed by the in vitro co-cultured mesenchymal stem cell (MSC) [64]. Moreover, the age-related variation of Wnt signaling in IVD cells may limit regeneration by depleting the progenitors and attenuating the expansion of chondrocyte-like cells [65]. During IDD, CEP gradually calcified and the osteogenic differentiation was increased [66]. Cartilage endplate stem cells (CESCs) are essential for IDD by regulating chondrogenesis and osteogenesis in the CEP [67]. Downregulation of WNT5A was proved to inhibit IDD via downregulating the osteogenic differentiation of CESCs [68]. Exosomes derived from CESCs, however, can activate HIF-1α/Wnt signaling via autocrine mechanisms to increase the expression of GATA4 and TGF-β1, thereby promoting the migration of CESCs into the IVD and the transformation of CESCs into NP cells and inhibiting IDD [69]. Therefore, the activation of the Wnt signaling pathway in IVD stem cells may also reveal its alleviating effects in IDD. For example, the Wnt/-catenin pathway in IVD can be activated by bone marrow mesenchymal stem cells (BMSCs)-derived extracellular vesicles, leading to the suppression of cellular apoptosis, ECM degradation, and IDD progression [70]. Notably, the overexpression of Wnt11 in adipose-derived stem cells (ADSCs) induces the ADSCs cells differentiating to the NP cells, which may have a potential utility for the treatment of IDD [71] (Figure 1).

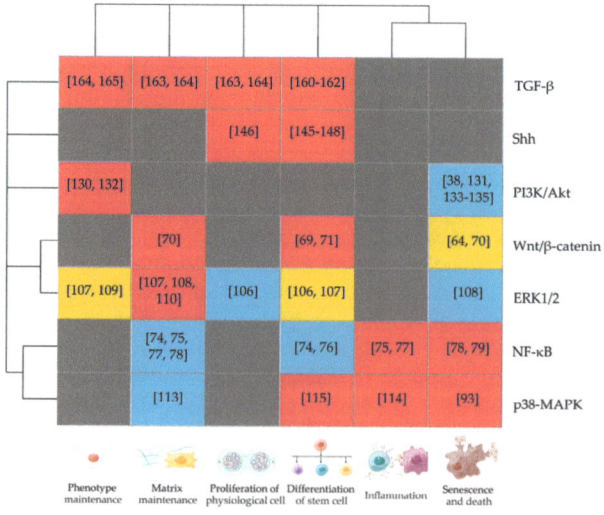

Figure 1. Effects of stem cell treatment and roles of related signaling pathways on IDD progression.

Red module: positive relations between the activations of signaling pathway and corresponding biological processes. Blue module: negative relations between the activations of signaling pathway and corresponding biological processes. Yellow module: relations between the activations of signaling pathways and corresponding biological processes varied in different studies. Grey module: lack of relevant evidence. (The figure was created with Figdraw and the OmicStudio tools at https://www.omicstudio.cn on 25 August 2023).

3. NF-κB Signaling Pathway

NF-κB protein, initially found in B lymphocyte extracts, binds to enhancer regions of immunoglobulin light chain genes [72]. In the classical NF-κB signaling pathway, IκB kinase (IKK) regulated the IκB proteins' phosphorylation [73]. For IVD, NF-κB nuclear translocation upregulation accelerates IDD [29]. For example, HMGB1, a pro-inflammatory factor, upregulates the NF-κB signaling pathway in IVD cells to induce inflammatory cytokines and matrix metalloproteinases [20]. Additionally, in degenerative IVD, the neuropeptide CGRP and its receptors are overexpressed, which inhibits cellular growth and promotes apoptosis and inflammation by upregulating the NF-κB signaling pathway [28]. Notably, inflammatory mediators and chemokines produced by the NF-κB signaling pathway activation formed a vicious cycle in the IDD process [23]. For example, the NF-κB pathway activation by IL-1β would also promote the IL-1β precursors expression, accelerating IVD degeneration [24]. Another study showed that IL-1β could also regulate the miR-133a-5p/FBXO6 axis expression through the NF-κB pathway, which would regulate the proliferation of IVD cells and apoptosis [25].

Besides regulating the inflammatory responses [25], the NF-κB signaling pathway upregulation can also deteriorate IDD by promoting matrix metalloproteinases and destructing the cellular matrix of IVD [20]. For instance, the inflammatory chemokine N-Ac-PGP promotes NF-κB and MAPK signaling pathways in NP cells to generate pro-inflammatory cytokines and matrix catabolic enzymes [21]. Moreover, the increase in neovascularization in aging IVD would exacerbate the oxidative stress for this tissue. Upregulation of reactive oxygen species (ROS) would induce catabolic and inflammatory expression in IVD cells by stimulating the NF-κB pathway [22]. Moreover, the oxygen-sensing proteins would induce apoptosis, matrix degradation, and the inflammatory response for NP cells by NF-κB signaling pathway activation [26]. NF-κB can enhance oxidative stress, generating another vicious cycle between IDD and the oxidative stress [27]. Thus, NF-κB signaling pathway activation promotes IVD apoptosis, inflammatory response, matrix breakdown, and oxidative stress, which worsens IDD.

Studies have revealed the use of BMSCs in tissue-engineering treatments to slow or reverse IDD. The coculturing of BMSCs with disc-native NP cells promotes the matrix production of NP cells and the differentiation of BMSCs into NP-like cells through downregulating NF-κB pathway [74]. Moreover, TNF-α-stimulated gene 6 secreted by BMSCs can attenuate inflammation factors production, matrix degeneration, and IDD by inhibiting the NF-κB signaling pathway [75]. Interestingly, inflammation factors also revealed positive roles for stem cells in recent degenerative disease studies. Tumor necrosis factor-α (TNF-α) is critical for accelerating IDD. While with a relatively low concentration (0.1–10 ng/mL), TNF-α promotes the proliferation and migration of NP mesenchymal stem cells (NPMSCs) but inhibits their differentiation toward NP cells. Moreover, the NF-κB signaling pathway is activated during the TNF-α-inhibited differentiation of NPMSCs, and the NF-κB signal inhibitor can partially counteract the adverse effect of TNF-α on the differentiation of NPMSCs [76]. Moreover, TGF-β1 is a strong immune suppressor, whose increase would inhibit IκB phosphorylation and NF-κB activation. Co-culturing of NP cells with BMSCs significantly increases TGF-β1 in NP, leading to anti-inflammatory effects via the inhibition of NF-κB, and ameliorating IDD due to increased collagen II and aggrecan in the degenerative disc [77]. Cellular senescence is another promotive factor for IDD. Upon TNF-α stimulation, NF-κB activation reveals pro-senescence effects in NP cells, while co-culturing with BMSCs reduces senescence-associated β-galactosidase, matrix metalloproteinase 9, and NF-κB signaling in senescent NP cells. Accordingly, Zinc metallopeptidase STE24, whose dysfunction is related to premature cell senescence and aging, is restored upon BMSC co-culture and inhibits the effects of NF-κB activation [78]. Moreover, ataxia-telangiectasia mutated kinase is a vital component for NF-κB-mediated cellular senescence, stem cell dysfunction, and aging. Inhibition of this kinase also reduces activation of NF-κB, improves the functions of muscle-derived stem/progenitor cells, and thus alleviates IDD [79].

4. MAPK Signaling Pathway

The mitogen-activated protein kinase (MAPK) cascade signaling pathway has three main sub-pathways: the extracellular signal-regulated kinase 1/2 (ERK1/2) pathway, the p38 kinase pathway, and the c-Jun amino-terminal kinase (JNK1–3) pathway. All three sub-pathways involved physiological and pathological processes such as cell proliferation, differentiation, apoptosis, stress, and inflammatory responses (Table 2). As mentioned in Figure 1, the promotion of inflammation, oxidative stress, senescence, and death processes deteriorate IDD, while the activations of stem cell differentiation, proliferation of physiological cells, phenotype maintenance, and matrix maintenance mitigate this pathological process.

Table 2. Effects of the MAPK signaling pathway activation for cells in IVD.

Sub-Pathways in MAPK Pathway	Inflammation	Oxidative Stress	Senescence and Death	Proliferation	Phenotype Maintenance	Matrix Maintenance
ERK1/2 signaling pathway	↑[80]	↑[22]	↓[81]↑[22]	↑[82–84]	↑[85–87]↓[88]	↑[84]↓[54,80]
p38-MAPK signaling pathway	↑[57,89–94]	↑[94,95]	↑[56,93,96,97]	↓[92]	↓[92,98]	↓[57]
JNK signaling pathway	↑[59,62,99]	↑[100]	↑[55,60,61,101]	↑[102]	↓[58]	↓[60,62,99]

↑: Promoting effect. ↓: Inhibitory effect.

4.1. ERK1/2 Signaling Pathway

The MAPK/ERK pathway activation in AF and NP may have different or opposite roles [103]. MAPK/ERK pathway activation in AF helps IVD maintain its physiological phenotype, repair damage, and prevent tissue degeneration. For example, low-intensity pulsed ultrasound would enhance cell proliferation and collagen synthesis processes by activating the ERK pathway in AF, promoting the AF's repair and alleviating IDD [84]. Additionally, the ERK pathway activation can significantly enhance the proliferation and migration of AF cells, promoting IVD repair [82,83,104]. Moreover, ERK maintains IVD function in acidic and hyperosmotic microenvironments [87] and the activation of this pathway would also activate AF cell regeneration in 3D culture [81]. For phenotypic maintenance in AF cells, however, the activated MAPK-ERK pathway revealed opposite roles in studies [86,88]. In NP tissue, MAPK/ERK pathway activation was linked to extracellular matrix breakdown, cellular senescence, apoptosis, inflammation, autophagy, and oxidative stress, worsening IDD pathology [105]. For example, the M1-type [80] and M2a-type [54] macrophages would promote the imbalance of extracellular matrix metabolism in NP cells by activating the ERK signaling pathway. Additionally, elevated oxygen tension-induced ROS in NP causes cell cycle arrest and senescence through ERK signaling pathway activation [22].

Both NPMSC and ADSC are used as candidate cells for IDD treatment. The ERK pathway is activated by the hyperosmolarity in the disc, which inhibits proliferation and chondrogenic differentiation of NPMSCs [106]. In another study, however, the activation of the MAPK/ERK signaling pathway leads to the enhancement of NPMSC viability, differentiation towards NP cells, and extracellular matrix biosynthesis in the disc [107].

Similarly, lithium, a common anti-depression drug, was found to promote ROS and ERK1/2 pathway, which enhances ADSC's survival and ECM deposits in the degenerative disc [108]. Recently, scaffolds for IDD tissue engineering were designed for the maintenance of stem cells in the acidic environment of the disc. For example, Sa12b-modified hydrogel enhances the biological activity of NPMSCs by inhibiting acid-sensing ion channels by inhibiting the ERK signaling pathway [109]. In addition, collagen type II hydrogel significantly promotes extracellular matrix synthesis by activating the ERK pathway [110].

4.2. p38-MAPK Signaling Pathway

The p38-MAPK signaling pathway also regulated inflammation, cellular stress, growth and development, and apoptosis in IVD. Growth factors, inflammatory cytokines, and environmental stresses trigger IVD's p38-MAPK signaling pathway, releasing inflammatory substances, and degrading the cellular matrix, thus accelerating IDD [111]. For example, non-physiological loading can stimulate apoptotic body production in AF cells by activating the p38-MAPK pathway, ultimately leading to the apoptosis and degeneration of IVD [96]. For chondrocytes in CEP, the p38-MAPK signaling pathway would also induce cellular apoptosis [56]. In recent years, the roles of resistin and endoplasmic reticulum stress have been revealed in multiple degenerative diseases. In IVD, these two variables activated the p38-MAPK pathway to produce pro-inflammatory effects [57,89].

Various research has proven the therapeutic effects of inhibiting the p38-MAPK pathway on IDD in recent years. All of the pulsed electromagnetic fields [90], tyrosine kinase inhibitors [91], and tanshinone IIA sulfonate [94] exert their anti-inflammatory activities for IVD cells by downregulating the p38-MAPK signaling pathway. Moreover, blocking the p38-MAPK pathway can greatly reduce the inflammatory consequences of non-physiological stress on IVD cells [97]. Moreover, the p38-MAPK pathway inhibition would protect NP cells against oxidative stress and mitochondrial dysfunction [95], prevent NP cells apoptosis by inhibiting M1-type macrophage polarization and promoting the release of anti-inflammatory factors from M2-type macrophages [93], and also increase the expression of IVD protective factors [98]. Additionally, ERK5 is another member of the MAPK family and regulates the maintenance of the extracellular matrix in IVD, and the suppression of ERK5 resulted in decreased type II collagen and aggrecan in NP cells, indicating the potential protective roles of MAPK family members in IDD [112].

In the disc, BMSC-derived extracellular vesicles have the potential to alleviate extracellular matrix degradation, apoptosis, and cell cycle arrest in IDD via downregulating phosphorylated p38 MAPK levels [93,113]. In addition, the suppression of p38 MAPK signaling with specific inhibitors also promotes the anti-inflammatory impact of MSCs and the alleviation of IDD [114]. The activation of the p38 signaling pathway, however, has also revealed its therapeutic potential for IDD by stimulating the differentiation of MSC in the disc. For example, TGF-β1 promotes the differentiation of MSC to NP-like cells in the disc's physiological hypoxia environment by activating ERK and p38 signaling pathways [115]. Notably, the therapeutic effect of intervertebral fusion for IDD is still unsatisfactory and the conditioned medium of BMSCs treated with electromagnetic fields can promote osteogenic differentiation of BMSCs by activating the p38 signaling pathway, which accelerates intervertebral fusion for IDD treatment [116,117].

4.3. JNK Signaling Pathway

In IVD, JNK activation causes inflammation and matrix breakdown [58]. For example, aberrant expression of pancreatic amyloid polypeptide would increase the secretion of IL-1, TNF-α, and matrix-degrading enzymes in IVD by activating this pathway [60]. Similarly, IL-17A can exert a pro-inflammatory effect by stimulating the p38 and JNK pathways, causing NP cells to produce more COX2/PGE2 [59]. Recently, the endocrine function of adipose tissue was revealed. Visfatin, a protein secreted by adipose tissue, can induce IL-6 expression in NP cells by activating the JNK/ERK/p38-MAPK signaling pathway, thus promoting the inflammatory response and extracellular matrix degradation in IVD [62].

Increased JNK signaling pathway also upregulates IVD cell autophagy and apoptosis. Under mechanical stress stimulation, elevated ROS in rat NP cells activates the JNK signaling pathway and induces autophagy, thus accelerating IDD [55]. Moreover, IDD was also more common among people with diabetes than non-diabetics [118]. High glucose can lead to premature senescence of AF cells in young rats [101] and promote apoptosis of AF cells in a glucose concentration-dependent manner through activation of the JNK pathway [61]. Notably, JNK pathway suppression may also alleviate IDD. Crocin, the bioactive component of saffron, can alleviate the inflammatory and catabolic processes in IVD by JNK phosphorylation inhibition in NP cells [99]. Moreover, hinokitiol can also maintain the function of iron transport proteins and alleviate oxidative stress in NP cells by regulating the JNK pathway [100].

Inhibition of the JNK signaling pathway alleviates degeneration of stem cells derived from CEP, NP, and bone marrow [119]. For example, oxidative stress during the transplant of BMSC to degenerative discs may cause cell toxicity and poor survival of BMSCs. Mitophagy can maintain cellular homeostasis and defend against oxidative stress by eliminating dysfunctional or damaged mitochondria. Mechanically, oxidative stress facilitates mitophagy through the JNK signaling pathway at an early stage of IDD but decreases mitophagy and increases apoptosis at a late stage [120]. Moreover, excessive oxidative stress also induces apoptosis and senescence of NP stem cells. Heat shock protein 70 (HSP70), a cytoprotective and antioxidative protein, reveals its protective roles against apoptosis and senescence of NP stem cells by downregulating the JNK signaling pathway [121].

5. PI3K/Akt Signaling Pathway

PI3K/Akt also regulates cell survival, metabolism, and proliferation in numerous tissues [122]. IVD cells need PI3K/Akt pathway activation to survive hypoxic conditions [123]. A possible explanation for this role was proposed as the PI3K/Akt pathway activation would promote autophagy and inhibit apoptosis of NP-derived [38] and endplate-derived [36] stem cells, which protected IVD from oxidative damage and facilitated the repair of degenerative injury.

Moreover, PI3K/AKT signaling protected matrix production in NP cells, while inhibiting PI3K activity would decrease proteoglycans in the IVD matrix [30]. Specifically, the PI3K/Akt/FOXO3 signaling pathway activation would downregulate the MMP-3 expression and upregulate type II collagen and ACAN in NP cells [34]. Activating PI3K/AKT signaling reduces matrix breakdown and inflammation [32]. For example, PI3K/Akt signaling pathway activation by BMP2 [33] and the Apelin-13/APJ system [35] can not only promote the production of type II collagen, ACAN, SOX9, and downregulate matrix-degrading enzymes in IVD, but also significantly inhibit the inflammatory response and apoptosis of NP cells. As the key driver of the inflammatory cascade in IVD, IL-1β promotes NP cell death, inflammatory responses, extracellular matrix remodeling, endoplasmic reticulum stress responses, and mitochondrial dysfunction. The PI3K/Akt pathway inhibits these IDD-related activities [31,37].

Recently, drugs and physiotherapeutic means to alleviate the IDD process by modulating PI3K/Akt pathway activity have also emerged. As mentioned, high oxidative stress in NP cells would promote degenerative changes by increasing intracellular ROS production. While resveratrol can inhibit oxidative stress-related effects by PI3K/Akt pathway activation in NP cells [63]. For physiotherapeutic aspects, circulating mechanical traction [124] and low-intensity pulsed ultrasound [125] can also alleviate degenerative changes in the NP extracellular matrix by activating the PI3K/Akt pathway. For AF cells, PI3K/AKT signaling pathway activation would also alleviate the degenerative processes. For example, the activation of this pathway inhibits AF cell cadmium-induced apoptosis [126]. However, a recent study also revealed the promotive effects of the PI3K/AKT signaling pathway for angiogenesis in IVD [127]. Thus, the data suggest that PI3K/AKT signaling pathway activation may treat IDD.

Based on stem cell studies, promising tools and insights for PI3K/AKT pathway-related IDD therapeutics were offered in recent studies. Mechanically, disc-derived stem cells regulate the function of the disc by delivering exosomes. The CESC-derived exosomes inhibit apoptosis of NP cells and attenuated IDD in rats via activation of the PI3K/AKT pathway. Additionally, exosomes from normal CESC inhibit NP apoptosis and alleviate IDD more effectively than exosomes from degenerative CESC [38]. Moreover, CESCs overexpressing Sphk2-engineered exosomes activates the PI3K/p-AKT pathway as well as the intracellular autophagy of NP cells, which ultimately ameliorates IDD by balancing autophagy/senescence [128]. In addition, for NP progenitor cells (NPPCs), exosomes secreted by NPPCs derived from degenerative discs would even exacerbate AF degeneration by blocking the activation of the PI3K-Akt pathway [129]. Notably, NPPCs remain difficult to maintain in culture. Fibroblast growth factor (FGF) 2 and chimeric FGF, however, were reported to enhance the phenotype maintenance of NPPCs via PI3K/Akt and MEK/ERK signals [130]. In addition, $1,25(OH)_2D_3$ can also attenuate oxidative stress-induced apoptosis and mitochondrial dysfunction to NPPCs through PI3K/Akt pathway [131].

MSCs can also attenuate IDD by regulating cellular mechanical properties and apoptosis in the disc. For example, co-culture of degenerative NP cells with MSCs resulted in significantly decreased mechanical moduli and increased biological activity in degenerative NP by activating AKT signaling [132]. In addition, MSC-derived exosomes can prevent NP cells from TNF-α induced apoptosis and alleviate IDD by targeting phosphatase and tensin homolog by activating the PI3K-Akt pathway [133]. Through the AKT and ERK signaling pathways, exosomes from urine-derived stem cells can significantly inhibit endoplasmic reticulum (ER) stress-induced apoptosis and IDD under pressure conditions [134]. Similarly, exosomes from BMSCs can attenuate ER stress-induced apoptosis in degenerative discs by activating AKT and ERK signaling [135].

6. Hedgehog Signaling Pathway

Hedgehog signaling regulates skeletal development and repair [136]. Hedgehog proteins regulate IVD maturation, degradation, and calcification [137]. Hedgehog is highly expressed in young and healthy IVD cells, diminishes with notochord cell phenotypic loss, and increases again in late IDD [138]. Hedgehog contains three homologous proteins: Sonic hedgehog (Shh), Indian hedgehog (Ihh), and Desert hedgehog (Dhh). Among them, Shh and Ihh are closely related to the IDD process as described as follows.

6.1. Shh Signaling Pathway

IVD development and function require an appropriate Shh signaling pathway expression [139] and the deficiency of this pathway has been proven to be related to the aging phenotype of NP cells [140,141]. During the embryonic stage, the notochord eventually undergoes segmentation and forms IVD, and a notochord sheath must wrap it to retain its usual rod-shaped structure. The Shh signal loss in early embryonic stages would lead to structural abnormalities in the notochord sheath, leading to aberrant development of IVD and vertebrae [142,143].

Shh signaling influenced IVD growth and differentiation after birth. Without this signaling pathway, NP cells would lose their reticular network and collapse into IVD's core region, while AF cells would lose their polar layered structure. Mechanistically, blocking the Shh signal would lead to the downregulation of TGF-β signaling and the upregulation of BMP and Wnt signaling expression [140]. The IVD between the sacral vertebrae collapses and merges during childhood, forming a typical sacral structure. In addition, the collapse of the sacral IVD has been associated with the downregulation of Shh signaling in the NP cells. Conversely, Shh signaling activation in NP cells would reactivate dormant NP cells and initiate IVD regeneration [144].

The activation of the Shh signaling pathway was proved to facilitate the differentiation of pluripotent stem cells to notochordal cells [145]. As mentioned, ADSC-based therapy is a promising treatment for IDD, while the difficulty in inducing NP-like differentiation limits

its applications. Collagen type II promotes ADSC proliferation and differentiation toward an NP-like phenotype through the activation of the Shh signaling pathway [146] while the Shh signaling pathway inhibitor reduces the NP-like differentiation from ADSCs [147]. Similarly, the histone demethylase KDM4B also promotes the osmolarity-induced NP-like differentiation of ADSC by activating Shh signaling [148].

6.2. Ihh Signaling Pathway

The Ihh gene was first expressed in mesenchymal cells and chondrocytes of limbs. Ihh expression is confined to hypertrophic chondrocytes during skeletal growth plate development. Ihh inhibits chondrocyte maturation during long bone growth, and its dysregulation prevents proliferating chondrocytes from hypertrophic differentiation [149]. For example, mice carrying null mutations of the Ihh gene exhibit severe destruction of the growth plate at the embryonic stage with abnormalities in the proliferation and maturation of chondrocytes [150]. Additionally, conditional knockout of Ihh leads to reduced proliferation of chondroprogenitor cells and chondrocytes and the pathological processes in chondrocytes, including apoptosis, ectopic hypertrophy, and subchondral bone degeneration [151].

Moreover, blood vessels' premature infiltration, loss of normal columnar structure in growth plates, and ectopic hypertrophic chondrocyte formation were also revealed in neonatal Ihh-knockout mice. Then, after birth, Ihh knockout mice would exhibit disruption of the articular surface of long bones and premature fusion of growth plates, leading to dwarfism in the mice [152]. However, Ihh signaling also promotes chondrocyte development, according to research. For instance, Ihh-regulated parathyroid hormone-related protein (PTHrP) prevents premature growth plate cartilage hypertrophic differentiation. Meanwhile, Ihh can also stimulate the differentiation of periarticular chondrocytes to columnar chondrocytes through a PTHrP-independent pathway [153].

IVD research discovered that Ihh is significantly expressed in embryonic vertebrae endplate cartilage and chondrocytes [154]. Ihh pathway overexpression decreased chondrocytes and alterations in IVD extracellular matrix proteins. For example, upregulation of this pathway would promote the calcification in endplate cartilage and the degradation in the extracellular matrix, and inhibiting this pathway would reverse these degenerative processes [155]. In the NP, ROS would enhance Ihh expression and induce cellular apoptosis, and inhibiting the p-eIF2α/ATF4/Ihh signaling cascade axis reduces antioxidant enzyme degradation, ROS, and NP cell death [156]. Furthermore, microtubule-based cilia were found to be involved in regulating the developmental and degenerative processes of IVD. During IDD, the downregulation of intraflagellar transport protein 80 disrupts the transduction of the Ihh signaling pathway, resulting in apoptosis and disordered cellular proliferation and differentiation in IVD cells [157].

7. TGF-β Signaling Pathway

TGF-β1 is a ubiquitous growth factor that regulates various cells' proliferation, migration, differentiation, and survival. In skeletal tissues, TGF-β1 was proven to regulate osteochondral development and maintenance by affecting metabolism in cartilage and bone [158]. Notably, the TGF-β signaling pathway is critical for IVD growth and preserves IVD tissues by increasing matrix formation, limiting matrix disintegration, and reducing inflammatory responses [51]. For example, morphological deformities, including spinal kyphosis, the decreased height of endplate chondrocytes, and disordered arrangement, were revealed in Smad3 knockout mice. At the molecular expression level, the IVD in these mice exhibited a decrease in type II collagen, TGF-β1, and proteoglycan. These results also suggested a positive role of TGF-β1 in alleviating IDD [43]. Furthermore, TGF-β signaling also helps spine development during embryogenesis and IVD growth and maintenance after birth [159].

By generating glycosaminoglycan, NP cells preserve the matrix's water-binding capabilities, and activating the TGF-β-Smad3 axis would increase the synthesis of glycosaminoglycan in NP cells, thus maintaining the water content and organizational structure of IVD [45]. In inflammatory response regulation, TGF-β1 can act synergistically with the inflammatory factor inhibitor ML264 to alleviate the IL-1β-induced inflammatory response and matrix degradation in the NP tissue [49]. CCN2 is another matrix protein that has anti-inflammatory and homeostatic properties. In addition, TGF-β1 can induce CCN2 expression by activating Smad3 and AP-1 signaling pathways in NP cells, thus alleviating the IDD process [44]. TGF-β1 can also inhibit the pro-inflammatory factors expression, thus providing matrix protection and altering the NP cells' overall secretory phenotype [47].

For functional maintenance and damage repair, the TGF-β/SMAD signaling pathway can regulate the miR-455-5p/RUNX2 axis to prevent mechanically induced endplate chondrocyte degeneration [48]. Moreover, inflammation or degenerative stimulation would cause the increase in TGF-β1, which can down-regulate the expression of sodium channel proteins and thus stabilize the Na^+ flux and the proteoglycan metabolism of NP cells [42]. Similarly, scaffold protein caveolin-1 can promote IVD repair by enhancing TGF-β signal transduction [46]. Moreover, the parathyroid hormone can also activate the TGF-β/CCN2 signaling pathway expression in NP cells and maintain the height and homeostasis of IVD by enhancing the TGF-β1 activity and upregulating the ACAN level [50]. Contrarily, TGF-β1 upregulation would deteriorate the process of IDD, and inhibition of overexpressed TGF-β1 in degenerative IVD would promote the proliferation of NP cells and inhibit cellular senescence and apoptosis [41]. Regarding the cellular matrix, TGF-β1 can exacerbate the inflammatory and fibrotic manifestations of degenerating IVD [40]. Furthermore, the increased TGF-β1 activity can also increase the osmotic pressure of the extracellular environment and lead to IDD advancement [39].

The activation of the TGF-β signaling pathway can also alleviate IDD by increasing the differentiation of stem cells to NP-like cells [160]. For example, TGF-β pathway stimulation is a vital step in a protocol for directed in vitro differentiation of human pluripotent stem cells into notochord-like and NP-like cells of the disc [161]. TGF-β1 can also differentiate human ADSCs into NP cells, providing a new mechanism for its IDD-relieving effects [162]. Moreover, TGF-β signaling is also related to the homeostasis of cellularity and cellular matrix for the disc. For example, exosomal matrilin-3 from urine-derived stem cell exosomes promotes NP cell proliferation and extracellular matrix synthesis by activating TGF-β signaling [163]. Controlled release of TGF-β1 by pullulan microbeads can also lead to an increase in NP cellularity, collagen type II and aggrecan staining intensities, and the Tie^{2+} progenitor cell density in the disc [164]. Notably, the activation of the TGF-β signaling pathway can promote the pro-fibrotic effect of bleomycin on AF cells and BMSCs, which induces rapid fibrosis and height maintenance for IVD. Moreover, bleomycin-induced fibrosis also improves the stress tolerance of the degenerative disc [165].

8. Conclusions and Outlook

As mentioned above, there is a complex network among cellular signaling pathways for the IDD process. Stem cells, with regulatory roles in the signaling network, revealed great potential for biological cell-based treatment of IDD. As mentioned above, activation of PI3K/AKT, Shh, and TGF-β signaling pathways, and inhibition of NF-κB and JNK signaling pathways induce IDD remission with stem cell treatment, and the roles of Wnt/β-catenin, ERK1/2, and p38-MAPK pathways in stem-cell-treated IDD remain two-sided. Notably, IVD signaling pathway markers generally precede morphological alterations. A possible approach to improve the clinical practice of IDD-related diseases is to incorporate biomarkers in diagnosis, therapeutic intervention, and prognosis prediction. However, early IDD clinical markers were still lacking in practice. Thus, exploring biomarkers in specific signaling pathways for IDD, as well as stem cells with regulatory effects for these biomarkers, has a high potential value in clinical applications.

Author Contributions: Writing—original draft preparation, review, and editing, X.D. and H.S.; writing—review and editing, X.D., H.S. and K.L.; table preparation, S.D. All authors have read and agreed to the published version of the manuscript.

Funding: This research was funded by the Natural Science Foundation of China, grant number 82272465; the Health Science and Technology Program of Zhejiang Province, grant number 2021KY163; and the Zhejiang Provincial Natural Science Foundation of China, grant number LY20H060008.

Institutional Review Board Statement: Not applicable.

Informed Consent Statement: Not applicable.

Data Availability Statement: Not applicable.

Conflicts of Interest: The authors declare no conflict of interest.

References

1. Vos, T.; Allen, C.; Arora, M.; Barber, R.M.; Bhutta, Z.A.; Brown, A.; Carter, A.; Casey, D.C.; Charlson, F.J.; Chen, A.Z.; et al. Global, regional, and national incidence, prevalence, and years lived with disability for 310 diseases and injuries, 1990–2015: A systematic analysis for the Global Burden of Disease Study 2015. *Lancet* **2016**, *388*, 1545–1602. [CrossRef]
2. Clark, S.; Horton, R. Low back pain: A major global challenge. *Lancet* **2018**, *391*, 2302. [CrossRef] [PubMed]
3. Rogerson, A.; Aidlen, J.; Jenis, L.G. Persistent radiculopathy after surgical treatment for lumbar disc herniation: Causes and treatment options. *Int. Orthop.* **2019**, *43*, 969–973. [CrossRef] [PubMed]
4. Feng, Z.; Hu, X.; Zheng, Q.; Battié, M.; Chen, Z.; Wang, Y. Cartilaginous endplate avulsion is associated with modic changes and endplate defects, and residual back and leg pain following lumbar discectomy. *Osteoarthr. Cartil.* **2021**, *29*, 707–717. [CrossRef]
5. Francisco, V.; Pino, J.; González-Gay, M.; Lago, F.; Karppinen, J.; Tervonen, O.; Mobasheri, A.; Gualillo, O. A new immunometabolic perspective of intervertebral disc degeneration. *Nat. Rev. Rheumatol.* **2022**, *18*, 47–60. [CrossRef] [PubMed]
6. Lang, G.; Liu, Y.; Geries, J.; Zhou, J.; Kubosch, D.; Südkamp, N.; Richards, R.G.; Alini, M.; Grad, S.; Li, Z. An intervertebral disc whole organ culture system to investigate proinflammatory and degenerative disc disease condition. *J. Tissue Eng. Regen. Med.* **2018**, *12*, e2051–e2061. [CrossRef]
7. Li, Z.; Ye, D.; Dai, L.; Xu, Y.; Wu, H.; Luo, W.; Liu, Y.; Yao, X.; Wang, P.; Miao, H.; et al. Single-Cell RNA Sequencing Reveals the Difference in Human Normal and Degenerative Nucleus Pulposus Tissue Profiles and Cellular Interactions. *Front. Cell Dev. Biol.* **2022**, *10*, 910626. [CrossRef]
8. Costa, L.A.; Eiro, N.; Fraile, M.; Gonzalez, L.O.; Saá, J.; Garcia-Portabella, P.; Vega, B.; Schneider, J.; Vizoso, F.J. Functional heterogeneity of mesenchymal stem cells from natural niches to culture conditions: Implications for further clinical uses. *Cell. Mol. Life Sci.* **2021**, *78*, 447–467. [CrossRef]
9. Elashry, M.I.; Kinde, M.; Klymiuk, M.C.; Eldaey, A.; Wenisch, S.; Arnhold, S. The effect of hypoxia on myogenic differentiation and multipotency of the skeletal muscle-derived stem cells in mice. *Stem Cell Res. Ther.* **2022**, *13*, 56. [CrossRef]
10. Wu, Z.-L.; Xie, Q.-Q.; Liu, T.-C.; Yang, X.; Zhang, G.-Z.; Zhang, H.-H. Role of the Wnt pathway in the formation, development, and degeneration of intervertebral discs. *Pathol. Res. Pract.* **2021**, *220*, 153366. [CrossRef]
11. Colombier, P.; Halgand, B.; Chédeville, C.; Chariau, C.; François-Campion, V.; Kilens, S.; Vedrenne, N.; Clouet, J.; David, L.; Guicheux, J.; et al. NOTO Transcription Factor Directs Human Induced Pluripotent Stem Cell-Derived Mesendoderm Progenitors to a Notochordal Fate. *Cells* **2020**, *9*, 509. [CrossRef] [PubMed]
12. Kondo, N.; Yuasa, T.; Shimono, K.; Tung, W.; Okabe, T.; Yasuhara, R.; Pacifici, M.; Zhang, Y.; Iwamoto, M.; Enomoto-Iwamoto, M. Intervertebral disc development is regulated by Wnt/beta-catenin signaling. *Spine* **2011**, *36*, E513–E518. [CrossRef] [PubMed]
13. Hiyama, A.; Morita, K.; Sakai, D.; Watanabe, M. CCN family member 2/connective tissue growth factor (CCN2/CTGF) is regulated by Wnt-beta-catenin signaling in nucleus pulposus cells. *Arthritis Res. Ther.* **2018**, *20*, 217. [CrossRef] [PubMed]
14. Iwata, M.; Aikawa, T.; Hakozaki, T.; Arai, K.; Ochi, H.; Haro, H.; Tagawa, M.; Asou, Y.; Hara, Y. Enhancement of Runx2 expression is potentially linked to beta-catenin accumulation in canine intervertebral disc degeneration. *J. Cell. Physiol.* **2015**, *230*, 180–190. [CrossRef] [PubMed]
15. Wang, M.; Tang, D.; Shu, B.; Wang, B.; Jin, H.; Hao, S.; Dresser, K.A.; Shen, J.; Im, H.-J.; Sampson, E.R.; et al. Conditional activation of beta-catenin signaling in mice leads to severe defects in intervertebral disc tissue. *Arthritis Rheum.* **2012**, *64*, 2611–2623. [CrossRef]
16. Zhan, S.; Wang, K.; Song, Y.; Li, S.; Yin, H.; Luo, R.; Liao, Z.; Wu, X.; Zhang, Y.; Yang, C. Long non-coding RNA HOTAIR modulates intervertebral disc degenerative changes via Wnt/beta-catenin pathway. *Arthritis Res. Ther.* **2019**, *21*, 201. [CrossRef] [PubMed]
17. Hiyama, A.; Yokoyama, K.; Nukaga, T.; Sakai, D.; Mochida, J. A complex interaction between Wnt signaling and TNF-alpha in nucleus pulposus cells. *Arthritis Res. Ther.* **2013**, *15*, R189. [CrossRef]
18. Penkov, D.; Ni, R.; Else, C.; Piñol-Roma, S.; Ramirez, F.; Tanaka, S. Cloning of a human gene closely related to the genes coding for the c-myc single-strand binding proteins. *Gene* **2000**, *243*, 27–36. [CrossRef]
19. Wang, J.J.; Liu, X.Y.; Du, W.; Liu, J.Q.; Sun, B.; Zheng, Y.P. RBMS3 delays disc degeneration by inhibiting Wnt/beta-catenin signaling pathway. *Eur. Rev. Med. Pharmacol.* **2020**, *24*, 499–507. [CrossRef]
20. Fang, F.; Jiang, D. IL-1beta/HMGB1 signalling promotes the inflammatory cytokines release via TLR signalling in human intervertebral disc cells. *Biosci. Rep.* **2016**, *36*, e00379. [CrossRef]

21. Feng, C.; He, J.; Zhang, Y.; Lan, M.; Yang, M.; Liu, H.; Huang, B.; Pan, Y.; Zhou, Y. Collagen-derived N-acetylated proline-glycine-proline upregulates the expression of pro-inflammatory cytokines and extracellular matrix proteases in nucleus pulposus cells via the NF-kappaB and MAPK signaling pathways. *Int. J. Mol. Med.* **2017**, *40*, 164–174. [CrossRef]
22. Feng, C.; Zhang, Y.; Yang, M.; Lan, M.; Liu, H.; Huang, B.; Zhou, Y. Oxygen-Sensing Nox4 Generates Genotoxic ROS to Induce Premature Senescence of Nucleus Pulposus Cells through MAPK and NF-kappaB Pathways. *Oxid. Med. Cell. Longev.* **2017**, *2017*, 7426458. [CrossRef] [PubMed]
23. Shen, L.; Xiao, Y.; Wu, Q.; Liu, L.; Zhang, C.; Pan, X. TLR4/NF-kappaB axis signaling pathway-dependent up-regulation of miR-625-5p contributes to human intervertebral disc degeneration by targeting COL1A1. *Am. J. Transl. Res.* **2019**, *11*, 1374–1388. [PubMed]
24. Sun, Y.; Leng, P.; Song, M.; Li, D.; Guo, P.; Xu, X.; Gao, H.; Li, Z.; Li, C.; Zhang, H. Piezo1 activates the NLRP3 inflammasome in nucleus pulposus cell-mediated by Ca^{2+}/NF-kappaB pathway. *Int. Immunopharmacol.* **2020**, *85*, 106681. [CrossRef] [PubMed]
25. Du, X.-F.; Cui, H.-T.; Pan, H.-H.; Long, J.; Cui, H.-W.; Chen, S.-L.; Wang, J.-R.; Li, Z.-M.; Liu, H.; Huang, Y.-C.; et al. Role of the miR-133a-5p/FBXO6 axis in the regulation of intervertebral disc degeneration. *J. Orthop. Transl.* **2021**, *29*, 123–133. [CrossRef]
26. Guo, S.; Su, Q.; Wen, J.; Zhu, K.; Tan, J.; Fu, Q.; Sun, G. S100A9 induces nucleus pulposus cell degeneration through activation of the NF-kappaB signaling pathway. *J. Cell. Mol. Med.* **2021**, *25*, 4709–4720. [CrossRef]
27. Li, F.; Sun, X.; Zheng, B.; Sun, K.; Zhu, J.; Ji, C.; Lin, F.; Huan, L.; Luo, X.; Yan, C.; et al. Arginase II Promotes Intervertebral Disc Degeneration Through Exacerbating Senescence and Apoptosis Caused by Oxidative Stress and Inflammation via the NF-kappaB Pathway. *Front. Cell Dev. Biol.* **2021**, *9*, 737809. [CrossRef]
28. Sun, K.; Zhu, J.; Yan, C.; Li, F.; Kong, F.; Sun, J.; Sun, X.; Shi, J.; Wang, Y. CGRP Regulates Nucleus Pulposus Cell Apoptosis and Inflammation via the MAPK/NF-kappaB Signaling Pathways during Intervertebral Disc Degeneration. *Oxid. Med. Cell. Longev.* **2021**, *2021*, 2958584. [CrossRef]
29. Zhang, G.Z.; Liu, M.Q.; Chen, H.W.; Wu, Z.; Gao, Y.; Ma, Z.; He, X.; Kang, X. NF-kappaB signalling pathways in nucleus pulposus cell function and intervertebral disc degeneration. *Cell Prolif.* **2021**, *54*, e13057. [CrossRef]
30. Cheng, C.-C.; Uchiyama, Y.; Hiyama, A.; Gajghate, S.; Shapiro, I.M.; Risbud, M.V. PI3K/AKT regulates aggrecan gene expression by modulating Sox9 expression and activity in nucleus pulposus cells of the intervertebral disc. *J. Cell. Physiol.* **2009**, *221*, 668–676. [CrossRef]
31. Xu, D.; Jin, H.; Wen, J.; Chen, J.; Chen, D.; Cai, N.; Wang, Y.; Wang, J.; Chen, Y.; Zhang, X.; et al. Hydrogen sulfide protects against endoplasmic reticulum stress and mitochondrial injury in nucleus pulposus cells and ameliorates intervertebral disc degeneration. *Pharmacol. Res.* **2017**, *117*, 357–369. [CrossRef] [PubMed]
32. Yang, Y.; Wang, X.; Liu, Z.; Xiao, X.; Hu, W.; Sun, Z. Osteogenic protein-1 attenuates nucleus pulposus cell apoptosis through activating the PI3K/Akt/mTOR pathway in a hyperosmotic culture. *Biosci. Rep.* **2018**, *38*, BSR20181708. [CrossRef] [PubMed]
33. Tan, Y.; Yao, X.; Dai, Z.; Wang, Y.; Lv, G. Bone morphogenetic protein 2 alleviated intervertebral disc degeneration through mediating the degradation of ECM and apoptosis of nucleus pulposus cells via the PI3K/Akt pathway. *Int. J. Mol. Med.* **2019**, *43*, 583–592. [CrossRef] [PubMed]
34. Gao, X.-W.; Su, X.-T.; Lu, Z.-H.; Ou, J. 17beta-Estradiol Prevents Extracellular Matrix Degradation by Downregulating MMP3 Expression via PI3K/Akt/FOXO3 Pathway. *Spine* **2020**, *45*, 292–299. [CrossRef] [PubMed]
35. Liu, W.; Niu, F.; Sha, H.; Liu, L.D.; Lv, Z.S.; Gong, W.Q.; Yan, M. Apelin-13/APJ system delays intervertebral disc degeneration by activating the PI3K/AKT signaling pathway. *Eur. Rev. Med. Pharmacol.* **2020**, *24*, 2820–2828. [CrossRef]
36. Nan, L.-P.; Wang, F.; Liu, Y.; Wu, Z.; Feng, X.-M.; Liu, J.-J.; Zhang, L. 6-gingerol protects nucleus pulposus-derived mesenchymal stem cells from oxidative injury by activating autophagy. *World J. Stem Cells* **2020**, *12*, 1603–1622. [CrossRef]
37. Qi, W.; Ren, D.; Wang, P.; Song, Z.; Wu, H.; Yao, S.; Geng, L.; Su, Y.; Bai, X. Upregulation of Sirt1 by tyrosol suppresses apoptosis and inflammation and modulates extracellular matrix remodeling in interleukin-1beta-stimulated human nucleus pulposus cells through activation of PI3K/Akt pathway. *Int. Immunopharmacol.* **2020**, *88*, 106904. [CrossRef]
38. Luo, L.; Jian, X.; Sun, H.; Qin, J.; Wang, Y.; Zhang, J.; Shen, Z.; Yang, D.; Li, C.; Zhao, P.; et al. Cartilage endplate stem cells inhibit intervertebral disc degeneration by releasing exosomes to nucleus pulposus cells to activate Akt/autophagy. *Stem Cells* **2021**, *39*, 467–481. [CrossRef]
39. Bian, Q.; Ma, L.; Jain, A.; Crane, J.L.; Kebaish, K.; Wan, M.; Zhang, Z.; Guo, X.E.; Sponseller, P.D.; Séguin, C.A.; et al. Mechanosignaling activation of TGFbeta maintains intervertebral disc homeostasis. *Bone Res.* **2017**, *5*, 17008. [CrossRef]
40. Cui, L.; Wei, H.; Li, Z.M.; Dong, X.B.; Wang, P.Y. TGF-beta1 aggravates degenerative nucleus pulposus cells inflammation and fibrosis through the upregulation of angiopoietin-like protein 2 expression. *Eur. Rev. Med. Pharmacol.* **2020**, *24*, 12025–12033. [CrossRef]
41. Li, H.; Li, W.; Liang, B.; Wei, J.; Yin, D.; Fan, Q. Role of AP-2alpha/TGF-beta1/Smad3 axis in rats with intervertebral disc degeneration. *Life Sci.* **2020**, *263*, 118567. [CrossRef] [PubMed]
42. Uchiyama, Y.; Guttapalli, A.; Gajghate, S.; Mochida, J.; Shapiro, I.M.; Risbud, M.V. SMAD3 functions as a transcriptional repressor of acid-sensing ion channel 3 (ASIC3) in nucleus pulposus cells of the intervertebral disc. *J. Bone Miner. Res.* **2008**, *23*, 1619–1628. [CrossRef] [PubMed]
43. Li, C.-G.; Liang, Q.-Q.; Zhou, Q.; Menga, E.; Cui, X.-J.; Shu, B.; Zhou, C.-J.; Shi, Q.; Wang, Y.-J. A continuous observation of the degenerative process in the intervertebral disc of Smad3 gene knock-out mice. *Spine* **2009**, *34*, 1363–1369. [CrossRef]

44. Tran, C.M.; Markova, D.; Smith, H.E.; Susarla, B.; Ponnappan, R.K.; Anderson, D.G.; Symes, A.; Shapiro, I.M.; Risbud, M.V. Regulation of CCN2/connective tissue growth factor expression in the nucleus pulposus of the intervertebral disc: Role of Smad and activator protein 1 signaling. *Arthritis Rheum.* **2010**, *62*, 1983–1992. [CrossRef] [PubMed]
45. Wu, Q.; Wang, J.; Skubutyte, R.; Kepler, C.K.; Huang, Z.; Anderson, D.G.; Shapiro, I.M.; Risbud, M.V. Smad3 controls beta-1,3-glucuronosyltransferase 1 expression in rat nucleus pulposus cells: Implications of dysregulated expression in disc disease. *Arthritis Rheum.* **2012**, *64*, 3324–3333. [CrossRef] [PubMed]
46. Bach, F.C.; Zhang, Y.; Miranda-Bedate, A.; Verdonschot, L.C.; Bergknut, N.; Creemers, L.B.; Ito, K.; Sakai, D.; Chan, D.; Meij, B.P.; et al. Increased caveolin-1 in intervertebral disc degeneration facilitates repair. *Arthritis Res. Ther.* **2016**, *18*, 59. [CrossRef]
47. Tian, Y.; Yuan, W.; Li, J.; Wang, H.; Hunt, M.G.; Liu, C.; Shapiro, I.M.; Risbud, M.V. TGFbeta regulates Galectin-3 expression through canonical Smad3 signaling pathway in nucleus pulposus cells: Implications in intervertebral disc degeneration. *Matrix Biol.* **2016**, *50*, 39–52. [CrossRef]
48. Xiao, L.; Xu, S.; Xu, Y.; Liu, C.; Yang, B.; Wang, J.; Xu, H. TGF-beta/SMAD signaling inhibits intermittent cyclic mechanical tension-induced degeneration of endplate chondrocytes by regulating the miR-455-5p/RUNX2 axis. *J. Cell. Biochem.* **2018**, *119*, 10415–10425. [CrossRef]
49. Xie, Z.; Jie, Z.; Wang, G.; Sun, X.; Tang, P.; Chen, S.; Qin, A.; Wang, J.; Fan, S. TGF-beta synergizes with ML264 to block IL-1beta-induced matrix degradation mediated by Kruppel-like factor 5 in the nucleus pulposus. *Biochim. Biophys. Acta BBA-Mol. Basis Dis.* **2018**, *1864*, 579–589. [CrossRef]
50. Zheng, L.; Cao, Y.; Ni, S.; Qi, H.; Ling, Z.; Xu, X.; Zou, X.; Wu, T.; Deng, R.; Hu, B.; et al. Ciliary parathyroid hormone signaling activates transforming growth factor-beta to maintain intervertebral disc homeostasis during aging. *Bone Res.* **2018**, *6*, 21. [CrossRef]
51. Chen, S.; Liu, S.; Ma, K.; Zhao, L.; Lin, H.; Shao, Z. TGF-beta signaling in intervertebral disc health and disease. *Osteoarthr. Cartil.* **2019**, *27*, 1109–1117. [CrossRef] [PubMed]
52. Zhang, F.; Lin, F.; Xu, Z.; Huang, Z. Circular RNA ITCH promotes extracellular matrix degradation via activating Wnt/beta-catenin signaling in intervertebral disc degeneration. *Aging* **2021**, *13*, 14185–14197. [CrossRef]
53. Bai, M.; Yin, H.; Zhao, J.; Li, Y.; Wu, Y. Roles of TREM2 in degeneration of human nucleus pulposus cells via NF-kappaB p65. *J. Cell. Biochem.* **2018**, *119*, 8784–8796. [CrossRef] [PubMed]
54. Li, Y.; Wei, K.; Ding, Y.; Ahati, P.; Xu, H.; Fang, H.; Wang, H. M2a Macrophage-Secreted CHI3L1 Promotes Extracellular Matrix Metabolic Imbalances via Activation of IL-13Ralpha2/MAPK Pathway in Rat Intervertebral Disc Degeneration. *Front. Immunol.* **2021**, *12*, 666361. [CrossRef] [PubMed]
55. Li, Z.; Wang, J.; Deng, X.; Huang, D.; Shao, Z.; Ma, K. Compression stress induces nucleus pulposus cell autophagy by inhibition of the PI3K/AKT/mTOR pathway and activation of the JNK pathway. *Connect. Tissue Res.* **2021**, *62*, 337–349. [CrossRef]
56. Jiang, Z.; Zeng, Q.; Li, D.; Ding, L.; Lu, W.; Bian, M.; Wu, J. Long non-coding RNA MALAT1 promotes high glucose-induced rat cartilage endplate cell apoptosis via the p38/MAPK signalling pathway. *Mol. Med. Rep.* **2020**, *21*, 2220–2226. [CrossRef]
57. Liu, C.; Yang, H.; Gao, F.; Li, X.; An, Y.; Wang, J.; Jin, A. Resistin Promotes Intervertebral Disc Degeneration by Upregulation of ADAMTS-5 Through p38 MAPK Signaling Pathway. *Spine* **2016**, *41*, 1414–1420. [CrossRef]
58. Ge, J.; Cheng, X.; Yuan, C.; Qian, J.; Wu, C.; Cao, C.; Yang, H.; Zhou, F.; Zou, J. Syndecan-4 is a Novel Therapeutic Target for Intervertebral Disc Degeneration via Suppressing JNK/p53 Pathway. *Int. J. Biol. Sci.* **2020**, *16*, 766–776. [CrossRef]
59. Li, J.-K.; Nie, L.; Zhao, Y.-P.; Zhang, Y.-Q.; Wang, X.; Wang, S.-S.; Liu, Y.; Zhao, H.; Cheng, L. IL-17 mediates inflammatory reactions via p38/c-Fos and JNK/c-Jun activation in an AP-1-dependent manner in human nucleus pulposus cells. *J. Transl. Med.* **2016**, *14*, 77. [CrossRef]
60. Wu, X.; Song, Y.; Liu, W.; Wang, K.; Gao, Y.; Li, S.; Duan, Z.; Shao, Z.; Yang, S.; Yang, C. IAPP modulates cellular autophagy, apoptosis, and extracellular matrix metabolism in human intervertebral disc cells. *Cell Death Discov.* **2017**, *3*, 16107. [CrossRef]
61. Shan, L.; Yang, D.; Zhu, D.; Feng, F.; Li, X. High glucose promotes annulus fibrosus cell apoptosis through activating the JNK and p38 MAPK pathways. *Biosci. Rep.* **2019**, *39*, BSR20190853. [CrossRef]
62. Cui, H.; Du, X.; Liu, C.; Chen, S.; Cui, H.; Liu, H.; Wang, J.; Zheng, Z. Visfatin promotes intervertebral disc degeneration by inducing IL-6 expression through the ERK/JNK/p38 signalling pathways. *Adipocyte* **2021**, *10*, 201–215. [CrossRef]
63. Wang, W.; Li, P.; Xu, J.; Wu, X.; Guo, Z.; Fan, L.; Song, R.; Wang, J.; Wei, L.; Teng, H. Resveratrol attenuates high glucose-induced nucleus pulposus cell apoptosis and senescence through activating the ROS-mediated PI3K/Akt pathway. *Biosci. Rep.* **2018**, *38*, BSR20171454. [CrossRef]
64. Zhao, Y.T.; Qin, Y.; Yang, J.S.; Huang, D.G.; Hu, H.M.; Wang, X.D.; Wu, S.F.; Hao, D.J. Wharton's Jelly-derived mesenchymal stem cells suppress apoptosis of nucleus pulposus cells in intervertebral disc degeneration via Wnt pathway. *Eur. Rev. Med. Pharmacol.* **2020**, *24*, 9807–9814. [CrossRef]
65. Silva, M.J.; Holguin, N. Aging aggravates intervertebral disc degeneration by regulating transcription factors toward chondrogenesis. *FASEB J.* **2020**, *34*, 1970–1982. [CrossRef]
66. Sun, C.; Lan, W.; Li, B.; Zuo, R.; Xing, H.; Liu, M.; Li, J.; Yao, Y.; Wu, J.; Tang, Y.; et al. Glucose regulates tissue-specific chondro-osteogenic differentiation of human cartilage endplate stem cells via O-GlcNAcylation of Sox9 and Runx2. *Stem Cell Res. Ther.* **2019**, *10*, 357. [CrossRef]
67. Volleman, T.N.E.; Schol, J.; Morita, K.; Sakai, D.; Watanabe, M. Wnt3a and wnt5a as Potential Chondrogenic Stimulators for Nucleus Pulposus Cell Induction: A Comprehensive Review. *Neurospine* **2020**, *17*, 19–35. [CrossRef] [PubMed]

68. Chen, Y.; Chen, Q.; Zhong, M.; Xu, C.; Wu, Y.; Chen, R. miR-637 Inhibits Osteogenic Differentiation of Human Intervertebral Disc Cartilage Endplate Stem Cells by Targeting WNT5A. *J. Investig. Surg.* **2022**, *35*, 1313–1321. [CrossRef]
69. Luo, L.; Gong, J.; Zhang, H.; Qin, J.; Li, C.; Zhang, J.; Tang, Y.; Zhang, Y.; Chen, J.; Zhou, Y.; et al. Cartilage Endplate Stem Cells Transdifferentiate Into Nucleus Pulposus Cells via Autocrine Exosomes. *Front. Cell Dev. Biol.* **2021**, *9*, 648201. [CrossRef] [PubMed]
70. Wang, B.; Xu, N.; Cao, L.; Yu, X.; Wang, S.; Liu, Q.; Wang, Y.; Xu, H.; Cao, Y. miR-31 from Mesenchymal Stem Cell-Derived Extracellular Vesicles Alleviates Intervertebral Disc Degeneration by Inhibiting NFAT5 and Upregulating the Wnt/beta-Catenin Pathway. *Stem Cells Int.* **2022**, *2022*, 2164057. [CrossRef] [PubMed]
71. Chen, H.-T.; Huang, A.-B.; He, Y.-L.; Bian, J.; Li, H.-J. Wnt11 overexpression promote adipose-derived stem cells differentiating to the nucleus pulposus-like phenotype. *Eur. Rev. Med. Pharmacol.* **2017**, *21*, 1462–1470.
72. Sen, R.; Baltimore, D. Multiple nuclear factors interact with the immunoglobulin enhancer sequences. *Cell* **1986**, *46*, 705–716. [CrossRef] [PubMed]
73. Yu, H.; Lin, L.; Zhang, Z.; Zhang, H.; Hu, H. Targeting NF-kappaB pathway for the therapy of diseases: Mechanism and clinical study. *Signal Transduct. Target. Ther.* **2020**, *5*, 209. [CrossRef]
74. Cao, C.; Zou, J.; Liu, X.; Shapiro, A.; Moral, M.; Luo, Z.; Shi, Q.; Liu, J.; Yang, H.; Ebraheim, N. Bone marrow mesenchymal stem cells slow intervertebral disc degeneration through the NF-kappaB pathway. *Spine J.* **2015**, *15*, 530–538. [CrossRef] [PubMed]
75. Yang, H.; Tian, W.; Wang, S.; Liu, X.; Wang, Z.; Hou, L.; Ge, J.; Zhang, X.; He, Z.; Wang, X. TSG-6 secreted by bone marrow mesenchymal stem cells attenuates intervertebral disc degeneration by inhibiting the TLR2/NF-kappaB signaling pathway. *Lab. Investig.* **2018**, *98*, 755–772. [CrossRef]
76. Cheng, S.; Li, X.; Jia, Z.; Lin, L.; Ying, J.; Wen, T.; Zhao, Y.; Guo, Z.; Zhao, X.; Li, D.; et al. The inflammatory cytokine TNF-alpha regulates the biological behavior of rat nucleus pulposus mesenchymal stem cells through the NF-kappaB signaling pathway in vitro. *J. Cell. Biochem.* **2019**, *120*, 13664–13679. [CrossRef] [PubMed]
77. Yang, H.; Cao, C.; Wu, C.; Yuan, C.; Gu, Q.; Shi, Q.; Zou, J. TGF-beta1 Suppresses Inflammation in Cell Therapy for Intervertebral Disc Degeneration. *Sci. Rep.* **2015**, *5*, 13254. [CrossRef]
78. Li, X.; Wu, A.; Han, C.; Chen, C.; Zhou, T.; Zhang, K.; Yang, X.; Chen, Z.; Qin, A.; Tian, H.; et al. Bone marrow-derived mesenchymal stem cells in three-dimensional co-culture attenuate degeneration of nucleus pulposus cells. *Aging* **2019**, *11*, 9167–9187. [CrossRef]
79. Zhao, J.; Zhang, L.; Lu, A.; Han, Y.; Colangelo, D.; Bukata, C.; Scibetta, A.; Yousefzadeh, M.J.; Li, X.; Gurkar, A.U.; et al. ATM is a key driver of NF-kappaB-dependent DNA-damage-induced senescence, stem cell dysfunction and aging. *Aging* **2020**, *12*, 4688–4710. [CrossRef]
80. Ni, L.; Zheng, Y.; Gong, T.; Xiu, C.; Li, K.; Saijilafu; Li, B.; Yang, H.; Chen, J. Proinflammatory macrophages promote degenerative phenotypes in rat nucleus pulpous cells partly through ERK and JNK signaling. *J. Cell. Physiol.* **2019**, *234*, 5362–5371. [CrossRef]
81. Pratsinis, H.; Kletsas, D. Organotypic Cultures of Intervertebral Disc Cells: Responses to Growth Factors and Signaling Pathways Involved. *BioMed Res. Int.* **2015**, *2015*, 427138. [CrossRef] [PubMed]
82. Pratsinis, H.; Kletsas, D. PDGF, bFGF and IGF-I stimulate the proliferation of intervertebral disc cells in vitro via the activation of the ERK and Akt signaling pathways. *Eur. Spine J.* **2007**, *16*, 1858–1866. [CrossRef]
83. Pratsinis, H.; Constantinou, V.; Pavlakis, K.; Sapkas, G.; Kletsas, D. Exogenous and autocrine growth factors stimulate human intervertebral disc cell proliferation via the ERK and Akt pathways. *J. Orthop. Res.* **2012**, *30*, 958–964. [CrossRef] [PubMed]
84. Chen, M.-H.; Sun, J.-S.; Liao, S.-Y.; Tai, P.-A.; Li, T.-C.; Chen, M.-H. Low-intensity pulsed ultrasound stimulates matrix metabolism of human annulus fibrosus cells mediated by transforming growth factor beta1 and extracellular signal-regulated kinase pathway. *Connect. Tissue Res.* **2015**, *56*, 219–227. [CrossRef]
85. Risbud, M.V.; Guttapalli, A.; Albert, T.J.; Shapiro, I.M. Hypoxia activates MAPK activity in rat nucleus pulposus cells: Regulation of integrin expression and cell survival. *Spine* **2005**, *30*, 2503–2509. [CrossRef] [PubMed]
86. Risbud, M.V.; Di Martino, A.; Guttapalli, A.; Seghatoleslami, R.; Denaro, V.; Vaccaro, A.R.; Albert, T.J.; Shapiro, I.M. Toward an optimum system for intervertebral disc organ culture: TGF-beta 3 enhances nucleus pulposus and anulus fibrosus survival and function through modulation of TGF-beta-R expression and ERK signaling. *Spine* **2006**, *31*, 884–890. [CrossRef] [PubMed]
87. Uchiyama, Y.; Cheng, C.-C.; Danielson, K.G.; Mochida, J.; Albert, T.J.; Shapiro, I.M.; Risbud, M.V. Expression of acid-sensing ion channel 3 (ASIC3) in nucleus pulposus cells of the intervertebral disc is regulated by p75NTR and ERK signaling. *J. Bone Miner. Res.* **2007**, *22*, 1996–2006. [CrossRef]
88. Saiyin, W.; Li, L.; Zhang, H.; Lu, Y.; Qin, C. Inactivation of FAM20B causes cell fate changes in annulus fibrosus of mouse intervertebral disc and disc defects via the alterations of TGF-beta and MAPK signaling pathways. *Biochim. Biophys. Acta BBA-Mol. Basis Dis.* **2019**, *1865*, 165555. [CrossRef]
89. Krupkova, O.; Sadowska, A.; Kameda, T.; Hitzl, W.; Nic Hausmann, O.; Klasen, J.; Wuertz-Kozak, K. p38 MAPK Facilitates Crosstalk between Endoplasmic Reticulum Stress and IL-6 Release in the Intervertebral Disc. *Front. Immunol.* **2018**, *9*, 1706. [CrossRef]
90. Tang, X.; Coughlin, D.; Ballatori, A.; Berg-Johansen, B.; Waldorff, E.I.; Zhang, N.; Ryaby, J.T.; Aliston, T.; Lotz, J.C. Pulsed Electromagnetic Fields Reduce Interleukin-6 Expression in Intervertebral Disc Cells Via Nuclear Factor-kappabeta and Mitogen-Activated Protein Kinase p38 Pathways. *Spine* **2019**, *44*, E1290–E1297. [CrossRef]

91. Ge, J.; Zhou, Q.; Cheng, X.; Qian, J.; Yan, Q.; Wu, C.; Chen, Y.; Yang, H.; Zou, J. The protein tyrosine kinase inhibitor, Genistein, delays intervertebral disc degeneration in rats by inhibiting the p38 pathway-mediated inflammatory response. *Aging* **2020**, *12*, 2246–2260. [CrossRef] [PubMed]
92. Wu, Y.-D.; Guo, Z.-G.; Deng, W.-J.; Wang, J.-G. SD0006 promotes nucleus pulposus cell proliferation via the p38MAPK/HDAC4 pathway. *Eur. Rev. Med. Pharmacol.* **2020**, *24*, 10966–10974. [CrossRef]
93. Cui, S.; Zhang, L. microRNA-129-5p shuttled by mesenchymal stem cell-derived extracellular vesicles alleviates intervertebral disc degeneration via blockade of LRG1-mediated p38 MAPK activation. *J. Tissue Eng.* **2021**, *12*, 1758511983. [CrossRef] [PubMed]
94. Dai, S.; Shi, X.; Qin, R.; Zhang, X.; Xu, F.; Yang, H. Sodium Tanshinone IIA Sulfonate Ameliorates Injury-Induced Oxidative Stress and Intervertebral Disc Degeneration in Rats by Inhibiting p38 MAPK Signaling Pathway. *Oxid. Med. Cell. Longev.* **2021**, *2021*, 5556122. [CrossRef] [PubMed]
95. Xiang, Q.; Cheng, Z.; Wang, J.; Feng, X.; Hua, W.; Luo, R.; Wang, B.; Liao, Z.; Ma, L.; Li, G.; et al. Allicin Attenuated Advanced Oxidation Protein Product-Induced Oxidative Stress and Mitochondrial Apoptosis in Human Nucleus Pulposus Cells. *Oxid. Med. Cell. Longev.* **2020**, *2020*, 6685043. [CrossRef]
96. Rannou, F.; Lee, T.-S.; Zhou, R.-H.; Chin, J.; Lotz, J.C.; Mayoux-Benhamou, M.-A.; Barbet, J.P.; Chevrot, A.; Shyy, J.Y.-J. Intervertebral disc degeneration: The role of the mitochondrial pathway in annulus fibrosus cell apoptosis induced by overload. *Am. J. Pathol.* **2004**, *164*, 915–924. [CrossRef]
97. Pang, L.; Li, P.; Zhang, R.; Xu, Y.; Song, L.; Zhou, Q. Role of p38-MAPK pathway in the effects of high-magnitude compression on nucleus pulposus cell senescence in a disc perfusion culture. *Biosci. Rep.* **2017**, *37*, BSR20170718. [CrossRef]
98. Chen, X.; Zhang, P.; Ma, X. Rab7 delays intervertebral disc degeneration through the inhibition of the p38MAPK pathway. *Biochem. Biophys. Res. Commun.* **2019**, *514*, 835–841. [CrossRef]
99. Li, K.; Li, Y.; Ma, Z.; Zhao, J. Crocin exerts anti-inflammatory and anti-catabolic effects on rat intervertebral discs by suppressing the activation of JNK. *Int. J. Mol. Med.* **2015**, *36*, 1291–1299. [CrossRef]
100. Lu, S.; Song, Y.; Luo, R.; Li, S.; Li, G.; Wang, K.; Liao, Z.; Wang, B.; Ke, W.; Xiang, Q.; et al. Ferroportin-Dependent Iron Homeostasis Protects against Oxidative Stress-Induced Nucleus Pulposus Cell Ferroptosis and Ameliorates Intervertebral Disc Degeneration In Vivo. *Oxid. Med. Cell. Longev.* **2021**, *2021*, 6670497. [CrossRef]
101. Park, J.-B.; Park, I.-J.; Park, E.-Y. Accelerated premature stress-induced senescence of young annulus fibrosus cells of rats by high glucose-induced oxidative stress. *Int. Orthop.* **2014**, *38*, 1311–1320. [CrossRef]
102. Veras, M.A.; Tenn, N.A.; Kuljanin, M.; Lajoie, G.A.; Hammond, J.R.; Dixon, S.J.; Séguin, C.A. Loss of ENT1 increases cell proliferation in the annulus fibrosus of the intervertebral disc. *J. Cell. Physiol.* **2019**, *234*, 13705–13719. [CrossRef] [PubMed]
103. Chen, Z.; Zhang, W.; Zhang, N.; Zhou, Y.; Hu, G.; Xue, M.; Liu, J.; Li, Y. Down-regulation of insulin-like growth factor binding protein 5 is involved in intervertebral disc degeneration via the ERK signalling pathway. *J. Cell. Mol. Med.* **2019**, *23*, 6368–6377. [CrossRef] [PubMed]
104. Liu, W.; Liu, D.; Zheng, J.; Shi, P.; Chou, P.-H.; Oh, C.; Chen, D.; An, H.S.; Chee, A. Annulus fibrosus cells express and utilize C-C chemokine receptor 5 (CCR5) for migration. *Spine J.* **2017**, *17*, 720–726. [CrossRef] [PubMed]
105. Zhang, H.-J.; Liao, H.-Y.; Bai, D.-Y.; Wang, Z.-Q.; Xie, X.-W. MAPK /ERK signaling pathway: A potential target for the treatment of intervertebral disc degeneration. *Biomed. Pharmacother.* **2021**, *143*, 112170. [CrossRef]
106. Li, H.; Wang, J.; Li, F.; Chen, G.; Chen, Q. The Influence of Hyperosmolarity in the Intervertebral Disc on the Proliferation and Chondrogenic Differentiation of Nucleus Pulposus-Derived Mesenchymal Stem Cells. *Cells Tissues Organs* **2018**, *205*, 178–188. [CrossRef] [PubMed]
107. Tao, Y.; Zhou, X.; Liang, C.; Li, H.; Han, B.; Li, F.; Chen, Q. TGF-beta3 and IGF-1 synergy ameliorates nucleus pulposus mesenchymal stem cell differentiation towards the nucleus pulposus cell type through MAPK/ERK signaling. *Growth Factors* **2015**, *33*, 326–336. [CrossRef]
108. Zhu, Z.; Xing, H.; Tang, R.; Qian, S.; He, S.; Hu, Q.; Zhang, N. The preconditioning of lithium promotes mesenchymal stem cell-based therapy for the degenerated intervertebral disc via upregulating cellular ROS. *Stem Cell Res. Ther.* **2021**, *12*, 239. [CrossRef]
109. Han, L.; Wang, Z.; Chen, H.; Li, J.; Zhang, S.; Zhang, S.; Shao, S.; Zhang, Y.; Shen, C.; Tao, H. Sa12b-Modified Functional Self-Assembling Peptide Hydrogel Enhances the Biological Activity of Nucleus Pulposus Mesenchymal Stem Cells by Inhibiting Acid-Sensing Ion Channels. *Front. Cell Dev. Biol.* **2022**, *10*, 822501. [CrossRef]
110. Tao, Y.; Zhou, X.; Liu, D.; Li, H.; Liang, C.; Li, F.; Chen, Q. Proportion of collagen type II in the extracellular matrix promotes the differentiation of human adipose-derived mesenchymal stem cells into nucleus pulposus cells. *Biofactors* **2016**, *42*, 212–223.
111. Studer, R.K.; Aboka, A.M.; Gilbertson, L.G.; Georgescu, H.; Sowa, G.; Vo, N.; Kang, J.D. p38 MAPK inhibition in nucleus pulposus cells: A potential target for treating intervertebral disc degeneration. *Spine* **2007**, *32*, 2827–2833. [CrossRef] [PubMed]
112. Liang, W.; Fang, D.; Ye, D.; Zou, L.; Shen, Y.; Dai, L.; Xu, J. Differential expression of extracellular-signal-regulated kinase 5 (ERK5) in normal and degenerated human nucleus pulposus tissues and cells. *Biochem. Biophys. Res. Commun.* **2014**, *449*, 466–470. [CrossRef]
113. Qi, L.; Wang, R.; Shi, Q.; Yuan, M.; Jin, M.; Li, D. Umbilical cord mesenchymal stem cell conditioned medium restored the expression of collagen II and aggrecan in nucleus pulposus mesenchymal stem cells exposed to high glucose. *J. Bone Miner. Metab.* **2019**, *37*, 455–466. [CrossRef] [PubMed]

114. Zhao, Y.; Qin, Y.; Wu, S.; Huang, D.; Hu, H.; Zhang, X.; Hao, D. Mesenchymal stem cells regulate inflammatory milieu within degenerative nucleus pulposus cells via p38 MAPK pathway. *Exp. Ther. Med.* **2020**, *20*, 22. [CrossRef] [PubMed]
115. Risbud, M.V.; Albert, T.J.; Guttapalli, A.; Vresilovic, E.J.; Hillibrand, A.S.; Vaccaro, A.R.; Shapiro, I.M. Differentiation of mesenchymal stem cells towards a nucleus pulposus-like phenotype in vitro: Implications for cell-based transplantation therapy. *Spine* **2004**, *29*, 2627–2632. [CrossRef] [PubMed]
116. Li, W.; Huang, C.; Ma, T.; Wang, J.; Liu, W.; Yan, J.; Sheng, G.; Zhang, R.; Wu, H.; Liu, C. Low-frequency electromagnetic fields combined with tissue engineering techniques accelerate intervertebral fusion. *Stem Cell Res. Ther.* **2021**, *12*, 143. [CrossRef]
117. Wang, T.; Zhao, H.; Jing, S.; Fan, Y.; Sheng, G.; Ding, Q.; Liu, C.; Wu, H.; Liu, Y. Magnetofection of miR-21 promoted by electromagnetic field and iron oxide nanoparticles via the p38 MAPK pathway contributes to osteogenesis and angiogenesis for intervertebral fusion. *J. Nanobiotechnol.* **2023**, *21*, 27. [CrossRef]
118. Cannata, F.; Vadalà, G.; Ambrosio, L.; Fallucca, S.; Napoli, N.; Papalia, R.; Pozzilli, P.; Denaro, V. Intervertebral disc degeneration: A focus on obesity and type 2 diabetes. *Diabetes Metab. Res. Rev.* **2020**, *36*, e3224. [CrossRef]
119. Zhang, Y.; Liu, C.; Li, Y.; Xu, H. Mechanism of the Mitogen-Activated Protein Kinases/Mammalian Target of Rapamycin Pathway in the Process of Cartilage Endplate Stem Cell Degeneration Induced by Tension Load. *Glob. Spine J.* **2022**, 1270943190. [CrossRef]
120. Fan, P.; Yu, X.-Y.; Xie, X.-H.; Chen, C.-H.; Zhang, P.; Yang, C.; Peng, X.; Wang, Y.-T. Mitophagy is a protective response against oxidative damage in bone marrow mesenchymal stem cells. *Life Sci.* **2019**, *229*, 36–45. [CrossRef]
121. Zhang, S.; Liu, W.; Wang, P.; Hu, B.; Lv, X.; Chen, S.; Wang, B.; Shao, Z. Activation of HSP70 impedes tert-butyl hydroperoxide (t-BHP)-induced apoptosis and senescence of human nucleus pulposus stem cells via inhibiting the JNK/c-Jun pathway. *Mol. Cell. Biochem.* **2021**, *476*, 1979–1994. [CrossRef] [PubMed]
122. Fruman, D.A.; Chiu, H.; Hopkins, B.D.; Bagrodia, S.; Cantley, L.C.; Abraham, R.T.; Fruman, D.A.; Chiu, H.; Hopkins, B.D.; Bagrodia, S.; et al. The PI3K Pathway in Human Disease. *Cell* **2017**, *170*, 605–635. [CrossRef] [PubMed]
123. Risbud, M.V.; Fertala, J.; Vresilovic, E.J.; Albert, T.J.; Shapiro, I.M. Nucleus pulposus cells upregulate PI3K/Akt and MEK/ERK signaling pathways under hypoxic conditions and resist apoptosis induced by serum withdrawal. *Spine* **2005**, *30*, 882–889. [CrossRef] [PubMed]
124. Wang, D.; Chen, Y.; Cao, S.; Ren, P.; Shi, H.; Li, H.; Xie, L.; Huang, W.; Shi, B.; Han, J. Cyclic Mechanical Stretch Ameliorates the Degeneration of Nucleus Pulposus Cells through Promoting the ITGA2/PI3K/AKT Signaling Pathway. *Oxid. Med. Cell. Longev.* **2021**, *2021*, 6699326. [CrossRef] [PubMed]
125. Zhang, X.; Hu, Z.; Hao, J.; Shen, J. Low Intensity Pulsed Ultrasound Promotes the Extracellular Matrix Synthesis of Degenerative Human Nucleus Pulposus Cells Through FAK/PI3K/Akt Pathway. *Spine* **2016**, *41*, E248–E254. [CrossRef]
126. Jing, D.; Wu, W.; Deng, X.; Peng, Y.; Yang, W.; Huang, D.; Shao, Z.; Zheng, D. FoxO1a mediated cadmium-induced annulus fibrosus cells apoptosis contributes to intervertebral disc degeneration in smoking. *J. Cell. Physiol.* **2021**, *236*, 677–687. [CrossRef]
127. Zhang, H.; Wang, P.; Zhang, X.; Zhao, W.; Ren, H.; Hu, Z. SDF1/CXCR4 axis facilitates the angiogenesis via activating the PI3K/AKT pathway in degenerated discs. *Mol. Med. Rep.* **2020**, *22*, 4163–4172. [CrossRef]
128. Luo, L.; Gong, J.; Wang, Z.; Liu, Y.; Cao, J.; Qin, J.; Zuo, R.; Zhang, H.; Wang, S.; Zhao, P.; et al. Injectable cartilage matrix hydrogel loaded with cartilage endplate stem cells engineered to release exosomes for non-invasive treatment of intervertebral disc degeneration. *Bioact. Mater.* **2022**, *15*, 29–43. [CrossRef]
129. Zhuang, Y.; Song, S.; Xiao, D.; Liu, X.; Han, X.; Du, S.; Li, Y.; He, Y.; Zhang, S. Exosomes Secreted by Nucleus Pulposus Stem Cells Derived From Degenerative Intervertebral Disc Exacerbate Annulus Fibrosus Cell Degradation via Let-7b-5p. *Front. Mol. Biosci.* **2021**, *8*, 766115. [CrossRef]
130. Sako, K.; Sakai, D.; Nakamura, Y.; Schol, J.; Matsushita, E.; Warita, T.; Horikita, N.; Sato, M.; Watanabe, M. Effect of Whole Tissue Culture and Basic Fibroblast Growth Factor on Maintenance of Tie2 Molecule Expression in Human Nucleus Pulposus Cells. *Int. J. Mol. Sci.* **2021**, *22*, 4723. [CrossRef]
131. Wang, J.-W.; Zhu, L.; Shi, P.-Z.; Wang, P.-C.; Dai, Y.; Wang, Y.-X.; Lu, X.-H.; Cheng, X.-F.; Feng, X.-M.; Zhang, L. 1,25(OH)2D3 Mitigates Oxidative Stress-Induced Damage to Nucleus Pulposus-Derived Mesenchymal Stem Cells through PI3K/Akt Pathway. *Oxid. Med. Cell. Longev.* **2022**, *2022*, 1427110. [CrossRef] [PubMed]
132. Liu, M.-H.; Bian, B.-S.; Cui, X.; Liu, L.-T.; Liu, H.; Huang, B.; Cui, Y.-H.; Bian, X.-W.; Zhou, Y. Mesenchymal stem cells regulate mechanical properties of human degenerated nucleus pulposus cells through SDF-1/CXCR4/AKT axis. *Biochim. Biophys. Acta* **2016**, *1863*, 1961–1968. [CrossRef]
133. Cheng, X.; Zhang, G.; Zhang, L.; Hu, Y.; Zhang, K.; Sun, X.; Zhao, C.; Li, H.; Li, Y.M.; Zhao, J. Mesenchymal stem cells deliver exogenous miR-21 via exosomes to inhibit nucleus pulposus cell apoptosis and reduce intervertebral disc degeneration. *J. Cell. Mol. Med.* **2018**, *22*, 261–276. [CrossRef] [PubMed]
134. Xiang, H.; Su, W.; Wu, X.; Chen, W.; Cong, W.; Yang, S.; Liu, C.; Qiu, C.; Yang, S.-Y.; Wang, Y.; et al. Exosomes Derived from Human Urine-Derived Stem Cells Inhibit Intervertebral Disc Degeneration by Ameliorating Endoplasmic Reticulum Stress. *Oxid. Med. Cell. Longev.* **2020**, *2020*, 6697577. [CrossRef]
135. Liao, Z.; Luo, R.; Li, G.; Song, Y.; Zhan, S.; Zhao, K.; Hua, W.; Zhang, Y.; Wu, X.; Yang, C. Exosomes from mesenchymal stem cells modulate endoplasmic reticulum stress to protect against nucleus pulposus cell death and ameliorate intervertebral disc degeneration in vivo. *Theranostics* **2019**, *9*, 4084–4100. [CrossRef] [PubMed]
136. Zhou, H.; Zhang, L.; Chen, Y.; Zhu, C.; Chen, F.; Li, A. Research progress on the hedgehog signalling pathway in regulating bone formation and homeostasis. *Cell Prolif.* **2022**, *55*, e13162. [CrossRef]

137. Haraguchi, R.; Kitazawa, R.; Kohara, Y.; Ikedo, A.; Imai, Y. Recent Insights into Long Bone Development: Central Role of Hedgehog Signaling Pathway in Regulating Growth Plate. *Int. J. Mol. Sci.* **2019**, *20*, 5840. [CrossRef]
138. Bach, F.C.; de Rooij, K.M.; Riemers, F.M.; Snuggs, J.W.; Jong, W.A.M.; Zhang, Y.; Creemers, L.B.; Chan, D.; Le Maitre, C.; Tryfonidou, M.A. Hedgehog proteins and parathyroid hormone-related protein are involved in intervertebral disc maturation, degeneration, and calcification. *JOR Spine* **2019**, *2*, e1071. [CrossRef]
139. Rajesh, D.; Dahia, C.L. Role of Sonic Hedgehog Signaling Pathway in Intervertebral Disc Formation and Maintenance. *Curr. Mol. Biol. Rep.* **2018**, *4*, 173–179. [CrossRef]
140. Dahia, C.L.; Mahoney, E.; Wylie, C. Shh signaling from the nucleus pulposus is required for the postnatal growth and differentiation of the mouse intervertebral disc. *PLoS ONE* **2012**, *7*, e35944. [CrossRef]
141. Winkler, T.; Mahoney, E.J.; Sinner, D.; Wylie, C.C.; Dahia, C.L. Wnt signaling activates Shh signaling in early postnatal intervertebral discs, and re-activates Shh signaling in old discs in the mouse. *PLoS ONE* **2014**, *9*, e98444. [CrossRef] [PubMed]
142. Choi, K.S.; Harfe, B.D. Hedgehog signaling is required for formation of the notochord sheath and patterning of nuclei pulposi within the intervertebral discs. *Proc. Natl. Acad. Sci. USA* **2011**, *108*, 9484–9489. [CrossRef] [PubMed]
143. Choi, K.S.; Lee, C.; Harfe, B.D. Sonic hedgehog in the notochord is sufficient for patterning of the intervertebral discs. *Mech. Dev.* **2012**, *129*, 255–262. [CrossRef] [PubMed]
144. Bonavita, R.; Vincent, K.; Pinelli, R.; Dahia, C.L. Formation of the sacrum requires down-regulation of sonic hedgehog signaling in the sacral intervertebral discs. *Biol. Open* **2018**, *7*, bio035592. [CrossRef] [PubMed]
145. Diaz-Hernandez, M.E.; Khan, N.M.; Trochez, C.M.; Yoon, T.; Maye, P.; Presciutti, S.M.; Gibson, G.; Drissi, H. Derivation of notochordal cells from human embryonic stem cells reveals unique regulatory networks by single cell-transcriptomics. *J. Cell. Physiol.* **2020**, *235*, 5241–5255. [CrossRef]
146. Zhou, X.; Tao, Y.; Chen, E.; Wang, J.; Fang, W.; Zhao, T.; Liang, C.; Li, F.; Chen, Q. Genipin-cross-linked type II collagen scaffold promotes the differentiation of adipose-derived stem cells into nucleus pulposus-like cells. *J. Biomed. Mater. Res. Part A* **2018**, *106*, 1258–1268. [CrossRef]
147. Zhou, X.; Ma, C.; Hu, B.; Tao, Y.; Wang, J.; Huang, X.; Zhao, T.; Han, B.; Li, H.; Liang, C.; et al. FoxA2 regulates the type II collagen-induced nucleus pulposus-like differentiation of adipose-derived stem cells by activation of the Shh signaling pathway. *FASEB J.* **2018**, *32*, fj201800373R. [CrossRef]
148. Zhang, Y.; Wang, Y.; Zhou, X.; Wang, J.; Shi, M.; Wang, J.; Li, F.; Chen, Q. Osmolarity controls the differentiation of adipose-derived stem cells into nucleus pulposus cells via histone demethylase KDM4B. *Mol. Cell. Biochem.* **2020**, *472*, 157–171. [CrossRef]
149. Vortkamp, A.; Lee, K.; Lanske, B.; Segre, G.V.; Kronenberg, H.M.; Tabin, C.J. Regulation of rate of cartilage differentiation by Indian hedgehog and PTH-related protein. *Science* **1996**, *273*, 613–622. [CrossRef]
150. St-Jacques, B.; Hammerschmidt, M.; McMahon, A.P. Indian hedgehog signaling regulates proliferation and differentiation of chondrocytes and is essential for bone formation. *Genes Dev.* **1999**, *13*, 2072–2086. [CrossRef]
151. Kurio, N.; Saunders, C.; Bechtold, T.E.; Salhab, I.; Nah, H.-D.; Sinha, S.; Billings, P.C.; Pacifici, M.; Koyama, E. Roles of Ihh signaling in chondroprogenitor function in postnatal condylar cartilage. *Matrix Biol.* **2018**, *67*, 15–31. [CrossRef] [PubMed]
152. Maeda, Y.; Nakamura, E.; Nguyen, M.-T.; Suva, L.J.; Swain, F.L.; Razzaque, M.S.; Mackem, S.; Lanske, B. Indian Hedgehog produced by postnatal chondrocytes is essential for maintaining a growth plate and trabecular bone. *Proc. Natl. Acad. Sci. USA* **2007**, *104*, 6382–6387. [CrossRef]
153. Kobayashi, T.; Soegiarto, D.W.; Yang, Y.; Lanske, B.; Schipani, E.; McMahon, A.P.; Kronenberg, H.M. Indian hedgehog stimulates periarticular chondrocyte differentiation to regulate growth plate length independently of PTHrP. *J. Clin. Investig.* **2005**, *115*, 1734–1742. [CrossRef] [PubMed]
154. Dipaola, C.P.; Farmer, J.C.; Manova, K.; Niswander, L.A. Molecular signaling in intervertebral disk development. *J. Orthop. Res.* **2005**, *23*, 1112–1119. [CrossRef]
155. Wang, S.; Yang, K.; Chen, S.; Wang, J.; Du, G.; Fan, S.; Wei, L. Indian hedgehog contributes to human cartilage endplate degeneration. *Eur. Spine J.* **2015**, *24*, 1720–1728. [CrossRef] [PubMed]
156. Bao, J.; Qian, Z.; Liu, L.; Hong, X.; Che, H.; Wu, X. Pharmacological Disruption of Phosphorylated Eukaryotic Initiation Factor-2alpha/Activating Transcription Factor 4/Indian Hedgehog Protects Intervertebral Disc Degeneration via Reducing the Reactive Oxygen Species and Apoptosis of Nucleus Pulposus Cells. *Front. Cell Dev. Biol.* **2021**, *9*, 675486. [CrossRef]
157. Li, X.; Han, L.; Mao, K.; Yang, S. Ciliary IFT80 is essential for intervertebral disc development and maintenance. *FASEB J.* **2020**, *34*, 6741–6756. [CrossRef]
158. Janssens, K.; ten Dijke, P.; Janssens, S.; Van Hul, W. Transforming growth factor-beta1 to the bone. *Endocr. Rev.* **2005**, *26*, 743–774. [CrossRef]
159. Jin, H.; Shen, J.; Wang, B.; Wang, M.; Shu, B.; Chen, D. TGF-beta signaling plays an essential role in the growth and maintenance of intervertebral disc tissue. *FEBS Lett.* **2011**, *585*, 1209–1215. [CrossRef]
160. Yang, S.; Li, Z.; Li, S.; Liu, X.; Nie, Y.; Yang, L.; Zhang, C.; Guo, Y. Psoralidin Induced Differentiation from Adipose-derived Stem Cells to Nucleus Pulposus-like Cells by TGF-beta/Smad Signaling. *Curr. Mol. Med.* **2023**, *23*, 688–697. [CrossRef]
161. Zhang, Y.; Zhang, Z.; Chen, P.; Ma, C.Y.; Li, C.; Au, T.Y.; Tam, V.; Peng, Y.; Wu, R.; Cheung, K.M.C.; et al. Directed Differentiation of Notochord-like and Nucleus Pulposus-like Cells Using Human Pluripotent Stem Cells. *Cell Rep.* **2020**, *30*, 2791–2806. [CrossRef] [PubMed]

162. Colombier, P.; Clouet, J.; Boyer, C.; Ruel, M.; Bonin, G.; Lesoeur, J.; Moreau, A.; Fellah, B.-H.; Weiss, P.; Lescaudron, L.; et al. TGF-beta1 and GDF5 Act Synergistically to Drive the Differentiation of Human Adipose Stromal Cells toward Nucleus Pulposus-like Cells. *Stem Cells* **2016**, *34*, 653–667. [CrossRef] [PubMed]
163. Guo, Z.; Su, W.; Zhou, R.; Zhang, G.; Yang, S.; Wu, X.; Qiu, C.; Cong, W.; Shen, N.; Guo, J.; et al. Exosomal MATN3 of Urine-Derived Stem Cells Ameliorates Intervertebral Disc Degeneration by Antisenescence Effects and Promotes NPC Proliferation and ECM Synthesis by Activating TGF-beta. *Oxid. Med. Cell. Longev.* **2021**, *2021*, 5542241. [CrossRef] [PubMed]
164. Frapin, L.; Clouet, J.; Chédeville, C.; Moraru, C.; Samarut, E.; Henry, N.; André, M.; Bord, E.; Halgand, B.; Lesoeur, J.; et al. Controlled release of biological factors for endogenous progenitor cell migration and intervertebral disc extracellular matrix remodelling. *Biomaterials* **2020**, *253*, 120107. [CrossRef]
165. Yang, X.; Chen, Z.; Chen, C.; Han, C.; Zhou, Y.; Li, X.; Tian, H.; Cheng, X.; Zhang, K.; Qin, A.; et al. Bleomycin induces fibrotic transformation of bone marrow stromal cells to treat height loss of intervertebral disc through the TGFbetaR1/Smad2/3 pathway. *Stem Cell Res. Ther.* **2021**, *12*, 34. [CrossRef]

Disclaimer/Publisher's Note: The statements, opinions and data contained in all publications are solely those of the individual author(s) and contributor(s) and not of MDPI and/or the editor(s). MDPI and/or the editor(s) disclaim responsibility for any injury to people or property resulting from any ideas, methods, instructions or products referred to in the content.

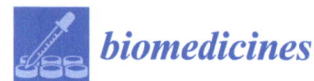 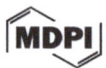

Review

Immune Evasion in Stem Cell-Based Diabetes Therapy—Current Strategies and Their Application in Clinical Trials

Razik Bin Abdul Mu-u-min [1,*], Abdoulaye Diane [1], Asma Allouch [2] and Heba Hussain Al-Siddiqi [1]

[1] Diabetes Research Center, Qatar Biomedical Research Institute (QBRI), Hamad Bin Khalifa University (HBKU), Qatar Foundation (QF), Doha P.O. Box 34110, Qatar; adiane@hbku.edu.qa (A.D.); halsiddiqi@hbku.edu.qa (H.H.A.-S.)

[2] College of Health and Life Sciences (CHLS), Hamad Bin Khalifa University (HBKU), Qatar Foundation (QF), Doha P.O. Box 34110, Qatar; aallouch@hbku.edu.qa

* Correspondence: raabdulmuumin@hbku.edu.qa

Academic Editor: Aline Yen Ling Wang

Received: 2 January 2025
Revised: 28 January 2025
Accepted: 3 February 2025
Published: 6 February 2025

Citation: Mu-u-min, R.B.A.; Diane, A.; Allouch, A.; Al-Siddiqi, H.H. Immune Evasion in Stem Cell-Based Diabetes Therapy—Current Strategies and Their Application in Clinical Trials. *Biomedicines* 2025, 13, 383. https://doi.org/10.3390/biomedicines13020383

Copyright: © 2025 by the authors. Licensee MDPI, Basel, Switzerland. This article is an open access article distributed under the terms and conditions of the Creative Commons Attribution (CC BY) license (https://creativecommons.org/licenses/by/4.0/).

Abstract: Background/Objectives: Human pancreatic islet transplantation shows promise for long-term glycemic control in diabetes patients. A shortage of healthy donors and the need for continuous immunosuppressive therapy complicates this. Enhancing our understanding of the immune tolerance mechanisms related to graft rejection is crucial to generate safer transplantation strategies. This review will examine advancements in immune protection strategies for stem cell-derived islet therapy and discuss key clinical trials involving stem cell-derived β-cells and their protective strategies against the host immune system. **Methods**: A comprehensive literature search was performed on peer-reviewed publications on Google Scholar, Pubmed, and Scopus up to September 2024 to extract relevant studies on the various strategies of immune evasion of stem cell-derived β-cells in humans. The literature search was extended to assimilate all relevant clinical studies wherein stem cell-derived β-cells are transplanted to treat diabetes. **Results**: Our analysis highlighted the importance of human pluripotent stem cells (hPSCs) as a potentially unlimited source of insulin-producing β-cells. These cells can be transplanted as an effective source of insulin in diabetes patients if they can be protected against the host immune system. Various strategies of immune protection, such as encapsulation and genetic manipulation, are currently being studied and clinically tested. **Conclusions**: Investigating immune tolerance in hPSC-derived islets may help achieve a cure for diabetes without relying on exogenous insulin. Although reports of clinical trials show promise in reducing insulin dependency in patients, their safety and efficacy needs to be further studied to promote their use as a long-term solution to cure diabetes.

Keywords: β-cells; diabetes; immune evasion; stem cells; transplantation

1. Introduction

Diabetes mellitus constitutes a group of chronic and metabolic disorders characterized by prolonged elevated blood glucose levels. The primary mechanism attributed to the onset and impact of the disease is insulin deficiency, resulting in impaired glucose metabolism. The International Diabetes Federation (IDF) reported that, as of 2021, 537 million adults are living with diabetes, a number that is projected to rise to 783 million by 2045. Additionally, 6.7 million deaths were attributed to diabetes-related comorbidities (www.idf.org). The American Diabetes Association (ADA) classifies diabetes into two main categories: Type 1 diabetes (T1DM) and Type 2 diabetes (T2DM) [1]. T1DM stems from the immune-mediated destruction of pancreatic β-cells, causing a near-complete deficiency in insulin production. While T1DM constitutes only 5–10% of diabetes cases, it represents 80–90% of cases in children and adolescents [2–4]. Conversely, T2DM occurs when individuals experience insulin resistance and a relative insulin deficiency due to β-cell dysfunction, accounting for 90–95% of all diabetes cases [5]. Other diabetes types encompass gestational diabetes mellitus (GDM), neonatal diabetes, and maturity-onset diabetes of the young (MODY) [6]. It is widely recognized that all forms of diabetes share a commonality in dysfunctional pancreatic β cells negatively affecting insulin secretion. Diabetes is associated with additional health burdens, manifesting in macrovascular complications such as stroke, peripheral artery disease, coronary heart diseases, and myocardial infarctions, as well as microvascular complications like neuropathy, retinopathy, and nephropathy. These complications lead to a reduced quality of life and premature death [7]. The treatment and management of T2DM involves a multifaceted approach combining lifestyle adjustments such as dietary habits, physical activity, sufficient sleep, and pharmacological interventions [8–12]. The current approach to treating T1DM involves managing glycemia through daily insulin supplementation, administered either via insulin injections or insulin pumps equipped with integrated glucose monitors [13,14]. Despite being lifesaving, these invasive treatment methods have limitations, often leading to acute hypoglycemia, which, in turn, can contribute to heart and kidney failures. An alternative treatment for T1DM is cadaveric islet transplantation using the Edmonton protocol. This approach offers the potential for temporary exogenous insulin independence [15]. However, its feasibility is increasingly hindered for the growing T1DM patient population due to factors such as a shortage of donors, and, importantly, the potential risk of graft rejection, necessitating lifelong use of immunosuppressive drugs [16,17].

1.1. Graft Rejection/Immune Protection in Islet Transplantation

Graft rejection or progressive loss of islet function in transplanted pancreatic islets occurs due to autoimmune and alloimmune reactions. Graft rejection occurs primarily through "direct" and "indirect" pathways in the host system. The direct pathway is mediated by the host (recipient) T cells, as T cells are activated via T cell receptor (TCR) recognition of antigenic peptides presented by major histocompatibility complexes (MHCs) expressed on the donor cells. This results in a direct attack by recipient T cells on the transplanted cells, leading to graft destruction. In the indirect pathway of graft rejection, donor specific MHCs are recognized by recipient antigen presenting cells (APC), such as B cells, macrophages, and dendritic cells, and broken down into fragments which are then presented on the recipient APCs, thus triggering the recipient T cells. The rejection of transplanted cells can be due to either direct or indirect pathways and could work in cohorts to effect graft rejection [18–22]. Treatment strategies designed to circumvent graft rejection generally involve an immunosuppression program. In transplantation attempts, notably in the 1990s, graft rejection was prevented by treating the patients with an induction of immunosuppressive agent targeting T lymphocytes, followed by a three-pronged immunosuppression strategy consisting of a calcineurin inhibitor, a DNA antimetabolite, and steroids. However, all these agents demonstrated, in varying degrees, β-cell toxicity or diabetogenicity [23]. The pioneering work of the Edmonton protocol introduced a steroid-free regimen that improved graft survival and insulin independence in T1DM patients. The treatment consisted of the anti-interleukin-2 receptor antibody 'daclizumab' to inhibit inflammation, the mammalian target of rapamycin inhibitor 'sirolimus' to deplete T cells, and the calcineurin inhibitor 'tacrolimus' to block T cell proliferation [15]. Although patients were able to sustain insulin independence for half a decade, immunosuppression-mediated side effects were prominent [24]. Multiple combinations of immunosuppressive treatment strategies were developed subsequently, with varying degrees of success. A study used an antibody-based approach where anti-thymocyte globulin, daclizumab, and etanercept were used for the induction phase; followed by mycophenolate mofetil to inhibit T cell proliferation; and lymphocyte adhesion molecules, sirolimus, and either no or low-dose tacrolimus for maintenance. Patients administered with this treatment regimen managed to retain insulin independence for over a year [25]. Other strategies of immunosuppression involved using hOKT3γ, an anti-CD3 antibody, to reduce T cell expression for the induction phase, followed by sirolimus- and tacrolimus-based immunosuppression [26]. Studies have also highlighted the success of an effective calcineurin inhibitor-free immunosuppression protocol using the co-stimulation blocker belatacept, and patients were able to achieve long-term insulin independence [27]. The major pitfalls in most immunosuppressive regimens include β-cell endoplasmic reticulum (ER) stress, faulty revascularization of grafts, impaired β-cell replication, impaired glucose-stimulated insulin secretion (GSIS), and reduced insulin sensitivity [28–31]. Moreover, patients are at risk of developing infections and tumors as immunosuppression compromises their immune system [22].

1.2. The Promise of Stem Cells in Regenerative Cell Therapy in Diabetic Patients

Advancements in regenerative medicine have recently highlighted the development of transplantable functional pancreatic β-cells derived from human pluripotent stem cells (hPSCs), both human embryonic stem cells (hESCs) and induced pluripotent stem cells (hiPSCs), as a potential diabetes treatment. These patient-specific-derived β-cells, also referred to as autologous PSC-derived β-cells, offer a promising solution to address challenges like insufficient islet availability by serving as an unlimited source of β-cells for diabetes therapy and graft rejection by using patient-specific stem cell lines. Additionally, patient-specific stem cell-derived β-cells in vitro are being used to study diabetes-related mutations, including inherited monogenic diabetes, and explore disease progression [32,33]. Efforts are underway across the world to differentiate hPSCs efficiently and reproducibly into insulin-producing β-cells using multistage directed differentiated protocols (Figure 1). Directed differentiation of stem cells attempts to mimic the embryonic development of pancreatic β-cells by emulating growth stages through the sequential addition of small molecules and growth factors. The success of these protocols is typically gauged by how closely the resulting cells resemble their in vivo counterparts in terms of maturity and functional efficiency. Over the years, numerous research laboratories have established protocols featuring optimized culture conditions, differentiation media, and small molecules, and these protocols are applicable to multiple hPSC cell lines, leading to an improved efficiency in differentiation and an enhanced functionality of β-cells [34–36]. The transplantation of hPSC-derived β-cell islet-like clusters into mice has been shown to improve maturation and functionality, thereby providing evidence for the possibility of using them for human transplantation [37].

In this review, we briefly present various strategies devised to overcome immune rejection following transplantation, with particular emphasis on the promise and progress of using hPSCs to achieve this goal. An insight is provided into various clinical trials that employ stem cell-derived pancreatic progenitors/beta-like cells for transplantation and their outcome.

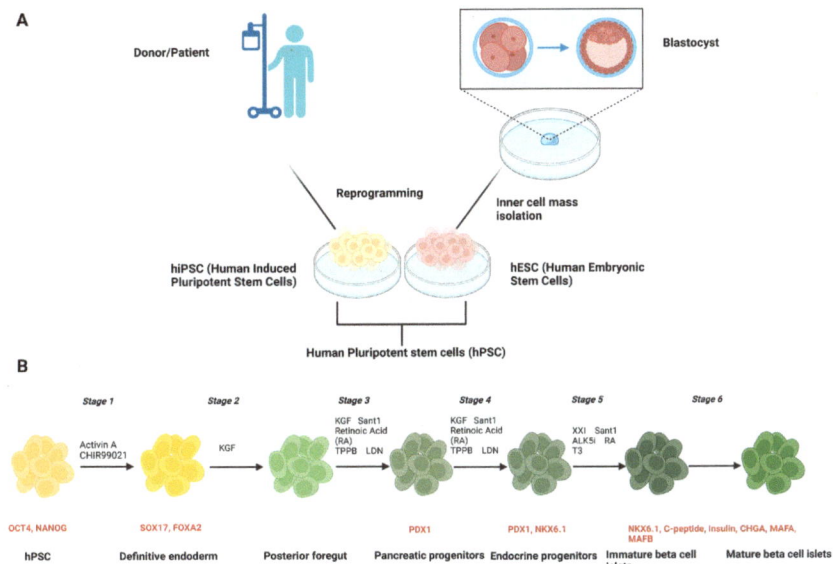

Figure 1. Schematic of the generation of stem cell-derived pancreatic β-cell islets. (**A**) hESCs are extracted from the inner cell mass of blastocyst stage of developing embryo and cultured to proliferate indefinitely. hiPSCs are generated through direct reprogramming of somatic cells from a donor to pluripotent stem cells. (**B**) A general protocol outlining the differentiation stages of the generation of pancreatic β-cell islets from hPSCs. The resulting cell stages are labelled in black and the quality control markers to track the efficiency (by flow cytometry or immunocytochemistry) of differentiation at each stage are labelled in red. This illustration was created with "BioRender.com".

2. Immune Protection Using Encapsulation

Cell encapsulation has been considered an attractive addendum to the current transplantation techniques to avoid graft rejection post-transplantation by bypassing the need for an immunosuppressive drugs regimen. Transplanted cells are encased by semi-permeable biomaterials that block immune cells' entry while being permeable to oxygen, nutrients, and the diffusion of metabolites. The two types of encapsulation strategies are microencapsulation, wherein a few cells are encased by microspheres of less than 1000 µm, and macroencapsulation, wherein millions of cells are encased in macroscopic polymeric devices [38]. The ideal islet encapsulation device design requires several considerations such as the capsule size, mode of surgery, and implantation site, among others [39].

2.1. Microencapsulation

The most used material for microencapsulation is alginate, a naturally occurring polysaccharide found in brown algae. The main components of alginate are the liner β-D-mannuronate and α-L-guluronate. Microcapsules are generated by crosslinking the polymer with divalent cations (e.g.,: calcium and barium). This forms a gel matrix suitable for encapsulating cells. The smaller size of the microcapsules as compared to macrocapsules provides them with a high surface-to-volume ratio that improves the diffusion of oxygen and other agents that are essential for β-cell survival [38,40]. Key alginate microcapsule factors, such as stability, pore size, immunogenicity, and cell-binding domains, can be manipulated by combining alginate with various compounds such as collagen, poly-L-lysine, pluronic F127, and immunomodulators such as dexamethasone and stromal cell-derived factor 1α (CXCL12) [41–44]. Studies have experimented with microencapsulation of β-cells followed by their transplantation. A 2016 study implanted hPSC-derived β-cells encased in barium–triazole–thiomorpholine dioxide alginate microcapsules into STZ-induced diabetic mice without immunosuppression. The implanted β-cells showed glucose responsiveness for 174 days, after which the retrieved implant still contained viable insulin producing cells [45]. Another study used an innovative technique which involved incorporating CXCL12 into sodium alginate microcapsules. hESC-derived β-cells encapsulated in these microcapsules showed enhanced insulin secretion in diabetic mice. Additionally, these cells were able to evade the foreign body response of cells wherein implanted materials are affected by fibroblast recruitment followed by collagen deposition around the implants, thereby affecting cell survival [46]. The cells were able to regulate hyperglycemia and maintain functionality for over 150 days without immunosuppression [47]. Microencapsulation isolates the cells from the host system with thick barriers that hinder the efficient diffusion of oxygen and essential metabolites, and could lead to delayed GSIS and islet necrosis due to a lack of oxygen supply [48,49]. A strategy devised to alleviate this issue is the encapsulation of cells in a conformal coating which has a much-reduced thickness in the order of tens of micrometers. Enhanced diffusion can be permitted in this setup while maintaining a barrier to the host immune system. A study created a polyethyleneglycol-based conformal coating to encapsulate human stem cells-derived islets which were then transplanted into diabetic non-obese diabetic/severe combined immunodeficiency (NOD-SCID) mice. The transplanted cells were able to reverse diabetes and maintain normal euglycemia for more than 80 days [50].

2.2. Macroencapsulation

In macroencapsulation, a large number of cells are generally encased in a perforated pouch or a large hydrogel over 1 mm long. Macroencapsulation devices provide good chemical and mechanical stability, in addition to the advantage of being retrievable post-transplantation in case of failure or malignant alteration of transplanted cells. Macroencapsulation techniques consist of hydrogel scaffold-based devices, membrane-controlled release systems, or microneedle array patches [51,52]. Several studies over the past decade have attempted to generate potential therapeutic applications of macroencapsulation devices combined with stem cell-derived β-cells. Earlier studies used a planar pouch-like encapsulation device using a bilaminar polytetrafluoroethylene membrane system (TheraCyte) which showed promising immunoprotection in transplanted cells in mice and primates [53–55]. The technology was later applied to hESC-derived pancreatic progenitors which were transplanted into mice. The cells achieved maturation within the macroencapsulation device and promoted insulin production with no change in biomass within the capsule for up to 150 days, suggesting high immunoprotection [55]. A 2017 study created a flexible and durable polycaprolactone-based 10 μm thick nanoporous thin-film cell-encapsulation device capable of neovascularization formation with minimal foreign body response and teratoma confinement, which increased the safety of the use of stem cell-derived β-cells. The membrane was also shown to exclude proinflammatory cytokines while promoting glucose and insulin exchange. The transplantation of the device encasing hESC-derived β-cells into immunocompetent mice showed long term biocompatibility as glucose responsiveness and cell viability were seen 6 months post-transplantation [56]. A recent study created a durable zwitterionically modified alginate hydrogel capable of evading foreign body responses. Stem cell-derived β-cells were encased in these macrocapsules and inserted into diabetic mice, which exhibited significantly better glucose clearance for over 230 days. Due to improved biocompatibility, mass transfer, and low fibrotic reactions, the device was capable of long-term cell engraftment [57]. Conventional macroencapsulation devices suffer from slow GSIS due to their reliance on diffusion of oxygen and metabolites. A recent study designed a convection-enhanced macroencapsulation device that enabled improved nutrient transfer across the device membrane, enabling a near 10-fold higher cell loading capacity. The polytetrafluoroethylene-based membrane chamber encased stem cell-derived β-cells suspended in matrigel, which enabled a homogenous cell distribution, prevention of aggregates, and lowered the shear stress during loading. Transplantation of the device into immunocompetent hyperglycemic rats demonstrated early improvement in hyperglycemia, improved GSIS, and reduced fibrosis [58]. An important consideration for the creation of micro and macroencapsulation devices is their ability to overcome a foreign body response. Various techniques have been adopted to manage a foreign body response evoked by encapsulation devices. These generally involve altering the device's surface chemistry (e.g., charge, composition, hydrophobicity), coating the device to alter its topography, and manipulating its shape and porosity [59]. Although advances have been made in encapsulation technologies, efficient oxygenation still remains a challenge for the long-term survival of the grafts due to the lack of vascularization of intraislet capillaries as compared to native islets. Recent strategies devised the use of encapsulation materials that promote graft revascularization. Encapsulation devices with direct vascularization developed by ViaCyte Inc. and Sernova are undergoing clinical trials to evaluate their safety and efficacy. The disadvantage of such devices is the loss of immunoprotection for grafts and the requirement of a systemic immunosuppression regimen to prevent rejection.

Several clinical trials over the past decade have studied the transplantation of hPSC-derived pancreatic progenitor/β-cells protected by various encapsulation devices. A summary of relevant clinical trials and their outcomes is outlined in a later section of this review.

3. Genetically Modified hiPSC-Derived β-Cells for Immune Evasion

hiPSC technology holds a great promise in precision medicine powered by personalized treatment designed using one's own somatic cells such as peripheral blood cells. The key advantage of using this technology is the production of patient-specific cells designed for autologous transplantation, thereby bypassing immune-driven organ rejection, and improving cell survival after transplantation [60]. Currently, the cost and time required to produce autologous hiPSC-derived β-cells hinder the effectiveness of this treatment strategy, although inroads are being made to better streamline the technology. Recognition of the cell surface markers MHC, also known as human leukocyte antigens (HLAs), by T cells is one of the most important criteria of allogeneic transplant rejection in humans. The genes encoding HLAs are classified into class I, comprising HLA-A, -B, -C, -D, -E, -F and -G; class II, comprising HLA-DR, -DP, -DQ, -DM, -DN, and -DO; and class III, which encodes for proteins of the complement system and the TNF family genes. HLA-A, -B, -DR, -DP, and -DQ are believed to contribute the most to immune rejection. Attempts have been made to generate HLA homozygous hiPSC lines which can potentially be used to transplant into patients to prevent HLA-mediated allorejection. hiPSCs from donors with homozygous HLA-A, -B, and -DR have been selectively generated and cryopreserved for their potential future use to generate β-cells which could be less reactive to the host immune system. However, a much larger scale study needs to be performed to account for genetic diversity in the population to create universal hiPSC lines that can be used globally. Also, this is not a complete solution to dealing with immune rejection, since the HLA haplotypes HLA-DR4-DQ8 and HLA-DR3-DQ2 have been implicated in immune responses wherein insulin is presented as antigens to activated T cells [61–63]. MHC expression in stem cells is generally low and the cells are therefore protected from immune responses. However, differentiation stimulates MHC expression and renders the cells vulnerable to immune system [64]. Stem cell-derived β-cells generally express class I antigens which are upregulated under inflammatory stress. A study reported that stem cell-derived β-cells largely express HLA-C, while native β-cells express all class I MHCs. The authors suggested that the difference in the cell properties with respect to MHC expression might be due to the immaturity of stem cell-derived β-cells as compared to native β-cells [65]. Another important candidate for immune response regulation is the immune checkpoint inhibitor programmed death-ligand 1 (PD-L1), which is upregulated as a protection agent in response to pro-inflammatory cytokines. Gene manipulation strategies to circumvent immune responses in transplanted cells are discussed below.

Genome editing, a powerful tool to create gene knockouts and knock-ins, is finding stronger footing in improving our understanding of the underlying genetic mechanisms of diseases. Genome editing tools work under the premise where a nuclease identifies a target sequence, induces a double-stranded DNA break (DSB), and activates endogenous cellular DNA repair mechanisms such as homologous recombination or non-homologous end-joining. In the field of diabetic research, genome editing has already been used to create models of diabetes subtypes from hESCs and hiPSCs [66,67]. Commonly used gene editing systems include zinc finger nucleases (ZFN), transcription activator-like effector nuclease (TALEN), and the promising Clustered Regularly Interspaced-Short Palindromic Repeats (CRISPR)/Cas9 technology. ZFNs are based on zinc finger proteins, a cohort of transcription factors fused on a restriction endonuclease *Fok*I that effects gene edits [68]. TALENs take advantage of the proteins 'transcription activator-like effectors (TALEs)' to provide high specificity to gene editing, while maintaining a lower cytotoxicity and simpler design structure as compared to ZFNs [67,69]. The CRISPR/Cas9 system utilizes short noncoding guide RNAs (sgRNA) to identify specific target DNA sequences and is combined with the enzyme CRISPR-associated protein 9 (Cas9) to effect gene cleavage [70].

Based on our current understanding of the immune responses on hPSC-derived β-cells post-transplantation, strategies can be developed to genetically engineer functional hPSC-derived β-cells which are immune evasive and thereby improve β-cell survival and functionality in diabetes patients. One approach for genetically modifying hPSC-derived β-cells is to prevent HLA expression and therefore avoid T cell responses. Beta-2 microglobulin (B2M) is responsible for the proper folding and cell surface expression of HLA class I proteins and therefore its deletion would abolish HLA class I expression, as demonstrated by a study. In this study, a B2M gene knockout (KO) cell line was generated using CRISPR-Cas9 in hPSCs and showed that wildtype hPSC-derived β-cells induced higher levels of T cell activation as compared to the B2M knockout model [65]. In another study, CRISPR-Cas9 was used to disrupt B2M gene in hiPSCs-derived from T1DM patients. A co-culture of PBMCs with wildtype beta-like cells and HLA class I deficient beta-like cells showed a reduction in the expression of immune markers CD25 and CD69 in autologous $CD8^+$ T cells, providing further evidence that HLA expression disruption can decrease immune responses [71]. Although preventing HLA class I antigens can prevent T cell-mediated immune responses, according to the "missing self" hypothesis, in the absence of all HLA-presenting antigens, natural killer cell-mediated lysis will be activated due to the lack of inhibitory signals on the target cells [72]. This effect was reported in studies which target-removed B2M in hPSCs, as cells became vulnerable in varying degrees to natural killer cell-mediated immune responses [73,74]. However, the targeted inactivation of HLA-A, -B, and -C genes while maintaining HLA-E expression alone, or in cohorts with HLA-G, CD47, and PD-L1, has proven to protect hPSCs from natural killer cell responses [75–77].

Another avenue for genetically engineering stem cells to evade immune responses is through PD-L1 overexpression. Cancer cells are known to evade T cell rejection by expressing the immune checkpoint molecule PD-L1, related to the T cell inhibitory receptor programmed death 1 (PD-1) [78]. Previous studies have shown that PD-L1 expression in islets protects against immune responses in the transplantation of syngeneic islets into diabetic recipients. PD-L1 also inhibited self-reactive CD4$^+$ T cell-mediated tissue destruction and effector cytokine production [79,80]. Another study highlighted the importance of PD-L1 with respect to islet transplantation. The authors noticed that though a PD-L1 deficiency in donor hearts does not evoke immune rejection, PD-L1-deficient islets heightened allograft rejection, thereby emphasizing the importance of PD-L1 in islet function and immune responses. The transplantation of islets from PD-L1-deficient mice into STZ-induced diabetic mice induced graft rejection. They attributed the islet rejection to enhanced T cell activation and inflammatory cell infiltration [81]. Studies have explored the idea of overexpression of PD-L1 in stem cells to protect stem cell-derived islets from immune rejection. A study used CRISPR technology to overexpress PD-L1 stem cells and reported that stem cell-derived functional beta-like cells were partially protected from T cell responses [82]. A more recent study generated functional beta-like islets from hiPSCs, which were genetically modified using a lentiviral system to overexpress PD-L1. The transplantation of these stem cell-derived islet-like cells restored glycemic control in immune competent diabetic mice and maintained glucose homeostasis for over 50 days when compared to islet-like cells which did not overexpress PD-L1. Recovered grafts showed a decrease in T cell and NK cells in PD-L1-overexpressed cells [83]. Another recent study used a TALEN-mediated overexpression of PD-L1 on hiPSCs, which were then target-differentiated into beta-like cells. The authors reported that the overexpression of PD-L1 reduced the activation of β-cell destruction-inducing diabetogenic CD8 T cells, as observed through a significant decrease in interleukin-2 secretion. When combined with a CRISPR-based mutation of the B2M gene, there was a further reduction in interleukin-2 secretion, highlighting the possible advantage of combining multiple gene targets to enhance immunoprotection [65].

An important consideration of gene editing of hPSCs is the precision and safety of the gene editing process. In CRISPR-based gene editing, off-target editing could occur when DNA cleavage and repair happens at sites containing similar sequences as the target editing site. Though the chances of such inaccurate edits are relatively low, they could lead to significant safety issues such as the inhibition of tumor suppressor genes or the activation of oncogenes [84,85]. However, there are strategies designed to curb the chances of inaccurate off-target edits, such as improving the specificity of gene targeting by using a combination of sgRNA and high-fidelity Cas9 variants, or the use of multiple sgRNAs to target the same gene [86,87]. A crucial factor in the use of genetically modified β-cells to evade the immune system is the potential to be undetected by other immune mechanisms in the event of infections or tumor formations. Careful consideration and further studies need to be performed to validate the safety of these technologies as long-term solutions to treat diabetes.

A comparison of the various immune evasion strategies and their relative strengths and weaknesses are summarized in Table 1.

Table 1. A comparison of various immune evasion strategies, highlighting advantages and potential safety concerns.

Immune Evasion Strategy	Mechanism	Advantages	Safety Concerns	References
Immunosuppressive drug therapy	β-cells are protected by inducing a general suppression of the immune system (e.g., anti-rejection drugs)	- Broad suppression of immune activity can reduce both innate and adaptive immune responses. - Readily available and well-studied agents.	Risk of infection, autoreactivity, cancer	[25,88]

Table 1. Cont.

Immune Evasion Strategy	Mechanism	Advantages	Safety Concerns	References
Encapsulation	β-cells are encapsulated in biocompatible materials that prevent immune cells from attacking them.	- Provides a physical barrier against immune cells and antibodies. - Reduces reliance on systemic immunosuppression.	Fibrotic responses, hypoxia, graft revascularization issues	[54,89,90]
Genetically engineered hPSC-derived β-cells	Modifies beta cells to express less immunogenicity or altered antigens (e.g., HLA knockout) to reduce immune recognition.	- Tailored to specific immune pathways, enabling precise modulation. - Can be combined with other therapies for synergistic effects.	Potential risks related to off-target effects or unintended gene modifications, which may lead to tumorigenesis or immune responses	[65,83]

4. Stem Cell-Based Clinical Trials for the Treatment of Diabetes

As a potentially unlimited source of β-cells of autogenic origin, stem cells can reduce the dependence on organ donors and the associated complications for the treatment of diabetes, and this aspect of stem cells has been explored in several clinical trials in recent years. The source of stem cells that have been used in clinical trials is mesenchymal stem cells (MSCs), or pluripotent stem cells including hESCs or hiPSCs.

MSCs are adult multipotent stem cells capable of differentiating into osteoblasts (bone cells), chondrocytes (cartilage cells), myocytes (muscle cells), and adipocytes (fat cells). They are found in bone marrow, umbilical cord, or adipose tissues [91,92]. MSCs pose attractive qualities, such as an increased biosafety profile and a lower tumorgenicity risk, that render them an interesting choice for a potential diabetes treatment [93]. Additionally, they have regenerative properties, lack immunogenicity due to the absence of MHC class II, and have also been shown to support damaged islets [94–96]. Clinical trials have explored using MSCs in different settings to understand the best therapeutic method for the treatment of T1DM. The different hypotheses tested are (i) using undifferentiated MSCs to improve islet health and survival without differentiating into pancreatic progenitors, (ii) using MSC-derived pancreatic progenitors that differentiate into functional β-cells, and (iii) transplanting undifferentiated MSCs with the goal of in vivo transdifferentiation into functional β-cells [97,98]. One of the earliest clinical studies was developed to test the effect of autologous bone marrow MSCs using intravenous transplantation in T1DM patients. During the first year, an increased C-peptide response to mixed meal tolerance test (MMTT) was noted, and no apparent side effects were observed (NCT01068951) [99]. Another study assessed the long-term effects of an intravenous implantation of Wharton's jelly-derived MSCs in newly diagnosed T1DM patients who were followed up for 21 months. The study concluded that patients with MSC treatment significantly improved HbA1c and C-peptide values as compared to pretreatment or control patients [100]. A study focused on the co-infusion of autologous adipose tissue-derived MSC-differentiated insulin-secreting cells and hematopoietic stem cells. Over a follow up period of over 31 months, the treatment improved mean C-peptide levels [101]. A recent pilot clinical study investigated the combined immunomodulatory effects of using MSCs and vitamin D in T1DM patients (NCT03920397). Patients were treated with intravenous MSC (allogenic) infusion, combined with oral cholecalciferol (vitamin D), and followed up for six months. An increase in basal C-peptide levels, which were stable for six months, was observed [102]. Another recent phase I/II clinical trial assessed the safety and efficacy of intravenous injection of MSCs in newly diagnosed T1DM patients who were followed up for at least one year post-transplant (NCT04078308). The study reported promising results where glycated hemoglobin (HbA1c) and C-peptide levels improved and shifted pro-inflammatory cytokines into anti-inflammatory cytokines. They suggested that an early transplantation of MSCs is favorable as compared to a late transplantation [96]. Several other clinical trials using MSCs have been completed with promising T1DM treatment observations [103–105].

Though MSC-based treatment strategies show promise in clinical settings, several weaknesses in the studies have been observed. The limited sample size of patients enrolled in most studies makes it difficult to draw concrete conclusions of the efficacy of MSC in T1DM treatment. Another valid point is that several clinical studies enrolled only patients who were recently diagnosed with T1DM. These studies reported high positive outcomes for the treatment and one study recommended early-stage T1DM intervention as compared to late-stage intervention. An interesting aspect of these clinical study designs is that the patients would be in the "honeymoon phase of diabetes", wherein the patient would require only minimal insulin or have near-normal blood glucose levels without the need for insulin treatment. Successful treatment at this condition is not representative of the efficacy of the treatment on all T1DM patients. Clinical trials with a larger scope of patient enrollment with an increased sample size, diverse populations, and recent- and late-onset T1DM patients is necessary [96,106]. Although clinical studies of the use of MSC in T1DM treatment were inconclusive, excellent results have been observed for its use in T2DM treatment. A systematic review analyzing the results of 10 MSC-based clinical trials reported its effectiveness in improving β-cell function in T2DM. A positive outcome in stimulated C-peptide levels, HbA1c values, and the reduction in exogenous insulin requirement showed promise for the use of MSCs in β-cell therapy [107].

Human pluripotent stem cells are another promising route for the use of stem cells for the potential treatment of diabetes by utilizing hESCs and hiPSCs. The current clinical trials using hPSCs consider two schools of thought as to at what stage of β-cell differentiation cells can be transplanted. The first option is transplanting pancreatic progenitor cells that co-express PDX1 and NKX6.1. The co-expression of these two factors is critical in the generation of functional and monohormonal β-cells, as cells that do not co-express these transcription factors generally follow an alternative differentiation path resulting in non-functional, polyhormonal, or non-β-cells [108,109]. The first clinical trial using hESCs was performed in 2014 on 19 candidates by combining pancreatic progenitor cells [PEC-01] and an immunoprotective macroencapsulation device (PEC-Encap), produced by the clinical-stage regenerative medicine company, ViaCyte. The purpose of this study was to test whether the combination product, named VC-01, can be implanted subcutaneously in T1DM subjects and maintained safely for two years (NCT02239354). The macroencapsulation device was designed to prevent allogeneic and autoimmune rejection by protecting the pancreatic progenitor cells from the immune system, thereby excluding a dependence on immunosuppressive drugs. This was achieved by having a semipermeable membrane which allowed the diffusion of molecules but restricted the movement of cells. The study observed that the macroencapsulation device was affected by a foreign body response that prevented vascularization, leading to inconsistent cell survival, and no evidence of insulin secretion was found [97,110,111]. The findings from this study necessitated the need for an updated design for the encapsulation device to overcome immune response issues. ViaCyte initiated a second clinical trial in 2017 with an updated macroencapsulation device which was not immunoprotective but was designed to enable direct capillary vascular permeation into the encapsulation device. The system, named PEC-Direct, combined PEC-01 with the updated macroencapsulation device VC-02 (NCT03163511). In this study, 17 patients between the ages 22 and 57 with T1DM were recruited. Following subcutaneous transplantation, 63% of candidates responded to the treatment as presented by successful engraftment and increased insulin positive cells at 3–12 months post-transplantation. Approximately 35% of candidates showed the ability to secrete C-peptide 6 months post-transplantation. The observed side-effects were related to surgical implant/explant procedures or to immunosuppression [112]. A 1-year follow-up study on the recipients showed the absence of teratoma formation or severe graft-rejection. Patients showed increased fasting and glucose responsive C-peptide levels and developed mixed meal-stimulated C-peptide secretion. Also, explanted grafts contained mature β-cell phenotype and were immunoreactive for insulin, MAFA and islet amyloid polypeptide, suggesting post-transplantation maturation of the pancreatic progenitors [110]. Recently, an interim report was published for this clinical study which analyzed 1 year outcome for a study group that received 2–3-fold higher cell doses with an enhanced perforation pattern of the encapsulation device. It was observed that out of ten patients, three were able to achieve improved C-peptide levels and reduced insulin dosing from six months onwards. The authors attributed these positive changes to the formation of a larger β-cell mass due to a higher initial dose of transplanted cells. They also suggested that design changes in the encapsulation device might have improved capillary ingrowth in the implanted cell mass, thereby improving β-cell maturation [113]. Further optimization of the PEC-Direct device was done by ViaCyte in collaboration with CRISPR therapeutics to use genetically edited cells to circumvent immune responses and rejection. This was achieved by modifying several genes in pancreatic endoderm cells (PEC210A) using CRSIPR/Cas9 technology, including the deletion of β2-microglobulin gene and transgenic expression of PD-L1. In a 2022 clinical trial (NCT05210530), the combination product VCTX210A was used, which contained PEC210A cells encased in a durable and removable perforated encapsulation device designed to deliver and retain PEC210A cells. Findings from the 1-year study have yet to be published. In a 2019 clinical study, Viacyte revisited their PEC-encap technology in collaboration the material science company Gore to create a modified PEC-encap device which aims to eliminate the need for immunosuppression while promoting vascularization (NCT04678557). The two-year study with 49 candidates has recently reached its conclusion, and detailed results from this study are awaited [114].

The above clinical studies used pancreatic progenitors for transplantation as they are less likely to be affected by inflammation due to transplantation and post-transplantation maturation is expected to occur over time [55,97]. However, a second option of transplantable cells considered are hPSC-derived islet-like organoids. These organoids consist of fully differentiated and glucose responsive hPSC-derived β-cells and upon transplantation, they are quicker to achieve glycemic control as compared to pancreatic progenitors, thereby, making them an attractive source for the treatment of diabetes [115,116]. Currently, Vertex Pharmaceuticals has entered phase I/II clinical trial with hPSC-derived β-cells (VX-880) generated by Melton group (NCT04786262). The cells, which lack any encapsulation devices, are transplanted into the patients via the hepatic portal vein. Although the lack of encapsulation requires immune suppression of the patient, early reports of the treatment's efficacy have been remarkably positive. Data collected 90 days post-transplant showed a 91% decrease in insulin requirement, mixed meal test-responsive elevation in circulating C-peptide and a reduction in HbA1c values [117]. Vertex is also actively recruiting candidates for a new phase I/II clinical trial in which patients are transplanted with hPSC-derived β-cells encapsulated in an immunoprotective device, thereby potentially bypassing immunosuppressive treatments (NCT05791201) [118]. Sigilon therapeutics, a subsidiary of the pharmaceutical company Eli Lilly and Company, has their encapsulated hiPSC-derived insulin-producing β-cells approaching clinical trials in the near future [97,112].

An important aspect of the successful transplantation of hPSC-derived pancreatic progenitors/β-cells is the cell delivery system employed. For a successful cell therapy treatment, cells should be both immunoprotected and have sufficient oxygen supply. Some of the hPSC-based clinical trials discussed above have used encapsulation devices to enhance cell survival and function. More methods of cell delivery have been developed and used in both preclinical and clinical trials using non-hPSC-based beta-cell transplantation. Alginate microencapsulation was the first cell delivery system used to protect transplanted β-cells. Clinical studies have used calcium/barium-alginate capsules to protect transplanted β-cells. Even though this encapsulation method prevented immune rejection, it was unable to significantly improve insulin release [119,120]. The biotech company Beta-02 Technologies has developed the Beta-air device, a "bioartificial pancreas" in which cells are placed in a slab of alginate and protected from the environment using a PTFE-based semipermeable membrane. A clinical trial using a subcutaneously transplanted "Beta-air" device produced small amounts of insulin, but not enough to reduce insulin dependency (NCT02064309). The disadvantage of this system was the need to continuously provide oxygen from an external source to maintain islet health and survival. An improved variant of the Beta-air device is being generated for hPSC-derived β-cells [51,97]. Cell Pouch^{TM}, developed by the biotech company Sernova, is another cell delivery device being used in clinical trials for islet transplantation. Cell Pouch^{TM} is a polypropylene membrane-based rectangular microporous pouch with multiple parallel chambers filled with PTFE. After transplantation, the PTFE plugs are removed, and islets are introduced into the void. A 2018 clinical study utilizing this technology reported promising results in terms of vascularization and β-cell function (NCT03513939). Although this device currently does not prevent immunosuppression, Sernova is considering hydrogel capsules to protect the cells from the host immune system [121]. The Shielded Living Therapeutics^{TM} sphere by Sigilon is another cell delivery candidate that shows promise. The sphere contains an external coating of alginate modified with the triazole–thiomorphaline dioxide and an internal core of modified alginate matrix housing cell clusters. This design of the sphere provides it with immune protection that is lacking in most other devices. Sigilon used this device in a clinical trial (NCT04541628) for hemophilia patients, but the study was terminated following safety concerns [121]. In addition to the devices mentioned above that have achieved clinical testing, a number of other devices have been developed which are in the preclinical phase. TheraCyte^{TM} produced by TheraCyte, ceMED produced by Harvard-MIT Health Sciences and Technology, a bioengineered vascular bed by Technion, an oxygenation cell delivery device from Procyon Technologies, and an electrospun nanofibrous encapsulation device from Novo Nordisk are some examples of potential encapsulation devices that may reduce the dependency on immunosuppressive treatments in the future [58,122–125]. These novel technologies carry immense promise for the development of systems to transplant β-cells while holding the deleterious host immune responses at bay. These devices can be combined with hPSC- and MSC-based cell therapies for successful transplantation strategies to drive long-term treatment options with minimal side effects. A summary of recent clinical trials using stem cell derived pancreatic progenitors/β-cells is summarized in Table 2.

Table 2. Stem cell based clinical trials for the treatment of diabetes.

Clinical Study ID	Start Year	Sponsor	Stem Cell Source	Status	Purpose of Study	Treatment Method	Reported Outcomes	Sample Size
NCT01068951	2010	Uppsala University Hospital, Sweden	MSCs	Completed	Evaluate the safety and efficacy of autologous MSCs in treatment of recently diagnosed patients with T1DM.	Intravenous transplantation.	Increased C-peptide response to MMTT.	20
NCT03920397	2015	Federal University of Rio de Janerio, Brazil	MSCs	Completed	Investigate the safety and efficacy of MSCs + daily cholecalciferol (VIT D) for 6 months in patients with recent-onset T1DM.	Allogeneic transplantation of adipose-derived MSCs with Vitamin D supplementation.	Increased basal C-peptide levels stable for 6 months.	30
NCT04078308	2015	Royan Institute, Iran	MSCs	Unknown	Examine the safety and efficacy of transplantation of MSCs in new-onset T1DM patients.	Intravenous transplantation of bone marrow-derived autologous MSCs.	Glycated hemoglobin (HbA1c) and C-peptide levels improved and shifted pro-inflammatory cytokines into anti-inflammatory cytokines.	21
NCT02239354	2014	Viacyte	hPSC	Completed	Test if VC-01™ combination product can be implanted subcutaneously in subjects with T1DM and maintained safely for two years.	Tranplantation of pancreatic progenitor cells (PEC-01) in a macroencapsulation device (PEC-Encap).	The macroencapsulation device was impacted by the foreign body response, which hindered vascularization, resulting in inconsistent cell survival and the absence of insulin secretion.	19

Table 2. Cont.

Clinical Study ID	Start Year	Sponsor	Stem Cell Source	Status	Purpose of Study	Treatment Method	Reported Outcomes	Sample Size
NCT03163511	2017	Viacyte	hPSC	Completed	Test if VC-02™ combination product can be implanted subcutaneously in subjects with T1DM and Hypoglycemia Unawareness and maintained safely for up to two years.	Transplantation of PEC-01 cells with the updated macroencapsulation device (VC-02).	63% of candidates showed a positive response to the treatment, demonstrated by successful engraftment and an increase in insulin-positive cells between 3 to 12 months after transplantation. Around 35% of candidates were able to secrete C-peptide 6 months post-transplant.	17
NCT04786262	2021	Vertex Pharmaceuticals Incorporated	hPSC	Recruiting	Evaluate the safety, tolerability, and efficacy of VX-880 cells infusion in participants with T1DM and impaired awareness of hypoglycemia and severe hypoglycemia.	Transplantation of hESC-derived β-cells (VX-880) via hepatic portal vein.	91% decrease in insulin requirement, mixed meal test-responsive elevation in circulating C-peptide, and a reduction in HbA1c values after 90 days.	17
NCT05791201	2023	Vertex Pharmaceuticals Incorporated	hPSC	Recruiting	Evaluate the safety, tolerability, and efficacy of VX-264 in participants with T1DM.	Transplantation of hESC-derived β-cells encapsulated in an immunoprotective device.	N/A	17

Table 2. Cont.

Clinical Study ID	Start Year	Sponsor	Stem Cell Source	Status	Purpose of Study	Treatment Method	Reported Outcomes	Sample Size
NCT04678557	2019	Viacyte	hPSC	Terminated	Evaluate an experimental combination product, cell replacement therapy intended to provide a functional cure to subjects with T1DM.	Transplantation of PEC-01 cells with encapsulation device (VC-01).	Insufficient functional product engraftment.	31
NCT05210530	2022	Viacyte, CRISPR Therapeutics AG	hPSC	Completed	Evaluate the safety and tolerability of VCTX210A combination product in patients with T1DM.	Transplantation of CRISPR-based genetically modified pancreatic endoderm cells (PEC210A) encased in a durable and removable perforated encapsulation device designed to deliver and retain PEC210A cells.	N/A	7

5. Conclusions and Future Directions

In this review, we outlined the key challenges of β-cell islet transplantation with respect to graft-mediated host immune responses and emphasized the prospects of using hPSC-derived β-cells as a viable treatment strategy for diabetes. Immune-evasive hiPSC-derived β-cells hold promise as an autologous renewable cell source that can eliminate the necessity of cadaver islets for transplantation and can also reduce the dependence on immunosuppression regimens that compromise the host's immune system and make them prone to infections and tumors. The advantages of combining stem cell technology with material sciences to create efficient encapsulation devices and gene editing tools to create immune evasive cells presents great excitement for the future of diabetes treatment. Great strides are being made to achieve the goal of generating hPSC-derived β-cells that mimic native β-cells. A summary of the different techniques explored to render immunoprotection to transplanted beta cells is shown in Figure 2.

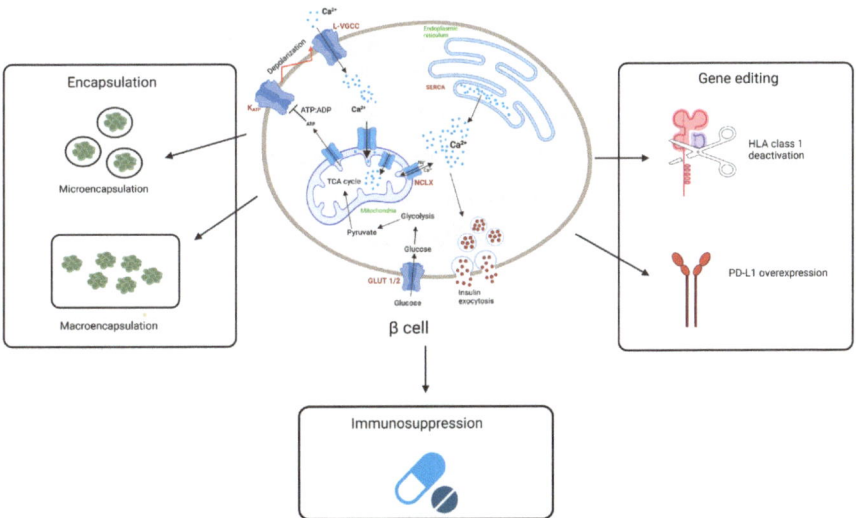

Figure 2. Schematic of the different approaches for the immunoprotection of hPSC-derived β-cell islets for transplantation. Encapsulation strategies involve microencapsulation and macroencapsulation, differentiated by the number of beta cells each method holds. Gene editing techniques include HLA class 1 deactivation using B2M gene knockout, and PD-L1 overexpression. Immunosuppression regimens follow several combinations of drugs to protect transplanted cells from host immune system. This illustration was created with "BioRender.com".

Acute stress immediately after transplantation is a cause for the loss of a large percentage of transplanted cells. Hypoxia, inflammatory cytokines, and hyperglycemia can lead to apoptosis or dysfunction via ER stress responses [126]. Also, instant blood-mediated inflammatory reaction (IBMIR), an inflammatory response to contact with blood leading to platelet encapsulation of the transplanted cells, reduces the diffusion of nutrients into the cells [127]. Research is ongoing to address these concerns while considering hPSC-derived β-cell transplantation. A notable strategy to overcome these issues includes considering alternative transplantation sites such as intramuscular space and omentum [128,129]. However, these techniques have yet to circumvent transplantation stress effectively and further research needs to be performed to improve the safety of transplantation. Research to improve the process of creating enhanced functional hPSC-derived islets that would improve transplantation is also ongoing. Different hPSC differentiation protocols generate varying efficiencies of β-cells and efficiencies also vary between different hPSC cell lines, making the adoption of an ideal differentiation protocol for clinical use difficult [34]. Also, making this therapy accessible to a large number of patients would involve efficient methods to produce transplantable cells at large scales, while keeping production and treatment costs affordable. Current techniques for hPSC differentiation involve small-scale 2D plates or 3D bioreactors. Although current differentiation techniques can produce relatively high-quality β-cells, the same might not be possible to achieve at large-scale production. Further research is imperative to bridge knowledge gaps in the field to seamlessly transfer lab technologies to clinical scales. Consistent improvements are also being made to encapsulation devices to better protect transplanted cells. Numerous trials are underway that closely monitor the application of these technologies in a clinical setting. Although initial reports of these trials show promise in reducing insulin dependency in patients, a closer look into their safety and efficacy needs to be studied to promote their use as a long-term solution to cure diabetes.

Author Contributions: H.H.A.-S. conceptualized the manuscript idea. R.B.A.M.-u.-m. performed the literature search and drafted the manuscript. A.D. and H.H.A.-S. reviewed and edited the manuscript. R.B.A.M.-u.-m. and A.A. prepared the figures. All authors have read and agreed to the published version of the manuscript.

Funding: This research received no external funding.

Institutional Review Board Statement: Not applicable.

Informed Consent Statement: Not applicable.

Data Availability Statement: No new data were created or analyzed in this study. Data sharing is not applicable to this article.

Conflicts of Interest: The authors declare no conflicts of interest.

Abbreviations

The following abbreviations are used in this manuscript:

T1DM	Type 1 diabetes mellitus
T2DM	Type 2 diabetes mellitus
hPSC	human pluripotent stem cells
IDF	International Diabetes Federation
ADA	American Diabetes Association
GDM	gestational diabetes mellitus
MODY	maturity-onset diabetes of the young
hESC	human embryonic stem cells
ER	Endoplasmic reticulum
hiPSC	human induced pluripotent stem cells
TCR	T cell receptor
MHC	Major histocompatibility complexes
APC	Antigen presenting cells
GSIS	glucose-stimulated insulin secretion
NOD-scid	non-obese diabeteic/severe combined immunodeficiency
HLA	human leukocyte antigens
PD-L1	Programmed death-ligand 1
PD-1	Programmed death 1
DSB	Double-stranded DNA break
ZFN	Zinc finger nucleases
TALEN	Transcription activator-like effector nuclease
CRISPR	Clustered Regularly interspaced-Short Palindromic Repeats

TALEs	Transcription activator-like effectors
sgRNA	short noncoding guide RNAs
Cas9	CRISPR-associated protein 9
B2M	Beta 2 microglobulin
KO	knockout
MSC	mesenchymal stem cells
MMTT	mixed meal tolerance test
IBMIR	Instant blood-mediated inflammatory reaction

References

1. American Diabetes Association. Diagnosis and classification of diabetes mellitus. *Diabetes Care* **2010**, *33* (Suppl. S1), S62–S69. [CrossRef] [PubMed]
2. Maahs, D.M.; West, N.A.; Lawrence, J.M.; Mayer-Davis, E.J. Epidemiology of type 1 diabetes. *Endocrinol. Metab. Clin. N. Am.* **2010**, *39*, 481–497. [CrossRef] [PubMed]
3. Craig, M.E.; Hattersley, A.; Donaghue, K.C. Definition, epidemiology and classification of diabetes in children and adolescents. *Pediatr. Diabetes* **2009**, *10* (Suppl. S12), 3–12. [CrossRef] [PubMed]
4. Dabelea, D.; Mayer-Davis, E.J.; Saydah, S.; Imperatore, G.; Linder, B.; Divers, J.; Bell, R.; Badaru, A.; Talton, J.W.; Crume, T.; et al. Prevalence of type 1 and type 2 diabetes among children and adolescents from 2001 to 2009. *JAMA* **2014**, *311*, 1778–1786. [CrossRef] [PubMed]
5. Eizirik, D.L.; Pasquali, L.; Cnop, M. Pancreatic beta-cells in type 1 and type 2 diabetes mellitus: Different pathways to failure. *Nat. Rev. Endocrinol.* **2020**, *16*, 349–362. [CrossRef]
6. American Diabetes Association. 2. Classification and Diagnosis of Diabetes: Standards of Medical Care in Diabetes-2021. *Diabetes Care* **2021**, *44* (Suppl. S1), S15–S33. [CrossRef]
7. Dal Canto, E.; Ceriello, A.; Ryden, L.; Ferrini, M.; Hansen, T.B.; Schnell, O.; Standl, E.; Beulens, J.W. Diabetes as a cardiovascular risk factor: An overview of global trends of macro and micro vascular complications. *Eur. J. Prev. Cardiol.* **2019**, *26*, 25–32. [CrossRef]
8. McNeil, J.; Doucet, E.; Chaput, J.P. Inadequate sleep as a contributor to obesity and type 2 diabetes. *Can. J. Diabetes* **2013**, *37*, 103–108. [CrossRef]
9. Marin-Penalver, J.J.; Martin-Timon, I.; Sevillano-Collantes, C.; Del Canizo-Gomez, F.J. Update on the treatment of type 2 diabetes mellitus. *World J. Diabetes* **2016**, *7*, 354–395. [CrossRef]
10. Song, R. Mechanism of Metformin: A Tale of Two Sites. *Diabetes Care* **2016**, *39*, 187–189. [CrossRef]
11. Eldor, R.; Raz, I. Diabetes therapy-focus on Asia: Second-line therapy debate: Insulin/secretagogues. *Diabetes Metab. Res. Rev.* **2012**, *28* (Suppl. S2), 85–89. [CrossRef] [PubMed]
12. Gerich, J.; Raskin, P.; Jean-Louis, L.; Purkayastha, D.; Baron, M.A. PRESERVE-beta: Two-year efficacy and safety of initial combination therapy with nateglinide or glyburide plus metformin. *Diabetes Care* **2005**, *28*, 2093–2099. [CrossRef] [PubMed]
13. Katsarou, A.; Gudbjornsdottir, S.; Rawshani, A.; Dabelea, D.; Bonifacio, E.; Anderson, B.J.; Jacobsen, L.M.; Schatz, D.A.; Lernmark, A. Type 1 diabetes mellitus. *Nat. Rev. Dis. Primers* **2017**, *3*, 17016. [CrossRef] [PubMed]
14. Miller, K.M.; Foster, N.C.; Beck, R.W.; Bergenstal, R.M.; DuBose, S.N.; DiMeglio, L.A.; Maahs, D.M.; Tamborlane, W.V.; Network, T.D.E.C. Current state of type 1 diabetes treatment in the U.S.: Updated data from the T1D Exchange clinic registry. *Diabetes Care* **2015**, *38*, 971–978. [CrossRef]
15. Shapiro, A.M.; Ricordi, C.; Hering, B.J.; Auchincloss, H.; Lindblad, R.; Robertson, R.P.; Secchi, A.; Brendel, M.D.; Berney, T.; Brennan, D.C.; et al. International trial of the Edmonton protocol for islet transplantation. *N. Engl. J. Med.* **2006**, *355*, 1318–1330. [CrossRef]
16. Diane, A.; Al-Shukri, N.A.; Bin Abdul Mu, U.M.R.; Al-Siddiqi, H.H. Beta-cell mitochondria in diabetes mellitus: A missing puzzle piece in the generation of hPSC-derived pancreatic beta-cells? *J. Transl. Med.* **2022**, *20*, 163. [CrossRef]
17. Sun, Z.Y.; Yu, T.Y.; Jiang, F.X.; Wang, W. Functional maturation of immature beta cells: A roadblock for stem cell therapy for type 1 diabetes. *World J. Stem Cells* **2021**, *13*, 193–207. [CrossRef]
18. Makhlouf, L.; Yamada, A.; Ito, T.; Abdi, R.; Ansari, M.J.; Khuong, C.Q.; Winn, H.J.; Auchincloss, H., Jr.; Sayegh, M.H. Allorecognition and effector pathways of islet allograft rejection in normal versus nonobese diabetic mice. *J. Am. Soc. Nephrol.* **2003**, *14*, 2168–2175. [CrossRef]
19. Brennan, T.V.; Jaigirdar, A.; Hoang, V.; Hayden, T.; Liu, F.C.; Zaid, H.; Chang, C.K.; Bucy, R.P.; Tang, Q.; Kang, S.M. Preferential priming of alloreactive T cells with indirect reactivity. *Am. J. Transplant.* **2009**, *9*, 709–718. [CrossRef]
20. Foulis, A.K.; Farquharson, M.A. Aberrant expression of HLA-DR antigens by insulin-containing beta-cells in recent-onset type I diabetes mellitus. *Diabetes* **1986**, *35*, 1215–1224. [CrossRef]

21. Hamilton-Williams, E.E.; Palmer, S.E.; Charlton, B.; Slattery, R.M. Beta cell MHC class I is a late requirement for diabetes. *Proc. Natl. Acad. Sci. USA* **2003**, *100*, 6688–6693. [CrossRef] [PubMed]
22. Sneddon, J.B.; Tang, Q.; Stock, P.; Bluestone, J.A.; Roy, S.; Desai, T.; Hebrok, M. Stem Cell Therapies for Treating Diabetes: Progress and Remaining Challenges. *Cell Stem Cell* **2018**, *22*, 810–823. [CrossRef] [PubMed]
23. Farney, A.C.; Sutherland, D.E.; Opara, E.C. Evolution of Islet Transplantation for the Last 30 Years. *Pancreas* **2016**, *45*, 8–20. [CrossRef] [PubMed]
24. Tekin, Z.; Garfinkel, M.R.; Chon, W.J.; Schenck, L.; Golab, K.; Savari, O.; Thistlethwaite, J.R.; Philipson, L.H.; Majewski, C.; Pannain, S.; et al. Outcomes of Pancreatic Islet Allotransplantation Using the Edmonton Protocol at the University of Chicago. *Transplant. Direct* **2016**, *2*, e105. [CrossRef] [PubMed]
25. Hering, B.J.; Kandaswamy, R.; Ansite, J.D.; Eckman, P.M.; Nakano, M.; Sawada, T.; Matsumoto, I.; Ihm, S.H.; Zhang, H.J.; Parkey, J.; et al. Single-donor, marginal-dose islet transplantation in patients with type 1 diabetes. *JAMA* **2005**, *293*, 830–835. [CrossRef]
26. Hering, B.J.; Kandaswamy, R.; Harmon, J.V.; Ansite, J.D.; Clemmings, S.M.; Sakai, T.; Paraskevas, S.; Eckman, P.M.; Sageshima, J.; Nakano, M.; et al. Transplantation of cultured islets from two-layer preserved pancreases in type 1 diabetes with anti-CD3 antibody. *Am. J. Transplant.* **2004**, *4*, 390–401. [CrossRef]
27. Posselt, A.M.; Szot, G.L.; Frassetto, L.A.; Masharani, U.; Tavakol, M.; Amin, R.; McElroy, J.; Ramos, M.D.; Kerlan, R.K.; Fong, L.; et al. Islet transplantation in type 1 diabetic patients using calcineurin inhibitor-free immunosuppressive protocols based on T-cell adhesion or costimulation blockade. *Transplantation* **2010**, *90*, 1595–1601. [CrossRef]
28. Johnson, J.D.; Ao, Z.; Ao, P.; Li, H.; Dai, L.J.; He, Z.; Tee, M.; Potter, K.J.; Klimek, A.M.; Meloche, R.M.; et al. Different effects of FK506, rapamycin, and mycophenolate mofetil on glucose-stimulated insulin release and apoptosis in human islets. *Cell Transplant.* **2009**, *18*, 833–845. [CrossRef]
29. Zhang, N.; Su, D.; Qu, S.; Tse, T.; Bottino, R.; Balamurugan, A.N.; Xu, J.; Bromberg, J.S.; Dong, H.H. Sirolimus is associated with reduced islet engraftment and impaired beta-cell function. *Diabetes* **2006**, *55*, 2429–2436. [CrossRef]
30. Zahr, E.; Molano, R.D.; Pileggi, A.; Ichii, H.; San Jose, S.; Bocca, N.; An, W.; Gonzalez-Quintana, J.; Fraker, C.; Ricordi, C.; et al. Rapamycin impairs beta-cell proliferation in vivo. *Transplant. Proc.* **2008**, *40*, 436–437. [CrossRef]
31. Fraenkel, M.; Ketzinel-Gilad, M.; Ariav, Y.; Pappo, O.; Karaca, M.; Castel, J.; Berthault, M.F.; Magnan, C.; Cerasi, E.; Kaiser, N.; et al. mTOR inhibition by rapamycin prevents beta-cell adaptation to hyperglycemia and exacerbates the metabolic state in type 2 diabetes. *Diabetes* **2008**, *57*, 945–957. [CrossRef] [PubMed]
32. Abdelalim, E.M.; Bonnefond, A.; Bennaceur-Griscelli, A.; Froguel, P. Pluripotent stem cells as a potential tool for disease modelling and cell therapy in diabetes. *Stem Cell Rev. Rep.* **2014**, *10*, 327–337. [CrossRef] [PubMed]
33. Maxwell, K.G.; Millman, J.R. Applications of iPSC-derived beta cells from patients with diabetes. *Cell Rep. Med.* **2021**, *2*, 100238. [CrossRef] [PubMed]
34. Hogrebe, N.J.; Maxwell, K.G.; Augsornworawat, P.; Millman, J.R. Generation of insulin-producing pancreatic beta cells from multiple human stem cell lines. *Nat. Protoc.* **2021**, *16*, 4109–4143. [CrossRef]
35. Rezania, A.; Bruin, J.E.; Arora, P.; Rubin, A.; Batushansky, I.; Asadi, A.; O'Dwyer, S.; Quiskamp, N.; Mojibian, M.; Albrecht, T.; et al. Reversal of diabetes with insulin-producing cells derived in vitro from human pluripotent stem cells. *Nat. Biotechnol.* **2014**, *32*, 1121–1133. [CrossRef]
36. Pagliuca, F.W.; Millman, J.R.; Gurtler, M.; Segel, M.; Van Dervort, A.; Ryu, J.H.; Peterson, Q.P.; Greiner, D.; Melton, D.A. Generation of functional human pancreatic beta cells in vitro. *Cell* **2014**, *159*, 428–439. [CrossRef]
37. Sui, L.; Danzl, N.; Campbell, S.R.; Viola, R.; Williams, D.; Xing, Y.; Wang, Y.; Phillips, N.; Poffenberger, G.; Johannesson, B.; et al. Beta-Cell Replacement in Mice Using Human Type 1 Diabetes Nuclear Transfer Embryonic Stem Cells. *Diabetes* **2018**, *67*, 26–35. [CrossRef]
38. Paez-Mayorga, J.; Lukin, I.; Emerich, D.; de Vos, P.; Orive, G.; Grattoni, A. Emerging strategies for beta cell transplantation to treat diabetes. *Trends Pharmacol. Sci.* **2022**, *43*, 221–233. [CrossRef]
39. Zhang, Q.; Gonelle-Gispert, C.; Li, Y.; Geng, Z.; Gerber-Lemaire, S.; Wang, Y.; Buhler, L. Islet Encapsulation: New Developments for the Treatment of Type 1 Diabetes. *Front. Immunol.* **2022**, *13*, 869984. [CrossRef]
40. Lee, K.Y.; Mooney, D.J. Alginate: Properties and biomedical applications. *Prog. Polym. Sci.* **2012**, *37*, 106–126. [CrossRef]
41. Neumann, M.; Arnould, T.; Su, B.L. Encapsulation of stem-cell derived beta-cells: A promising approach for the treatment for type 1 diabetes mellitus. *J. Colloid. Interface Sci.* **2023**, *636*, 90–102. [CrossRef] [PubMed]
42. Soltani, A.; Soleimani, M.; Ghiass, M.A.; Enderami, S.E.; Rabbani, S.; Jafarian, A.; Allameh, A. Treatment of diabetic mice by microfluidic system-assisted transplantation of stem cells-derived insulin-producing cells transduced with miRNA. *Life Sci.* **2021**, *274*, 119338. [CrossRef] [PubMed]
43. Kuncorojakti, S.; Rodprasert, W.; Yodmuang, S.; Osathanon, T.; Pavasant, P.; Srisuwatanasagul, S.; Sawangmake, C. Alginate/Pluronic F127-based encapsulation supports viability and functionality of human dental pulp stem cell-derived insulin-producing cells. *J. Biol. Eng.* **2020**, *14*, 23. [CrossRef] [PubMed]

44. Chaimov, D.; Baruch, L.; Krishtul, S.; Meivar-Levy, I.; Ferber, S.; Machluf, M. Innovative encapsulation platform based on pancreatic extracellular matrix achieve substantial insulin delivery. *J. Control Release* **2017**, *257*, 91–101. [CrossRef]
45. Vegas, A.J.; Veiseh, O.; Gurtler, M.; Millman, J.R.; Pagliuca, F.W.; Bader, A.R.; Doloff, J.C.; Li, J.; Chen, M.; Olejnik, K.; et al. Long-term glycemic control using polymer-encapsulated human stem cell-derived beta cells in immune-competent mice. *Nat. Med.* **2016**, *22*, 306–311. [CrossRef]
46. Kharbikar, B.N.; Chendke, G.S.; Desai, T.A. Modulating the foreign body response of implants for diabetes treatment. *Adv. Drug Deliv. Rev.* **2021**, *174*, 87–113. [CrossRef]
47. Alagpulinsa, D.A.; Cao, J.J.L.; Driscoll, R.K.; Sirbulescu, R.F.; Penson, M.F.E.; Sremac, M.; Engquist, E.N.; Brauns, T.A.; Markmann, J.F.; Melton, D.A.; et al. Alginate-microencapsulation of human stem cell-derived beta cells with CXCL12 prolongs their survival and function in immunocompetent mice without systemic immunosuppression. *Am. J. Transplant.* **2019**, *19*, 1930–1940. [CrossRef]
48. Buchwald, P. A local glucose-and oxygen concentration-based insulin secretion model for pancreatic islets. *Theor. Biol. Med. Model.* **2011**, *8*, 20. [CrossRef]
49. Williams, S.J.; Huang, H.H.; Kover, K.; Moore, W.; Berkland, C.; Singh, M.; Smirnova, I.V.; MacGregor, R.; Stehno-Bittel, L. Reduction of diffusion barriers in isolated rat islets improves survival, but not insulin secretion or transplantation outcome. *Organogenesis* **2010**, *6*, 115–124. [CrossRef]
50. Stock, A.A.; Manzoli, V.; De Toni, T.; Abreu, M.M.; Poh, Y.C.; Ye, L.; Roose, A.; Pagliuca, F.W.; Thanos, C.; Ricordi, C.; et al. Conformal Coating of Stem Cell-Derived Islets for beta Cell Replacement in Type 1 Diabetes. *Stem Cell Rep.* **2020**, *14*, 91–104. [CrossRef]
51. Carlsson, P.O.; Espes, D.; Sedigh, A.; Rotem, A.; Zimerman, B.; Grinberg, H.; Goldman, T.; Barkai, U.; Avni, Y.; Westermark, G.T.; et al. Transplantation of macroencapsulated human islets within the bioartificial pancreas betaAir to patients with type 1 diabetes mellitus. *Am. J. Transplant.* **2018**, *18*, 1735–1744. [CrossRef] [PubMed]
52. Liu, W.; Wang, Y.; Wang, J.; Lanier, O.L.; Wechsler, M.E.; Peppas, N.A.; Gu, Z. Macroencapsulation Devices for Cell Therapy. *Engineering* **2022**, *13*, 53–70. [CrossRef]
53. Sweet, I.R.; Yanay, O.; Waldron, L.; Gilbert, M.; Fuller, J.M.; Tupling, T.; Lernmark, A.; Osborne, W.R. Treatment of diabetic rats with encapsulated islets. *J. Cell. Mol. Med.* **2008**, *12*, 2644–2650. [CrossRef] [PubMed]
54. Kumagai-Braesch, M.; Jacobson, S.; Mori, H.; Jia, X.; Takahashi, T.; Wernerson, A.; Flodstrom-Tullberg, M.; Tibell, A. The TheraCyte device protects against islet allograft rejection in immunized hosts. *Cell Transplant.* **2013**, *22*, 1137–1146. [CrossRef]
55. Kirk, K.; Hao, E.; Lahmy, R.; Itkin-Ansari, P. Human embryonic stem cell derived islet progenitors mature inside an encapsulation device without evidence of increased biomass or cell escape. *Stem Cell Res.* **2014**, *12*, 807–814. [CrossRef]
56. Chang, R.; Faleo, G.; Russ, H.A.; Parent, A.V.; Elledge, S.K.; Bernards, D.A.; Allen, J.L.; Villanueva, K.; Hebrok, M.; Tang, Q.; et al. Nanoporous Immunoprotective Device for Stem-Cell-Derived beta-Cell Replacement Therapy. *ACS Nano* **2017**, *11*, 7747–7757. [CrossRef]
57. Liu, W.; Flanders, J.A.; Wang, L.H.; Liu, Q.; Bowers, D.T.; Wang, K.; Chiu, A.; Wang, X.; Ernst, A.U.; Shariati, K.; et al. A Safe, Fibrosis-Mitigating, and Scalable Encapsulation Device Supports Long-Term Function of Insulin-Producing Cells. *Small* **2022**, *18*, e2104899. [CrossRef]
58. Yang, K.; O'Cearbhaill, E.D.; Liu, S.S.; Zhou, A.; Chitnis, G.D.; Hamilos, A.E.; Xu, J.; Verma, M.K.S.; Giraldo, J.A.; Kudo, Y.; et al. A therapeutic convection-enhanced macroencapsulation device for enhancing beta cell viability and insulin secretion. *Proc. Natl. Acad. Sci. USA* **2021**, *118*, e2101258118. [CrossRef]
59. Claire, E.; Hilburger, M.J.R. Derfogail Delcassian. The type 1 diabetes immune niche: Immunomodulatory biomaterial design considerations for beta cell transplant therapies. *J. Immunol. Regen. Med.* **2022**, *17*, 100063. [CrossRef]
60. Bloor, A.J.C.; Patel, A.; Griffin, J.E.; Gilleece, M.H.; Radia, R.; Yeung, D.T.; Drier, D.; Larson, L.S.; Uenishi, G.I.; Hei, D.; et al. Production, safety and efficacy of iPSC-derived mesenchymal stromal cells in acute steroid-resistant graft versus host disease: A phase I, multicenter, open-label, dose-escalation study. *Nat. Med.* **2020**, *26*, 1720–1725. [CrossRef]
61. Umekage, M.; Sato, Y.; Takasu, N. Overview: An iPS cell stock at CiRA. *Inflamm. Regen.* **2019**, *39*, 17. [CrossRef] [PubMed]
62. Tahbaz, M.; Yoshihara, E. Immune Protection of Stem Cell-Derived Islet Cell Therapy for Treating Diabetes. *Front. Endocrinol.* **2021**, *12*, 716625. [CrossRef]
63. Soleimanpour, S.A.; Stoffers, D.A. The pancreatic beta cell and type 1 diabetes: Innocent bystander or active participant? *Trends Endocrinol. Metab.* **2013**, *24*, 324–331. [CrossRef] [PubMed]
64. Drukker, M.; Katz, G.; Urbach, A.; Schuldiner, M.; Markel, G.; Itskovitz-Eldor, J.; Reubinoff, B.; Mandelboim, O.; Benvenisty, N. Characterization of the expression of MHC proteins in human embryonic stem cells. *Proc. Natl. Acad. Sci. USA* **2002**, *99*, 9864–9869. [CrossRef] [PubMed]
65. Castro-Gutierrez, R.; Alkanani, A.; Mathews, C.E.; Michels, A.; Russ, H.A. Protecting Stem Cell Derived Pancreatic Beta-like Cells from Diabetogenic T Cell Recognition. *Front. Endocrinol.* **2021**, *12*, 707881. [CrossRef]

66. Millette, K.; Georgia, S. Gene Editing and Human Pluripotent Stem Cells: Tools for Advancing Diabetes Disease Modeling and Beta-Cell Development. *Curr. Diab. Rep.* **2017**, *17*, 116. [CrossRef]
67. George, M.N.; Leavens, K.F.; Gadue, P. Genome Editing Human Pluripotent Stem Cells to Model beta-Cell Disease and Unmask Novel Genetic Modifiers. *Front. Endocrinol.* **2021**, *12*, 682625. [CrossRef]
68. Chou, S.T.; Leng, Q.; Mixson, A.J. Zinc Finger Nucleases: Tailor-made for Gene Therapy. *Drugs Future* **2012**, *37*, 183–196. [CrossRef]
69. Cox, D.B.; Platt, R.J.; Zhang, F. Therapeutic genome editing: Prospects and challenges. *Nat. Med.* **2015**, *21*, 121–131. [CrossRef]
70. Zhang, Z.; Zhang, Y.; Gao, F.; Han, S.; Cheah, K.S.; Tse, H.F.; Lian, Q. CRISPR/Cas9 Genome-Editing System in Human Stem Cells: Current Status and Future Prospects. *Mol. Ther. Nucleic Acids* **2017**, *9*, 230–241. [CrossRef]
71. Leite, N.C.; Sintov, E.; Meissner, T.B.; Brehm, M.A.; Greiner, D.L.; Harlan, D.M.; Melton, D.A. Modeling Type 1 Diabetes In Vitro Using Human Pluripotent Stem Cells. *Cell Rep.* **2020**, *32*, 107894. [CrossRef] [PubMed]
72. Karre, K.; Ljunggren, H.G.; Piontek, G.; Kiessling, R. Selective rejection of H-2-deficient lymphoma variants suggests alternative immune defence strategy. *Nature* **1986**, *319*, 675–678. [CrossRef]
73. Xu, H.; Wang, B.; Ono, M.; Kagita, A.; Fujii, K.; Sasakawa, N.; Ueda, T.; Gee, P.; Nishikawa, M.; Nomura, M.; et al. Targeted Disruption of HLA Genes via CRISPR-Cas9 Generates iPSCs with Enhanced Immune Compatibility. *Cell Stem Cell* **2019**, *24*, 566–578 e567. [CrossRef] [PubMed]
74. Wang, D.; Quan, Y.; Yan, Q.; Morales, J.E.; Wetsel, R.A. Targeted Disruption of the beta2-Microglobulin Gene Minimizes the Immunogenicity of Human Embryonic Stem Cells. *Stem Cells Transl. Med.* **2015**, *4*, 1234–1245. [CrossRef] [PubMed]
75. Gornalusse, G.G.; Hirata, R.K.; Funk, S.E.; Riolobos, L.; Lopes, V.S.; Manske, G.; Prunkard, D.; Colunga, A.G.; Hanafi, L.A.; Clegg, D.O.; et al. HLA-E-expressing pluripotent stem cells escape allogeneic responses and lysis by NK cells. *Nat. Biotechnol.* **2017**, *35*, 765–772. [CrossRef]
76. Han, X.; Wang, M.; Duan, S.; Franco, P.J.; Kenty, J.H.; Hedrick, P.; Xia, Y.; Allen, A.; Ferreira, L.M.R.; Strominger, J.L.; et al. Generation of hypoimmunogenic human pluripotent stem cells. *Proc. Natl. Acad. Sci. USA* **2019**, *116*, 10441–10446. [CrossRef]
77. Shi, L.; Li, W.; Liu, Y.; Chen, Z.; Hui, Y.; Hao, P.; Xu, X.; Zhang, S.; Feng, H.; Zhang, B.; et al. Generation of hypoimmunogenic human pluripotent stem cells via expression of membrane-bound and secreted beta2m-HLA-G fusion proteins. *Stem Cells* **2020**, *38*, 1423–1437. [CrossRef]
78. Iwai, Y.; Ishida, M.; Tanaka, Y.; Okazaki, T.; Honjo, T.; Minato, N. Involvement of PD-L1 on tumor cells in the escape from host immune system and tumor immunotherapy by PD-L1 blockade. *Proc. Natl. Acad. Sci. USA* **2002**, *99*, 12293–12297. [CrossRef]
79. Keir, M.E.; Liang, S.C.; Guleria, I.; Latchman, Y.E.; Qipo, A.; Albacker, L.A.; Koulmanda, M.; Freeman, G.J.; Sayegh, M.H.; Sharpe, A.H. Tissue expression of PD-L1 mediates peripheral T cell tolerance. *J. Exp. Med.* **2006**, *203*, 883–895. [CrossRef]
80. Ansari, M.J.; Salama, A.D.; Chitnis, T.; Smith, R.N.; Yagita, H.; Akiba, H.; Yamazaki, T.; Azuma, M.; Iwai, H.; Khoury, S.J.; et al. The programmed death-1 (PD-1) pathway regulates autoimmune diabetes in nonobese diabetic (NOD) mice. *J. Exp. Med.* **2003**, *198*, 63–69. [CrossRef]
81. Ma, D.; Duan, W.; Li, Y.; Wang, Z.; Li, S.; Gong, N.; Chen, G.; Chen, Z.; Wan, C.; Yang, J. PD-L1 Deficiency within Islets Reduces Allograft Survival in Mice. *PLoS ONE* **2016**, *11*, e0152087. [CrossRef] [PubMed]
82. Ma, H.; Jeppesen, J.F.; Jaenisch, R. Human T Cells Expressing a CD19 CAR-T Receptor Provide Insights into Mechanisms of Human CD19-Positive beta Cell Destruction. *Cell Rep. Med.* **2020**, *1*, 100097. [CrossRef] [PubMed]
83. Yoshihara, E.; O'Connor, C.; Gasser, E.; Wei, Z.; Oh, T.G.; Tseng, T.W.; Wang, D.; Cayabyab, F.; Dai, Y.; Yu, R.T.; et al. Immune-evasive human islet-like organoids ameliorate diabetes. *Nature* **2020**, *586*, 606–611. [CrossRef] [PubMed]
84. Haapaniemi, E.; Botla, S.; Persson, J.; Schmierer, B.; Taipale, J. CRISPR-Cas9 genome editing induces a p53-mediated DNA damage response. *Nat. Med.* **2018**, *24*, 927–930. [CrossRef]
85. Ihry, R.J.; Worringer, K.A.; Salick, M.R.; Frias, E.; Ho, D.; Theriault, K.; Kommineni, S.; Chen, J.; Sondey, M.; Ye, C.; et al. p53 inhibits CRISPR-Cas9 engineering in human pluripotent stem cells. *Nat. Med.* **2018**, *24*, 939–946. [CrossRef]
86. Doench, J.G.; Fusi, N.; Sullender, M.; Hegde, M.; Vaimberg, E.W.; Donovan, K.F.; Smith, I.; Tothova, Z.; Wilen, C.; Orchard, R.; et al. Optimized sgRNA design to maximize activity and minimize off-target effects of CRISPR-Cas9. *Nat. Biotechnol.* **2016**, *34*, 184–191. [CrossRef]
87. Zhang, D.; Zhang, Z.; Unver, T.; Zhang, B. CRISPR/Cas: A powerful tool for gene function study and crop improvement. *J. Adv. Res.* **2021**, *29*, 207–221. [CrossRef]
88. Hering, B.J.; Clarke, W.R.; Bridges, N.D.; Eggerman, T.L.; Alejandro, R.; Bellin, M.D.; Chaloner, K.; Czarniecki, C.W.; Goldstein, J.S.; Hunsicker, L.G.; et al. Phase 3 Trial of Transplantation of Human Islets in Type 1 Diabetes Complicated by Severe Hypoglycemia. *Diabetes Care* **2016**, *39*, 1230–1240. [CrossRef]
89. Ludwig, B.; Rotem, A.; Schmid, J.; Weir, G.C.; Colton, C.K.; Brendel, M.D.; Neufeld, T.; Block, N.L.; Yavriyants, K.; Steffen, A.; et al. Improvement of islet function in a bioartificial pancreas by enhanced oxygen supply and growth hormone releasing hormone agonist. *Proc. Natl. Acad. Sci. USA* **2012**, *109*, 5022–5027. [CrossRef]

90. Soon-Shiong, P.; Heintz, R.E.; Merideth, N.; Yao, Q.X.; Yao, Z.; Zheng, T.; Murphy, M.; Moloney, M.K.; Schmehl, M.; Harris, M.; et al. Insulin independence in a type 1 diabetic patient after encapsulated islet transplantation. *Lancet* **1994**, *343*, 950–951. [CrossRef]
91. Kern, S.; Eichler, H.; Stoeve, J.; Kluter, H.; Bieback, K. Comparative analysis of mesenchymal stem cells from bone marrow, umbilical cord blood, or adipose tissue. *Stem Cells* **2006**, *24*, 1294–1301. [CrossRef] [PubMed]
92. Moreira, A.; Kahlenberg, S.; Hornsby, P. Therapeutic potential of mesenchymal stem cells for diabetes. *J. Mol. Endocrinol.* **2017**, *59*, R109–R120. [CrossRef] [PubMed]
93. Ra, J.C.; Shin, I.S.; Kim, S.H.; Kang, S.K.; Kang, B.C.; Lee, H.Y.; Kim, Y.J.; Jo, J.Y.; Yoon, E.J.; Choi, H.J.; et al. Safety of intravenous infusion of human adipose tissue-derived mesenchymal stem cells in animals and humans. *Stem Cells Dev.* **2011**, *20*, 1297–1308. [CrossRef] [PubMed]
94. Lee, R.H.; Seo, M.J.; Reger, R.L.; Spees, J.L.; Pulin, A.A.; Olson, S.D.; Prockop, D.J. Multipotent stromal cells from human marrow home to and promote repair of pancreatic islets and renal glomeruli in diabetic NOD/scid mice. *Proc. Natl. Acad. Sci. USA* **2006**, *103*, 17438–17443. [CrossRef]
95. Abdi, R.; Fiorina, P.; Adra, C.N.; Atkinson, M.; Sayegh, M.H. Immunomodulation by mesenchymal stem cells: A potential therapeutic strategy for type 1 diabetes. *Diabetes* **2008**, *57*, 1759–1767. [CrossRef]
96. Izadi, M.; Sadr Hashemi Nejad, A.; Moazenchi, M.; Masoumi, S.; Rabbani, A.; Kompani, F.; Hedayati Asl, A.A.; Abbasi Kakroodi, F.; Jaroughi, N.; Mohseni Meybodi, M.A.; et al. Mesenchymal stem cell transplantation in newly diagnosed type-1 diabetes patients: A phase I/II randomized placebo-controlled clinical trial. *Stem Cell Res. Ther.* **2022**, *13*, 264. [CrossRef]
97. de Klerk, E.; Hebrok, M. Stem Cell-Based Clinical Trials for Diabetes Mellitus. *Front. Endocrinol.* **2021**, *12*, 631463. [CrossRef]
98. Ghoneim, M.A.; Gabr, M.M.; El-Halawani, S.M.; Refaie, A.F. Current status of stem cell therapy for type 1 diabetes: A critique and a prospective consideration. *Stem Cell Res. Ther.* **2024**, *15*, 23. [CrossRef]
99. Carlsson, P.O.; Schwarcz, E.; Korsgren, O.; Le Blanc, K. Preserved beta-cell function in type 1 diabetes by mesenchymal stromal cells. *Diabetes* **2015**, *64*, 587–592. [CrossRef]
100. Hu, J.; Yu, X.; Wang, Z.; Wang, F.; Wang, L.; Gao, H.; Chen, Y.; Zhao, W.; Jia, Z.; Yan, S.; et al. Long term effects of the implantation of Wharton's jelly-derived mesenchymal stem cells from the umbilical cord for newly-onset type 1 diabetes mellitus. *Endocr. J.* **2013**, *60*, 347–357. [CrossRef]
101. Dave, S.D.; Vanikar, A.V.; Trivedi, H.L.; Thakkar, U.G.; Gopal, S.C.; Chandra, T. Novel therapy for insulin-dependent diabetes mellitus: Infusion of in vitro-generated insulin-secreting cells. *Clin. Exp. Med.* **2015**, *15*, 41–45. [CrossRef]
102. Dantas, J.R.; Araujo, D.B.; Silva, K.R.; Souto, D.L.; de Fatima Carvalho Pereira, M.; Luiz, R.R.; Dos Santos Mantuano, M.; Claudio-da-Silva, C.; Gabbay, M.A.L.; Dib, S.A.; et al. Adipose tissue-derived stromal/stem cells + cholecalciferol: A pilot study in recent-onset type 1 diabetes patients. *Arch. Endocrinol. Metab.* **2021**, *65*, 342–351. [CrossRef] [PubMed]
103. Lu, J.; Shen, S.M.; Ling, Q.; Wang, B.; Li, L.R.; Zhang, W.; Qu, D.D.; Bi, Y.; Zhu, D.L. One repeated transplantation of allogeneic umbilical cord mesenchymal stromal cells in type 1 diabetes: An open parallel controlled clinical study. *Stem Cell Res. Ther.* **2021**, *12*, 340. [CrossRef] [PubMed]
104. Thakkar, U.G.; Trivedi, H.L.; Vanikar, A.V.; Dave, S.D. Insulin-secreting adipose-derived mesenchymal stromal cells with bone marrow-derived hematopoietic stem cells from autologous and allogenic sources for type 1 diabetes mellitus. *Cytotherapy* **2015**, *17*, 940–947. [CrossRef] [PubMed]
105. Cai, J.; Wu, Z.; Xu, X.; Liao, L.; Chen, J.; Huang, L.; Wu, W.; Luo, F.; Wu, C.; Pugliese, A.; et al. Umbilical Cord Mesenchymal Stromal Cell with Autologous Bone Marrow Cell Transplantation in Established Type 1 Diabetes: A Pilot Randomized Controlled Open-Label Clinical Study to Assess Safety and Impact on Insulin Secretion. *Diabetes Care* **2016**, *39*, 149–157. [CrossRef] [PubMed]
106. Jayasinghe, M.; Prathiraja, O.; Perera, P.B.; Jena, R.; Silva, M.S.; Weerawarna, P.S.H.; Singhal, M.; Kayani, A.M.A.; Karnakoti, S.; Jain, S. The Role of Mesenchymal Stem Cells in the Treatment of Type 1 Diabetes. *Cureus* **2022**, *14*, e27337. [CrossRef]
107. Hwang, G.; Jeong, H.; Yang, H.K.; Kim, H.S.; Hong, H.; Kim, N.J.; Oh, I.H.; Yim, H.W. Efficacies of Stem Cell Therapies for Functional Improvement of the beta Cell in Patients with Diabetes: A Systematic Review of Controlled Clinical Trials. *Int. J. Stem Cells* **2019**, *12*, 195–205. [CrossRef]
108. Bruin, J.E.; Erener, S.; Vela, J.; Hu, X.; Johnson, J.D.; Kurata, H.T.; Lynn, F.C.; Piret, J.M.; Asadi, A.; Rezania, A.; et al. Characterization of polyhormonal insulin-producing cells derived in vitro from human embryonic stem cells. *Stem Cell Res.* **2014**, *12*, 194–208. [CrossRef]
109. Rezania, A.; Bruin, J.E.; Xu, J.; Narayan, K.; Fox, J.K.; O'Neil, J.J.; Kieffer, T.J. Enrichment of human embryonic stem cell-derived NKX6.1-expressing pancreatic progenitor cells accelerates the maturation of insulin-secreting cells in vivo. *Stem Cells* **2013**, *31*, 2432–2442. [CrossRef]
110. Ramzy, A.; Thompson, D.M.; Ward-Hartstonge, K.A.; Ivison, S.; Cook, L.; Garcia, R.V.; Loyal, J.; Kim, P.T.W.; Warnock, G.L.; Levings, M.K.; et al. Implanted pluripotent stem-cell-derived pancreatic endoderm cells secrete glucose-responsive C-peptide in patients with type 1 diabetes. *Cell Stem Cell* **2021**, *28*, 2047–2061 e2045. [CrossRef]

111. Henry, R.R.; Pettus, J.; Wilensky, J.O.N.; SHAPIRO, A.J.; Senior, P.A.; Roep, B.; Wang, R.; Kroon, E.J.; Scott, M.; D'Amour, K.; et al. Initial Clinical Evaluation of VC-01TM Combination Product—A Stem Cell–Derived Islet Replacement for Type 1 Diabetes (T1D). *Diabetes* **2018**, *67*, 138-OR. [CrossRef]
112. Shapiro, A.M.J.; Thompson, D.; Donner, T.W.; Bellin, M.D.; Hsueh, W.; Pettus, J.; Wilensky, J.; Daniels, M.; Wang, R.M.; Brandon, E.P.; et al. Insulin expression and C-peptide in type 1 diabetes subjects implanted with stem cell-derived pancreatic endoderm cells in an encapsulation device. *Cell Rep. Med.* **2021**, *2*, 100466. [CrossRef] [PubMed]
113. Keymeulen, B.; De Groot, K.; Jacobs-Tulleneers-Thevissen, D.; Thompson, D.M.; Bellin, M.D.; Kroon, E.J.; Daniels, M.; Wang, R.; Jaiman, M.; Kieffer, T.J.; et al. Encapsulated stem cell-derived beta cells exert glucose control in patients with type 1 diabetes. *Nat. Biotechnol.* **2023**, *42*, 1507–1514. [CrossRef] [PubMed]
114. Ramzy, A.; Belmonte, P.J.; Braam, M.J.S.; Ida, S.; Wilts, E.M.; Levings, M.K.; Rezania, A.; Kieffer, T.J. A Century-long Journey From the Discovery of Insulin to the Implantation of Stem Cell-derived Islets. *Endocr. Rev.* **2023**, *44*, 222–253. [CrossRef]
115. Memon, B.; Abdelalim, E.M. Toward Precision Medicine with Human Pluripotent Stem Cells for Diabetes. *Stem Cells Transl. Med.* **2022**, *11*, 704–714. [CrossRef]
116. Memon, B.; Abdelalim, E.M. Stem Cell Therapy for Diabetes: Beta Cells versus Pancreatic Progenitors. *Cells* **2020**, *9*, 283. [CrossRef]
117. Jones, P.M.; Persaud, S.J. beta-cell replacement therapy for type 1 diabetes: Closer and closer. *Diabet. Med.* **2022**, *39*, e14834. [CrossRef]
118. Parums, D.V. Editorial: First Regulatory Approval for Allogeneic Pancreatic Islet Beta Cell Infusion for Adult Patients with Type 1 Diabetes Mellitus. *Med. Sci. Monit.* **2023**, *29*, e941918. [CrossRef]
119. Tuch, B.E.; Keogh, G.W.; Williams, L.J.; Wu, W.; Foster, J.L.; Vaithilingam, V.; Philips, R. Safety and viability of microencapsulated human islets transplanted into diabetic humans. *Diabetes Care* **2009**, *32*, 1887–1889. [CrossRef]
120. Calafiore, R.; Basta, G.; Luca, G.; Lemmi, A.; Montanucci, M.P.; Calabrese, G.; Racanicchi, L.; Mancuso, F.; Brunetti, P. Microencapsulated pancreatic islet allografts into nonimmunosuppressed patients with type 1 diabetes: First two cases. *Diabetes Care* **2006**, *29*, 137–138. [CrossRef]
121. Dang, H.P.; Chen, H.; Dargaville, T.R.; Tuch, B.E. Cell delivery systems: Toward the next generation of cell therapies for type 1 diabetes. *J. Cell. Mol. Med.* **2022**, *26*, 4756–4767. [CrossRef] [PubMed]
122. Geller, R.L.; Loudovaris, T.; Neuenfeldt, S.; Johnson, R.C.; Brauker, J.H. Use of an immunoisolation device for cell transplantation and tumor immunotherapy. *Ann. N. Y. Acad. Sci.* **1997**, *831*, 438–451. [CrossRef] [PubMed]
123. Wang, X.; Maxwell, K.G.; Wang, K.; Bowers, D.T.; Flanders, J.A.; Liu, W.; Wang, L.H.; Liu, Q.; Liu, C.; Naji, A.; et al. A nanofibrous encapsulation device for safe delivery of insulin-producing cells to treat type 1 diabetes. *Sci. Transl. Med.* **2021**, *13*, eabb4601. [CrossRef] [PubMed]
124. Papas, K.K.; De Leon, H.; Suszynski, T.M.; Johnson, R.C. Oxygenation strategies for encapsulated islet and beta cell transplants. *Adv. Drug Deliv. Rev.* **2019**, *139*, 139–156. [CrossRef]
125. Kaufman-Francis, K.; Koffler, J.; Weinberg, N.; Dor, Y.; Levenberg, S. Engineered vascular beds provide key signals to pancreatic hormone-producing cells. *PLoS ONE* **2012**, *7*, e40741. [CrossRef]
126. Fonseca, S.G.; Gromada, J.; Urano, F. Endoplasmic reticulum stress and pancreatic beta-cell death. *Trends Endocrinol. Metab.* **2011**, *22*, 266–274. [CrossRef]
127. Nilsson, B.; Ekdahl, K.N.; Korsgren, O. Control of instant blood-mediated inflammatory reaction to improve islets of Langerhans engraftment. *Curr. Opin. Organ. Transplant.* **2011**, *16*, 620–626. [CrossRef]
128. Christoffersson, G.; Henriksnas, J.; Johansson, L.; Rolny, C.; Ahlstrom, H.; Caballero-Corbalan, J.; Segersvard, R.; Permert, J.; Korsgren, O.; Carlsson, P.O.; et al. Clinical and experimental pancreatic islet transplantation to striated muscle: Establishment of a vascular system similar to that in native islets. *Diabetes* **2010**, *59*, 2569–2578. [CrossRef]
129. Berman, D.M.; Molano, R.D.; Fotino, C.; Ulissi, U.; Gimeno, J.; Mendez, A.J.; Kenyon, N.M.; Kenyon, N.S.; Andrews, D.M.; Ricordi, C.; et al. Bioengineering the Endocrine Pancreas: Intraomental Islet Transplantation Within a Biologic Resorbable Scaffold. *Diabetes* **2016**, *65*, 1350–1361. [CrossRef]

Disclaimer/Publisher's Note: The statements, opinions and data contained in all publications are solely those of the individual author(s) and contributor(s) and not of MDPI and/or the editor(s). MDPI and/or the editor(s) disclaim responsibility for any injury to people or property resulting from any ideas, methods, instructions or products referred to in the content.

Morphological Signal Processing for Phenotype Recognition of Human Pluripotent Stem Cells Using Machine Learning Methods

Ekaterina Vedeneeva [1], Vitaly Gursky [2,3,*], Maria Samsonova [1] and Irina Neganova [2]

[1] Department of Physics and Mechanics & Mathematical Biology and Bioinformatics Laboratory, Peter the Great St. Petersburg Polytechnic University, 195251 Saint Petersburg, Russia; vedeneeva.ed@edu.spbstu.ru (E.V.); m.samsonova@spbstu.ru (M.S.)
[2] Laboratory of Molecular Medicine, Institute of Cytology, 194064 Saint Petersburg, Russia; irina.neganova@incras.ru
[3] Theoretical Department, Ioffe Institute, 194021 Saint Petersburg, Russia
* Correspondence: gursky@math.ioffe.ru

Abstract: Human pluripotent stem cells have the potential for unlimited proliferation and controlled differentiation into various somatic cells, making them a unique tool for regenerative and personalized medicine. Determining the best clone selection is a challenging problem in this field and requires new sensing instruments and methods able to automatically assess the state of a growing colony ('phenotype') and make decisions about its destiny. One possible solution for such label-free, non-invasive assessment is to make phase-contrast images and/or videos of growing stem cell colonies, process the morphological parameters ('morphological portrait', or signal), link this information to the colony phenotype, and initiate an automated protocol for the colony selection. As a step in implementing this strategy, we used machine learning methods to find an effective model for classifying the human pluripotent stem cell colonies of three lines according to their morphological phenotype ('good' or 'bad'), using morphological parameters from the previously published data as predictors. We found that the model using cellular morphological parameters as predictors and artificial neural networks as the classification method produced the best average accuracy of phenotype prediction (67%). When morphological parameters of colonies were used as predictors, logistic regression was the most effective classification method (75% average accuracy). Combining the morphological parameters of cells and colonies resulted in the most effective model, with a 99% average accuracy of phenotype prediction. Random forest was the most efficient classification method for the combined data. We applied feature selection methods and showed that different morphological parameters were important for phenotype recognition via either cellular or colonial parameters. Our results indicate a necessity for retaining both cellular and colonial morphological information for predicting the phenotype and provide an optimal choice for the machine learning method. The classification models reported in this study could be used as a basis for developing and/or improving automated solutions to control the quality of human pluripotent stem cells for medical purposes.

Keywords: human pluripotent stem cells; human embryonic stem cells; machine learning; best clone; morphological phenotype

1. Introduction

Assessment of the cellular morphology of biological samples has a long history, as it provides essential information on many underlying cellular processes and cellular states. In cell cultures, morphology is usually employed as a measure of cell classification; in clinical practice, morphological criteria are applied for diagnosis, prognosis, and treatment of human diseases. In recent years, quantification of cell morphology has seen great advances due to the development of new techniques and software that allow classification of cellular morphology from fluorescence or bright-field images at the single-cell level on both 2D and 3D cultures of cells on different substrates [1–4]. While fluorescent dyes may interfere with cellular functions, the live cell imaging under phase-contrast offers a great opportunity for label-free, non-invasive cell characterization and quantitative assessment of different parameters of cell morphology.

Nowadays, morphology-based high-content analysis of cellular phenotypes is increasingly recognized as a core methodology for the identification and analysis of cellular heterogeneity [1,5]. This is supported by the emergence of new software packages for high-dimensional image-based cell analysis with trained classifiers, such as CellProfiler Analyst, Enhanced Cell Classifier, and similar [5–8].

It has now been more than 15 years since machine learning (ML) and deep learning (DL) have granted us the computational power to understand questions in the field of cellular biology, drug development, medicine, etc. Without a doubt, research in the area of pluripotent stem cells, especially human embryonic stem cells (hESCs) and human induced pluripotent stem cells (hiPSCs), comprising human pluripotent stem cells (hPSCs), could benefit from the advances in ML and DL methods. These cells have the remarkable capability to differentiate to all the cell types of the human body, and these cells serve as a useful tool in regenerative medicine, disease modeling, drug testing, and the study of embryonic development. Two main types of hPSCs are very close in their morphology but have different origins. hESCs are derived from the inner cell mass of the preimplantation blastocysts, while hiPSCs originate through somatic cell reprogramming by overexpressing core pluripotency transcription factors [9,10]. Often, hPSCs are further differentiated into cell types that are useful for the researchers by subjecting them to a certain differentiation protocol. During this process, hPSCs undergo a global morphological transformation, in which the highly compact hPSC colonies give rise to more loosely organized cells with completely different morphological appearances and structures. Importantly, before the colonies from a single clone of the hiPSCs can be selected for further propagation followed by differentiation, these cells must be kept in culture in an undifferentiated state, without any signs of spontaneous differentiation.

Our group has a long-standing interest in developing an ML model for the best clone recognition based on the morphological parameters of the cells and colonies from hPSCs with different morphological phenotypes [11–13]. Although morphological changes can be quite evident to the trained human eye when colonies start to differentiate in an unwanted direction, this is inherently subjective and, thus, not applicable for the efficient translation of the laboratory methods to automated cell production for clinical purposes. Traditional manual cell culture is variable and labor-intensive, posing challenges for high-throughput applications. Moreover, the selection quality depends on the professional knowledge and practical experience of an expert, which limits the application of the manual feature selection method for cell culture assessment. In this regard, it is important to emphasize that the effective definition of morphological parameters and the evaluation of the extent of morphological heterogeneity within hPSC populations remain challenging.

Due to the huge expansion and wide use of hiPSCs in recent years [14], there is a need for new technologies to not only standardize the evaluation of iPSCs to allow the objective comparison of results across different groups, but also to ensure safe translation of these cells towards clinical use. Nowadays, regenerative medicine products are at the forefront of scientific research and clinical translation, but their reproducibility and large-scale production are compromised by poor automation, monitoring, and standardization issues, resulting in an increased batch-to-batch cell culture variability. To overcome these limitations, new technologies have been proposed at both software and hardware levels. Software solutions include algorithms and artificial intelligence models and are combined with imaging software and ML techniques, whereas hardware is presented by automated liquid handling devices, automated cell expansion bioreactor systems, automated colony-forming units, counting and characterization units, and scalable cell culture plates.

As an example of such technologies, we illustrate in Figure 1 a conceptual schema for a device designed to select the best clone by controlling the quality of the hPSCs. The experimental part ('hardware') contains a microscope making phase-contrast images or videos of growing hPSC colonies on a substrate. The software consists of two parts. The first part extracts informative morphological features of cells and colonies from the images or videos, thus providing the morphological portrait of a colony. The second software part processes this morphological signal by applying to it pretrained ML-based models, yielding the assessment of the colony phenotype. Finally, using this information, a decision is made about whether the colony should be kept in culture for further propagation or terminated. Our work contributes to an important step in this schema related to the development of the phenotype prediction models.

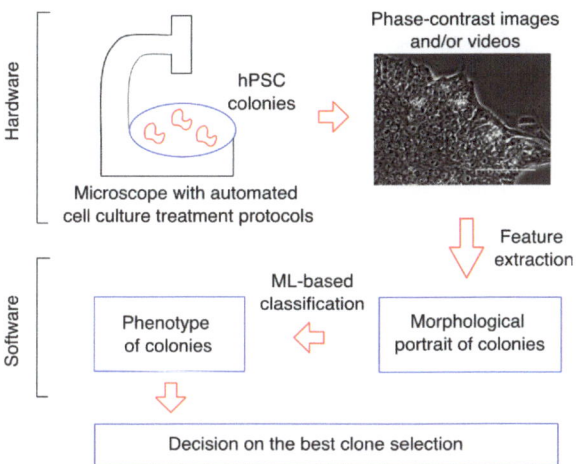

Figure 1. Schematic representation of a device designed for the automated best clone selection. Red arrows indicate the direction of information processing within the device.

There have been many efforts to utilize ML and DL methods to predict a hPSC phenotype and, thus, to provide the selection of the best clone [13]. These studies can roughly be split into two major classes. The first one comprises the phenotype classification models based on two-stage processing of the imaging data, in which biologically interpretable morphological features are first extracted from the hPSC images and then classification methods are applied with the extracted features as predictors [11,15–18]. Studies from the second class apply DL methods (e.g., convolutional neural networks) directly to the colony images to infer the phenotype, or some less biologically interpretable features are automatically extracted using image processing methods followed by ML-based classification with these features as predictors [12,19–24]. Despite the fact that the second approach often provides higher phenotype prediction accuracy, the first approach has an advantage in a clear biological interpretation of valuable morphological parameters found during this study, thus providing insights for possible new biological experiments. Various authors used different ML methods for phenotype prediction models, and their performance varies. Therefore, a search for a method that is optimal for a given datum is an important task.

The aim of our study was to identify the best classification method for predicting the hPSC colony phenotype based on morphological parameters of cells and colonies from three hPSC lines, given in the previously published data set [11,25]. As a further step, we proposed a model based on the combination of cellular and colonial parameters and showed that this model provided the best performance. Finally, we analyzed the importance of the morphological parameters in the resulting classification models.

2. Materials and Methods

2.1. Data

For model training, we used previously published data containing values of morphological parameters of cells and colonies extracted from phase-contrast images of three cell lines: human embryonic stem cell line H9 (WiCell, Madison, WI, USA), hiPSC line AD3, and patient-specific hiPSC line HPCASRi002-A (CaSR) [11,25]. The morphological parameters were as follows: area of the cell or colony ('Area'), length of the cell or colony boundary ('Perimeter'), length of the minor axis of the ellipse fitted to the cell or colony in the image ('Minor axis'), largest distance between two points on the cell or colony boundary ('Feret's diameter D'), smallest distance between two points on the cell or colony boundary ('Minimal Feret's diameter D'), area divided by squared perimeter and multiplied by 4π ('Shape factor', a measure of circularity and compactness), and total area of the free intercellular space in the colony ('Area of intercellular space', a measure of compact cell packing within a colony). These parameters could be considered as standard shape descriptors in 2D image analysis using ImageJ software, version 1.54g [26]. The parameter values were obtained for 53 colonies and 1602 cells of hESC line H9, 49 colonies and 1569 cells of control hiPSC line AD3, and 48 colonies and 1315 cells of patient-specific hiPSC line CaSR [11].

All colonies and cells in the data set contained binary phenotype score obtained via an expert analysis, as previously described [11]. The binary phenotype score can take one of two values, 'good' or 'bad', representing the pluripotency status of the colony. Colonies with the good phenotype demonstrate a high potential for proliferation, while colonies with the bad phenotype show signs of spontaneous differentiation.

2.2. Classification Models

We used the data set for training classification models to predict phenotype based on the morphological parameters as predictors. The following classification methods were tested: naïve Bayes classifier, k-nearest neighbors, logistic regression, random forest, support vector machines, and artificial neural networks. We analyzed the classification problem for the cellular and colonial data separately. In addition, we combined the cellular and colonial morphological parameters and phenotypic information into a separate data set, which we call a combined data set, and trained classification models on these data. The predictors in the models for the combined data included morphological parameters of a cell and morphological parameters of the colony containing that cell, and the phenotype of the colony containing that cell was used as the target for classification. All models were implemented using Python 3.8 (sklearn and keras libraries) and trained using the nested cross-validation, with 5 folds in both inner and outer cross-validation loops [27]. In each fold of the outer loop, data were split into training and test sets. Then, the selection of hyperparameters occurred in the inner loop using cross-validation on the training set from the outer loop. The classification accuracy of the best model from the inner loop was estimated on the test set in the fold of the outer loop, which we called the nested cross-validation accuracy. The mean nested cross-validation accuracy $\pm$ s.d. was recorded for test sets of all outer loop folds. The neural network configuration was tuned manually, and the hyperparameters of all other methods were selected using the grid search method [28].

In addition to the accuracy, we recorded the Area Under Curve (AUC) for the Receiver Operating Characteristic (ROC-curve) as another effective measure of binary classification for the best classification model of each classification method. This measure represents the area under the curve on a plane with the true positive rate on the ordinate axis and false positive rate on the abscissa axis, with AUC = 1 representing perfect classification and AUC = 0.5 representing random classification.

2.3. Feature Selection

We analyzed the importance of each feature as a predictor in the best classification models by applying the SHAP method (SHapley Additive exPlanations) [29]. The SHAP value for each feature represents the contribution of that feature to the prediction value of the selected model. SHAP are theoretically well justified and unify several previously suggested methods. This analysis was implemented using shap library in Python 3.8.

2.4. Statistical Methods

We compared the average nested accuracies of the classification models for different classification methods using t-test (ttest_rel function, stats module, scipy library in Python 3.8).

3. Results

3.1. Classification Models for Cellular and Colonial Data

To find out how various classification methods perform on the morphological data for hPSCs and colonies, we estimated the cross-validation accuracy of phenotype prediction for each method using the data containing all cell lines pooled together (Table 1).

Table 1. Classification model performance for cellular and colonial data and for various classification methods. Nested cross-validation accuracy and area under the ROC-curve (ROC AUC) are shown as measures of performance. Best performance values are highlighted in bold.

Method	Cellular Data		Colonial Data	
	Accuracy	ROC AUC	Accuracy	ROC AUC
Naïve Bayes	58 ± 2%	0.69	60 ± 14%	0.71
k-nearest neighbors	64 ± 3%	0.66	68 ± 12%	0.71
Logistic regression	59 ± 4%	0.63	**75 ± 12%**	**0.90**
Random forest	64 ± 2%	0.67	66 ± 10%	0.79
Support vector machines	64 ± 3%	0.68	68 ± 11%	0.86
Artificial neural networks	**67 ± 4%**	**0.70**	71 ± 12%	0.89

The results for cellular data showed a similar performance across various models, but the neural networks outperformed all the methods except the support vector machines ($p < 0.05$), with an average accuracy of 67%. Considering that the AUC measure was also the highest for this method, we can conclude that the neural networks method was the best model for predicting phenotype based on the morphological parameters of cells.

In the case of colonial data, the difference between methods was more pronounced, but also showed higher method-specific variation. Based on the average accuracy and the AUC value, logistic regression appeared to be the best classification method (75% accuracy) for predicting phenotype from the morphological parameters of colonies. Overall, the performance measures shown in Table 1 could be estimated as rather moderate, implying that either combining different cell-line-specific data in one data set or consideration of only cellular or colonial morphological parameters separately was possibly not an optimal strategy.

As the unification of various cell lines into one data set might create irrelevant variability, impeding the classification by phenotype, we tested whether the performance could be improved by considering each cell line separately. For this purpose, we trained classification models on the line-specific cellular and colonial data using the best classification methods from the analysis of the unified data (Table 2). These models incorporated the same morphological parameters as the models from Table 1 but were trained and analyzed on data of each cell line separately. The results showed an average performance for H9 that was either comparable to or higher than that for the unified data, but the models predicted the phenotype with less accuracy for other cell lines. Therefore, constraining the classification problem to the line-specific data did not improve the performance. These results showed that combining morphological data from different cell lines was justified, as it provided a larger data set without significantly degrading classification performance.

Table 2. Nested cross-validation accuracy in classification models trained on cell-line-specific data.

	Accuracy		
	hESC H9	hiPSC AD3	hiPSC CaSR
Cellular data (artificial neural networks)	73 ± 7%	60 ± 6%	64 ± 3%
Colonial data (logistic regression)	75 ± 18%	62 ± 20%	67 ± 17%

3.2. Classification Models for Combined Cellular and Colonial Data

Another way to improve the performance of the classification models in Table 1 was based on a biological hypothesis that colony phenotype could not be determined solely based on cellular or colonial morphological parameters. Cells differentiate irregularly within a colony, sometimes demonstrating a reverse behavior, so the phenotypic status is rather a collective property, also expressed in a change in the colony morphology. Under spontaneous differentiation, the morphological perturbations of both single cells and a colony as a whole should be considered as necessary elements of the true morphological portrait associated with the pluripotency potential.

Therefore, we tested the same classification methods but for the combined data set, in which predictors included morphological parameters of cells complemented with the parameters of the colony containing these cells. The results demonstrated a significant increase in performance for all methods (Table 3, Figure 2). The discrepancy between methods was also higher, with a more than 25% difference in the mean accuracy between the best and worst methods. Random forest and artificial neural networks showed the highest performance, which was clearly distinguishable from other methods ($p < 0.05$).

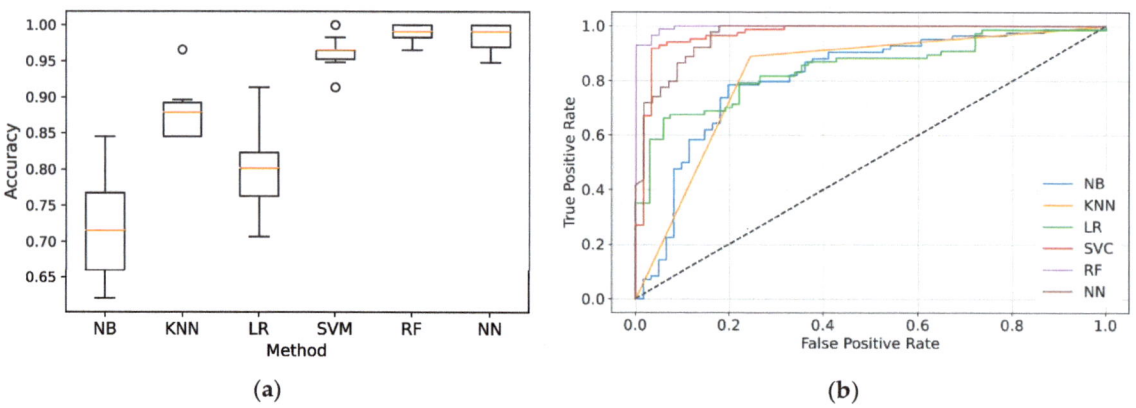

Figure 2. Performance of classification models trained on the combined cellular and colonial data: (**a**) Box plots for the nested cross-validation accuracy. Orange lines show the median accuracy values, boxes represent the interval between the lower and upper quartiles, whiskers mark the minimum and maximum accuracy values, and circles are outliers; (**b**) ROC-curves. The dashed line represents a random classifier, which assigns phenotypes randomly. NB: naïve Bayes; KNN: *k*-nearest neighbors; LR: logistic regression; SVM: support vector machines; RF: random forest; NN: neural networks.

Table 3. Classification model performance for combined cellular and colonial data and for various classification methods. Nested cross-validation accuracy and area under the ROC-curve (ROC AUC) are shown as measures of performance. Best performance values are highlighted in bold.

Method	Accuracy	ROC AUC
Naïve Bayes	72 ± 7%	0.815
k-nearest neighbors	88 ± 4%	0.818
Logistic regression	80 ± 6%	0.826
Random forest	**99 ± 2%**	**0.997**
Support vector machines	96 ± 2%	0.975
Artificial neural networks	98 ± 2%	0.956

3.3. Importance of Morphological Parameters in Classification Models

The classification models that we obtained can be used to understand which morphological characteristics of individual hPSCs and colonies are the most informative in representing the morphological signal as a manifestation of phenotype. We used the SHAP method to find the features that were the most important in all types of classification models. In the best cell-data-based model, two parameters clearly segregated from the others: Area and Perimeter (Figure 3a). In the best model based on the colonial parameters, Area and Area of intercellular space were the most important for phenotype prediction (Figure 3b). For the combined data, the analysis showed that the colonial parameters appeared to be more important in the best classification model than the cellular parameters (Figure 3c). The colonial Feret's D showed the highest impact on the classification, while other parameters exhibited a rather shallow distribution of their importance score. In other words, colonial Feret's D can be considered as the most influential parameter in the classification models on the combined data, but other parameters also contributed. The cellular area had the highest importance score among the cellular parameters in this case (Figure 3c).

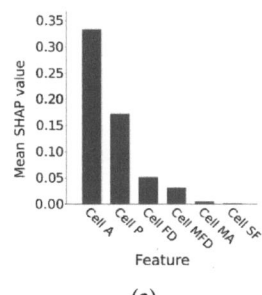
(a)

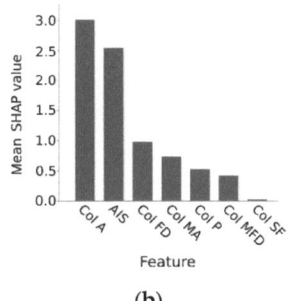
(b)

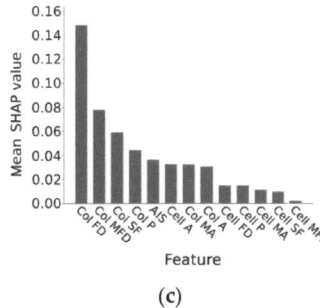
(c)

Figure 3. Mean SHAP values representing the importance of the morphological features in the best classification models based on (**a**) cell data, (**b**) colony data, and (**c**) combined data. Names of cellular parameters start with 'Cell', and names of colonial ones start with 'Col'. A: Area; P: Perimeter; MA: Minor axis; FD: Feret's diameter D; MFD: Minimal Feret's diameter D; SF: Shape factor; AIS: Area of intercellular space (only for colonies).

4. Discussion

For numerous cell types of the human body, their morphological appearance is mainly known and often described in terms of the cell size, cell form, its granularity, cytoskeletal architecture, etc. In many ways, these features of the cell morphology result from the spatiotemporally regulated activity of signaling proteins. However, the components of these signaling networks and the precise role they play in regulating the cell shape and other morphological parameters remain largely unclear. How and which signaling cascades govern the transition of the small pluripotent stem cell into a specialized and often much bigger cell type is still in question. In this regard, morphological profiling and identification of genes and clusters of genes which are important for maintaining hPSC morphological identity, as well as genes involved in the conversion of these cells into differentiated specialized cells, is undoubtedly important for both understanding hPSC biology and for the development of efficient protocols for directed differentiation. In this way, morphological data from our assay, together with novel computer-based assessment, can provide a further step toward discovering new biological connections that determine a hPSC's identity.

Our results showed that cellular and colonial data required different classification methods, emphasizing the inherent data dependency of ML approaches. The classification quality of artificial neural networks for the cellular data was comparable with a value previously obtained by us for the same data using a similar method [11]. However, in contrast to that study, we found that logistic regression was more efficient when the morphology of hPSC colonies was considered. For the combined cellular and colonial data, random forest appeared as a promising approach, and the resulting classification model showed the best performance. This indicates that the true morphological portrait associated directly with the hPSC pluripotency should be assembled from both the morphological parameters of pluripotent cells forming the colony and the parameters of the colony as a whole.

We demonstrated that parameters such as Area and Perimeter provided the most important and informative input in the phenotype classification based on cellular morphology. For classification based on the colonial data, we found that colonial Area and Area of intercellular space were the most informative. When the cellular and colonial parameters were combined, colonial Feret's diameter, colonial Minimal Feret's diameter, and colonial Shape factor had the greatest impact on classification.

This information can be used in two ways. Firstly, new biological knowledge can be obtained by focusing on the molecular mechanisms associated with the change in the important features under spontaneous differentiation. Secondly, simplified classification models can be trained to confine the predictors to only the important ones. This can be especially useful when a much larger amount of data are involved, so that the computational efficiency becomes a bottleneck.

The analysis of feature importance on the combined cellular and colonial data suggests that the morphological properties of colonies play a major role in assessing the phenotype. The shallow distribution of the importance score for cellular parameters in the best model based on the combined data indicates that each cellular morphological feature adds some information to the whole picture, but no single parameter can be singled out as drastically more informative.

The high classification accuracy of 98–99% that we have obtained approaches and sometimes exceeds the performance scores of previously reported classification models applied to pluripotent stem cells [11,12,15–24]. Morphological parameters of cells and colonies used as predictors in our models are biologically interpretable but require methods for their extraction from the images prior to classification. Other morphological characteristics, including morphological features of intracellular objects, have previously been considered and resulted in a classification accuracy of 80–89% [16,18]. Methods for automated feature extraction from images and videos of hPSCs with the subsequent application of supervised ML algorithms constitute another approach, with the reported classification accuracy values higher than 87% [19–21,24]. DL-based classification models applied directly to the images of hPSCs have been reported to perform at about 90% accuracy [12,23].

Despite the good performance shown by the classification models on the combined data, our approach has several limitations. We used data from three cell lines, and this number should be increased to make the models more applicable. This requires further studies on collecting morphological and phenotypic information for various hPSC lines, since previous efforts in developing classification models involved similar numbers of cell lines [13]. To make classification even more general, multiple hPSC growing conditions, including various experimental matrices and media, should also be tested. Another limitation concerns the necessity of extracting the morphological features prior to the application of our classification models, as this extraction is not a part of the models reported here. As a possible alternative, DL-based image classification can be utilized, in which no prior feature extraction is usually required [12,23].

Overall, our study confirms the utility of ML methods for the automated phenotype prediction for various hPSC lines. We consider our research as the first step towards developing software-guided analytical tools (Figure 1) that will automate the selection of the best iPSC clone for further research, namely for targeted differentiation of a patient-specific iPSC line towards the desired tissue-specific cell type. One of the bottlenecks in the use of iPSCs is the fact that not all obtained patient-specific clones are able to differentiate in the desired tissue-specific direction with equal efficiency. We previously showed the relationship between the morphological parameters of clones with different morphological phenotypes and the ability to differentiate along three germ layers [11]. In this study, we further refined our models to improve the efficiency of selecting the best clone. Based on these data, we are currently testing our model on clones that are unable to differentiate efficiently into mesenchymal stem cells and cardiomyocytes to improve model sensitivity.

Author Contributions: Conceptualization, I.N. and V.G.; methodology, E.V. and V.G.; investigation, E.V., I.N. and V.G.; data curation, I.N.; writing—original draft preparation, V.G. and I.N.; writing—review and editing, E.V. and M.S.; supervision, M.S. All authors have read and agreed to the published version of the manuscript.

Funding: Development of computational algorithms for training classification models was funded by the Ministry of Science and Higher Education of the Russian Federation as part of the World-class Research Center program: Advanced Digital Technologies (contract No. 075-15-2022-311 dated 20 April 2022). The Russian Science Foundation, grant number 21-75-20132 for I.N., funded the research of the classification models and model training results.

Institutional Review Board Statement: Not applicable.

Informed Consent Statement: Not applicable.

Data Availability Statement: Data with values of morphological parameters of cells and colonies extracted from phase-contrast images of three cell lines (H9, AD3, and HPCASRi002-A) were downloaded from the Zenodo public repository (https://doi.org/10.5281/zenodo.7150644, accessed on 1 February 2023) [25]. Programs implementing the classification models developed in this study were uploaded to the Zenodo public repository (https://zenodo.org/records/10052095, accessed on 30 October 2023).

Conflicts of Interest: The authors declare no conflict of interest. The funders had no role in the design of the study; in the collection, analyses, or interpretation of data; in the writing of the manuscript; or in the decision to publish the results.

References

1. Mousavikhamene, Z.; Sykora, D.J.; Mrksich, M.; Bagheri, N. Morphological Features of Single Cells Enable Accurate Automated Classification of Cancer from Non-Cancer Cell Lines. *Sci. Rep.* **2021**, *11*, 24375. [CrossRef] [PubMed]
2. Gosnell, M.E.; Anwer, A.G.; Mahbub, S.B.; Menon Perinchery, S.; Inglis, D.W.; Adhikary, P.P.; Jazayeri, J.A.; Cahill, M.A.; Saad, S.; Pollock, C.A.; et al. Quantitative Non-Invasive Cell Characterisation and Discrimination Based on Multispectral Autofluorescence Features. *Sci. Rep.* **2016**, *6*, 23453. [CrossRef]
3. Basu, S.; Kolouri, S.; Rohde, G.K. Detecting and Visualizing Cell Phenotype Differences from Microscopy Images Using Transport-Based Morphometry. *Proc. Natl. Acad. Sci. USA* **2014**, *111*, 3448–3453. [CrossRef]
4. Di, Z.; Klop, M.J.D.; Rogkoti, V.-M.; Le Dévédec, S.E.; van de Water, B.; Verbeek, F.J.; Price, L.S.; Meerman, J.H.N. Ultra High Content Image Analysis and Phenotype Profiling of 3D Cultured Micro-Tissues. *PLoS ONE* **2014**, *9*, e109688. [CrossRef]
5. Stanley, N.; Stelzer, I.A.; Tsai, A.S.; Fallahzadeh, R.; Ganio, E.; Becker, M.; Phongpreecha, T.; Nassar, H.; Ghaemi, S.; Maric, I.; et al. VoPo Leverages Cellular Heterogeneity for Predictive Modeling of Single-Cell Data. *Nat. Commun.* **2020**, *11*, 3738. [CrossRef]
6. Jones, T.R.; Carpenter, A.E.; Lamprecht, M.R.; Moffat, J.; Silver, S.J.; Grenier, J.K.; Castoreno, A.B.; Eggert, U.S.; Root, D.E.; Golland, P.; et al. Scoring Diverse Cellular Morphologies in Image-Based Screens with Iterative Feedback and Machine Learning. *Proc. Natl. Acad. Sci. USA* **2009**, *106*, 1826–1831. [CrossRef]
7. Misselwitz, B.; Strittmatter, G.; Periaswamy, B.; Schlumberger, M.C.; Rout, S.; Horvath, P.; Kozak, K.; Hardt, W.-D. Enhanced CellClassifier: A Multi-Class Classification Tool for Microscopy Images. *BMC Bioinform.* **2010**, *11*, 30. [CrossRef]

8. Singh, S.; Carpenter, A.E.; Genovesio, A. Increasing the Content of High-Content Screening: An Overview. *J. Biomol. Screen.* **2014**, *19*, 640–650. [CrossRef]
9. Thomson, J.A.; Itskovitz-Eldor, J.; Shapiro, S.S.; Waknitz, M.A.; Swiergiel, J.J.; Marshall, V.S.; Jones, J.M. Embryonic Stem Cell Lines Derived from Human Blastocysts. *Science* **1998**, *282*, 1145–1147. [CrossRef] [PubMed]
10. Takahashi, K.; Tanabe, K.; Ohnuki, M.; Narita, M.; Ichisaka, T.; Tomoda, K.; Yamanaka, S. Induction of Pluripotent Stem Cells from Adult Human Fibroblasts by Defined Factors. *Cell* **2007**, *131*, 861–872. [CrossRef]
11. Krasnova, O.A.; Gursky, V.V.; Chabina, A.S.; Kulakova, K.A.; Alekseenko, L.L.; Panova, A.V.; Kiselev, S.L.; Neganova, I.E. Prognostic Analysis of Human Pluripotent Stem Cells Based on Their Morphological Portrait and Expression of Pluripotent Markers. *Int. J. Mol. Sci.* **2022**, *23*, 12902. [CrossRef]
12. Mamaeva, A.; Krasnova, O.; Khvorova, I.; Kozlov, K.; Gursky, V.; Samsonova, M.; Tikhonova, O.; Neganova, I. Quality Control of Human Pluripotent Stem Cell Colonies by Computational Image Analysis Using Convolutional Neural Networks. *Int. J. Mol. Sci.* **2023**, *24*, 140. [CrossRef] [PubMed]
13. Gursky, V.; Krasnova, O.; Sopova, J.; Kovaleva, A.; Kulakova, K.; Tikhonova, O.; Neganova, I. *How Morphology of the Human Pluripotent Stem Cells Determines the Selection of the Best Clone*; IntechOpen: London, UK, 2023; ISBN 978-1-83769-262-0.
14. Ludwig, T.E.; Kujak, A.; Rauti, A.; Andrzejewski, S.; Langbehn, S.; Mayfield, J.; Fuller, J.; Yashiro, Y.; Hara, Y.; Bhattacharyya, A. 20 Years of Human Pluripotent Stem Cell Research: It All Started with Five Lines. *Cell Stem Cell* **2018**, *23*, 644–648. [CrossRef] [PubMed]
15. Wakao, S.; Kitada, M.; Kuroda, Y.; Ogura, F.; Murakami, T.; Niwa, A.; Dezawa, M. Morphologic and Gene Expression Criteria for Identifying Human Induced Pluripotent Stem Cells. *PLoS ONE* **2012**, *7*, e48677. [CrossRef] [PubMed]
16. Maddah, M.; Shoukat-Mumtaz, U.; Nassirpour, S.; Loewke, K. A System for Automated, Noninvasive, Morphology-Based Evaluation of Induced Pluripotent Stem Cell Cultures. *J. Lab. Autom.* **2014**, *19*, 454–460. [CrossRef]
17. Kato, R.; Matsumoto, M.; Sasaki, H.; Joto, R.; Okada, M.; Ikeda, Y.; Kanie, K.; Suga, M.; Kinehara, M.; Yanagihara, K.; et al. Parametric Analysis of Colony Morphology of Non-Labelled Live Human Pluripotent Stem Cells for Cell Quality Control. *Sci. Rep.* **2016**, *6*, 34009. [CrossRef]
18. Wakui, T.; Matsumoto, T.; Matsubara, K.; Kawasaki, T.; Yamaguchi, H.; Akutsu, H. Method for Evaluation of Human Induced Pluripotent Stem Cell Quality Using Image Analysis Based on the Biological Morphology of Cells. *J. Med. Imaging* **2017**, *4*, 044003. [CrossRef]
19. Tokunaga, K.; Saitoh, N.; Goldberg, I.G.; Sakamoto, C.; Yasuda, Y.; Yoshida, Y.; Yamanaka, S.; Nakao, M. Computational Image Analysis of Colony and Nuclear Morphology to Evaluate Human Induced Pluripotent Stem Cells. *Sci. Rep.* **2014**, *4*, 6996. [CrossRef]
20. Joutsijoki, H.; Haponen, M.; Rasku, J.; Aalto-Setälä, K.; Juhola, M. Machine Learning Approach to Automated Quality Identification of Human Induced Pluripotent Stem Cell Colony Images. *Comput. Math. Methods Med.* **2016**, *2016*, 3091039. [CrossRef]
21. Perestrelo, T.; Chen, W.; Correia, M.; Le, C.; Pereira, S.; Rodrigues, A.S.; Sousa, M.I.; Ramalho-Santos, J.; Wirtz, D. Pluri-IQ: Quantification of Embryonic Stem Cell Pluripotency through an Image-Based Analysis Software. *Stem Cell Rep.* **2017**, *9*, 697–709. [CrossRef]
22. Nishimura, K.; Ishiwata, H.; Sakuragi, Y.; Hayashi, Y.; Fukuda, A.; Hisatake, K. Live-Cell Imaging of Subcellular Structures for Quantitative Evaluation of Pluripotent Stem Cells. *Sci. Rep.* **2019**, *9*, 1777. [CrossRef] [PubMed]
23. Witmer, A.; Bhanu, B. Generative Adversarial Networks for Morphological-Temporal Classification of Stem Cell Images. *Sensors* **2021**, *22*, 206. [CrossRef]
24. Wakui, T.; Negishi, M.; Murakami, Y.; Tominaga, S.; Shiraishi, Y.; Carpenter, A.E.; Singh, S.; Segawa, H. Predicting Reprogramming-Related Gene Expression from Cell Morphology in Human Induced Pluripotent Stem Cells. *Mol. Biol. Cell* **2023**, *34*, ar45. [CrossRef]
25. Krasnova, O.A.; Gursky, V.V.; Chabina, A.S.; Kulakova, K.A.; Alekseenko, L.L.; Neganova, I.E. *Dataset with Values of Morphological Parameters and Phenotypes of Cells and Colonies from Three Human Pluripotent Stem Cell Lines*; Zenodo: Genève, Switzerland, 2022. [CrossRef]
26. Schneider, C.A.; Rasband, W.S.; Eliceiri, K.W. NIH Image to ImageJ: 25 Years of Image Analysis. *Nat. Methods* **2012**, *9*, 671–675. [CrossRef] [PubMed]
27. Krstajic, D.; Buturovic, L.J.; Leahy, D.E.; Thomas, S. Cross-Validation Pitfalls When Selecting and Assessing Regression and Classification Models. *J. Cheminform.* **2014**, *6*, 10. [CrossRef] [PubMed]
28. Zahedi, L.; Mohammadi, F.G.; Rezapour, S.; Ohland, M.W.; Amini, M.H. Search Algorithms for Automated Hyper-Parameter Tuning. *arXiv* **2021**, arXiv:2104.14677. [CrossRef]
29. Lundberg, S.; Lee, S.-I. A Unified Approach to Interpreting Model Predictions. *arXiv* **2017**, arXiv:1705.07874. [CrossRef]

Disclaimer/Publisher's Note: The statements, opinions and data contained in all publications are solely those of the individual author(s) and contributor(s) and not of MDPI and/or the editor(s). MDPI and/or the editor(s) disclaim responsibility for any injury to people or property resulting from any ideas, methods, instructions or products referred to in the content.

MDPI AG
Grosspeteranlage 5
4052 Basel
Switzerland
Tel.: +41 61 683 77 34

Biomedicines Editorial Office
E-mail: biomedicines@mdpi.com
www.mdpi.com/journal/biomedicines

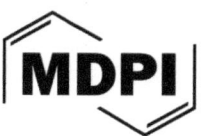

Disclaimer/Publisher's Note: The title and front matter of this reprint are at the discretion of the Guest Editor. The publisher is not responsible for their content or any associated concerns. The statements, opinions and data contained in all individual articles are solely those of the individual Editor and contributors and not of MDPI. MDPI disclaims responsibility for any injury to people or property resulting from any ideas, methods, instructions or products referred to in the content.

www.ingramcontent.com/pod-product-compliance
Lightning Source LLC
LaVergne TN
LVHW072347090526
838202LV00019B/2493